T0325854

Telemental Health

Telemental Health
Clinical, Technical, and Administrative Foundations for Evidence-Based Practice

Edited by

Kathleen Myers
Department of Psychiatry and Behavioral Sciences
University of Washington
Seattle, WA
USA

Carolyn L. Turvey
Department of Psychiatry
University of Iowa
Iowa, IA
USA

AMSTERDAM • BOSTON • HEIDELBERG • LONDON • NEW YORK • OXFORD
ELSEVIER   PARIS • SAN DIEGO • SAN FRANCISCO • SINGAPORE • SYDNEY • TOKYO

Elsevier
32 Jamestown Road, London NW1 7BY
225 Wyman Street, Waltham, MA 02451, USA

First edition 2013

Notices

Knowledge and best practice in this field are constantly changing. As new research and experience broaden our understanding, changes in research methods, professional practices, or medical treatment may become necessary.

Practitioners and researchers must always rely on their own experience and knowledge in evaluating and using any information, methods, compounds, or experiments described herein. In using such information or methods they should be mindful of their own safety and the safety of others, including parties for whom they have a professional responsibility.

To the fullest extent of the law, neither the Publisher nor the authors, contributors, or editors, assume any liability for any injury and/or damage to persons or property as a matter of products liability, negligence or otherwise, or from any use or operation of any methods, products, instructions, or ideas contained in the material herein.

British Library Cataloguing-in-Publication Data
A catalogue record for this book is available from the British Library

Library of Congress Cataloging-in-Publication Data
A catalog record for this book is available from the Library of Congress

ISBN: 978-0-12-416048-4

For information on all Elsevier publications
visit our website at store.elsevier.com

This book has been manufactured using Print On Demand technology. Each copy is produced to order and is limited to black ink. The online version of this book will show color figures where appropriate.

**Working together to grow
libraries in developing countries**

www.elsevier.com | www.bookaid.org | www.sabre.org

ELSEVIER   BOOK AID
             International   Sabre Foundation

Contents

Section Two   Developing a Therapeutic Space During Telemental Health   27

Section Three   Establishing a Telemental Health Practice   109

Section Four Improving Access for Special Populations Through Telemental Health   153

Acknowledgments

Kathleen Myers

I would like to acknowledge all of the families who have worked with me over time to patiently develop processes and techniques for telemental health care. I especially appreciate the collaboration with the primary care physicians who have welcomed telemental health into their communities. Four individuals at Seattle Children's Hospital have been especially crucial in the success of our telemental health service and research. My profound thanks to Phillip Busch, Audiovisual Team Supervisor, who is always knowledgeable, always available, and always helpful. Geraldine Rodriguez, Administrative Assistant, has had the grace and skills to see me through this and so many other academic tasks. Elizabeth McCauley PhD has been a long time role model who set me on this new career path. And, I am indebted to Ann Vander Stoep PhD, an inspiring academic partner who kept the dream alive.

I dedicate this book to my family, Len, Mary, Lenny, Karen, Jeffrey, and Jacqueline, for their ongoing love and support.

Carolyn L. Turvey

I would like to acknowledge my colleagues at the Department of Veterans Affairs and at the University of Iowa Carver College of Medicine. This includes members of the eHealth QUERI and the Office of Rural Health whose support helped me start my career in telemental health and who continue to assist me in the development of novel applications for telemedicine and eHealth.

I would also like to acknowledge Dawn Klein, my long-term senior research assistant. Though she did not contribute to this book specifically, she has tolerated my expansive professional goals and made their achievement possible through her quiet efficiency in managing my research lab.

This text would not have been possible without the continuous education I receive from my colleagues at the American Telemedicine Association. Their combination of experience, intelligence, innovativeness, humor, and practical wisdom has been critical to my development as a researcher and a practitioner of telemental health. I would like to acknowledge specifically Eugene Augusterfer, Elizabeth Brooks, Eve-Lynn Nelson, Terry Rabinowitz, Lisa Roberts, Peter Yellowlees, and especially Jay Shore.

I dedicate this book to my husband, Christopher Liebig, and my three daughters Mary, Sonja, and Erin – all of whom are far more skilled with technology than myself.

Contributors

Eugene F. Augusterfer Harvard Global Mental Health: Trauma and Recovery Program, McLean, VA, USA

Ashley B. Batastini Department of Psychology, Texas Tech University, Texas, USA

Caroline Bonham Center for Rural and Community Behavioral Health, University of New Mexico, Albuquerque, NM, USA

Elizabeth Brooks Centers for American Indian and Alaska Native Health, University of Colorado Denver, Aurora, CO, USA

L. Lee Carlisle Department of Psychiatry and Behavioral Sciences, Division of Child and Adolescent Psychiatry, University of Washington School of Medicine, Seattle, WA, USA

C. Munro Cullum University of Texas Southwestern Medical Center at Dallas, Dallas, TX, USA

Kathy Davis Pediatrics Department, University of Kansas Medical Center, Kansas City, KS, USA

Jennifer Dealy The Alpert Medical School of Brown University and Rhode Island Hospital, Providence, RI, USA

Angela Banitt Duncan KU Center for Telemedicine and Telehealth, University of Kansas Medical Center, Kansas City, KS, USA

Michael Flaum Department of Psychiatry, University of Iowa Carver College of Medicine, Iowa City, IA, USA

Dehra Glueck Department of Psychiatry, Washington University School of Medicine, St. Louis, MO, USA

Maria C. Grosch University of Texas Southwestern Medical Center at Dallas, Dallas, TX, USA

Benjamin Hidy UC Davis School of Medicine, Sacramento, CA, USA

Ashley Karr Iowa City VA Health Care System, Iowa City, IA, USA

Karen Kloezeman National Center for PTSD—Pacific Island Division, Department of Veterans Affairs Pacific Island Healthcare System, Honolulu, HI, USA

Greg M. Kramer National Center for Telehealth and Technology (T2), Tacoma, WA, USA

Avron Kriechman Center for Rural and Community Behavioral Health, University of New Mexico, Albuquerque, NM, USA

Teresa Lillis KU Center for Telemedicine and Telehealth, University of Kansas Medical Center, Kansas City, KS, USA

David D. Luxton National Center for Telehealth and Technology (T2), Tacoma, WA, USA

Brendan R. McDonald Department of Psychology, Texas Tech University, Texas, USA

Matt C. Mishkind National Center for Telehealth and Technology (T2), Tacoma, WA, USA

Robert D. Morgan Department of Psychology, Texas Tech University, Texas, USA

Leslie Morland National Center for PTSD—Pacific Island Division, Department of Veterans Affairs Pacific Island Healthcare System, Honolulu, HI, USA

Kathleen Myers Department of Psychiatry and Behavioral Sciences, University of Washington School of Medicine, Seattle, WA, USA

Eve-Lynn Nelson Pediatrics Department, University of Kansas Medical Center, Kansas City, KS; KU Center for Telemedicine and Telehealth, University of Kansas Medical Center, Kansas City, KS, USA

Patrick O'Neil Tulane University School of Medicine, New Orleans, LA, USA

Michelle Burke Parish UC Davis School of Medicine, Sacramento, CA, USA

Emily Porch UC Davis School of Medicine, Sacramento, CA, USA

Terry Rabinowitz University of Vermont College of Medicine, Fletcher Allen Health Care, Burlington, VT, USA

Sarah Reed UC Davis School of Medicine, Sacramento, CA, USA

Carol M. Rockhill Department of Psychiatry and Behavioral Sciences, University of Washington School of Medicine, Seattle, WA, USA

Thomas Sheeran The Alpert Medical School of Brown University and Rhode Island Hospital, Providence, RI, USA

Jay H. Shore Centers for American Indian and Alaska Native Health, University of Colorado Denver, Aurora, CO, USA

Garret Spargo Alaska Native Tribal Health Consortium, ANTHC, Anchorage, AK, USA

Carolyn L. Turvey Department of Psychiatry, University of Iowa Carver College of Medicine, Psychiatry Research-MEB, Iowa City, IA; Comprehensive Access and Delivery Research and Evaluation (CADRE) Center, Iowa City VA Healthcare System, Iowa City, IA, USA

Sarah E. Velasquez KU Center for Telemental Health and Telehealth, University of Kansas Medical Center, Kansas City, KS, USA

Peter Yellowlees UC Davis School of Medicine, Sacramento, CA, USA

Section One

Introduction to Telemental Health

1 Introduction[1]

Carolyn L. Turvey[a,b,*] and Kathleen Myers[c]

[a]Department of Psychiatry, University of Iowa Carver College of Medicine, Iowa City, IA, [b]Comprehensive Access and Delivery Research and Evaluation (CADRE) Center, Iowa City VA Healthcare System, Iowa City, IA, [c]Department of Psychiatry and Behavioral Sciences, University of Washington School of Medicine, Telemental Health Service, Seattle Children's Hospital, Seattle, WA

Introduction

The Telemental Health Imperative

Telemental health (TMH) has the potential to deliver needed care to millions of people struggling with mental disorders. A child suffering from autism who lives in a rural community of 500 can receive a teleconsultation at the local primary school and benefit from timely expert diagnosis and treatment. Timely diagnosis can help the child to remain in school and optimize both learning and socialization. An elderly woman in a nursing home, who was secluded because of disruptive behaviors, receives a videoconsultation and treatment recommendations from a psychiatrist located over 200 miles away. She is now able to control her temper, her mood is bright, and she interacts positively with other residents and staff. In response to Hurricane Katrina and the devastating earthquake in Haiti, the international community is coming together to develop strategies to provide mental health care even in conditions in which the technical infrastructure is devastated.

These success stories bring human faces to the statistics regarding mental health needs across the world and particularly for the disadvantaged. A study conducted by the World Health Organization ranked mental illness as a leading cause of disability in the United States, Canada, and Western Europe, more disabling than heart disease and cancer (Demyttenaere et al., 2004; World Health Organization, 2001). Mental illness accounts for 25% of all disability across major industrialized countries and the direct cost to the US economy is $79 billion annually

---

[1] The views expressed in this chapter are those of the authors and do not necessarily reflect the position or policy of the Department of Veterans Affairs or the US government.

* Corresponding author: Carolyn L. Turvey, Department of Psychiatry, University of Iowa Carver College of Medicine, Iowa City, IA 52242. Tel.: +1-319-353-5312, Fax: +1-319-353-3003, E-mail: carolyn-turvey@uiowa.edu

Telemental Health. DOI: http://dx.doi.org/10.1016/B978-0-12-416048-4.00001-4

(United States Public Health Service Office of the Surgeon General, 1999). Suicide, a tragic outcome closely tied to inadequately treated mental illness, is responsible for more deaths worldwide than homicide or war (Demyttenaere et al., 2004; World Health Organization, 2001). Nonetheless, the World Health Organization found that even in developed countries, 35–55% of people suffering serious mental illness did not receive care in the past 12 months (Demyttenaere et al., 2004). Many who do receive treatment receive inadequate care that does not comply with professional guidelines or evidence-based practice (Kessler, Berglund et al., 2001; Kessler, Demler et al., 2005). Unfortunately, the underserved are often children, the elderly, or disabled who must overcome considerable additional barriers to receive adequate mental health treatment.

Though there are many different barriers to mental health care, the most significant includes the shortage of mental health practitioners, poor access to specialty care, and financial barriers to care. TMH offers a way around each of these barriers. For example, currently there is a nationwide shortage of child psychiatrists. It is estimated that current practitioners can meet only 10–45% of the need in child mental health care (Thomas & Holzer, 2006). Most of this shortage occurs in rural communities. Programs like *Connected Kansas Kids*, a state-funded initiative, address this need by providing mental health services at rural primary schools through mental health providers located at the University of Kansas (Nelson, Barnard, & Cain, 2003). This collaboration allows children to receive mental health assessment and interventions in the naturalistic setting of their school and the mental health providers do not have to travel long distances at considerable disadvantage to their other clinical responsibilities and families. Both sites may benefit from lower financial costs associated with videoconferencing.

Current Trends Supporting the Broader Adoption of Telemental Health

The view that TMH can address many of the current woes facing the provision of mental health care is not new. TMH, the most commonly utilized aspect of telemedicine, has been practiced in some form or another since 1957 (Lewis, Martin, Over, & Tucker, 1957). Since this initial use, successive cohorts of clinicians and researchers have touted the benefits of TMH and predicted its certain widespread adoption. Though TMH has continued to grow slowly but steadily over the years, it remains outside the realm of mainstream clinical care. This pattern of expansive optimism about potential coupled with slow and, at times, disappointing adoption has drawn cynical comment that TMH has been "just around the corner for about 50 years." Thus confronted, we are faced with the challenge of arguing that the current wave of enthusiasm is somehow different from that of prior cohorts and that we are, in fact, on the brink of an exciting widespread expansion of the use of TMH into mainstream health care.

There are five critical developments in health care that just might make current conditions truly conducive to the broader adoption of TMH: (1) a growing shortage of mental health providers particularly for special populations such as children or the elderly; (2) advances in the quality and availability of desktop videoconferencing technologies; (3) improved reimbursement from Medicare combined with mandates in some states for private insurers to reimburse telemedicine equal to same-room care; (4) an increasingly large and sophisticated evidence base including randomized controlled trials demonstrating the effectiveness of TMH in the treatment of mental disorders; and finally (5) national-level mandates for health care reform. Throughout the chapters in this book, these issues are discussed with the aim of educating the reader about best practices in TMH and the research evidence supporting these practices.

The first critical development in health care that is influencing the adoption of TMH is a *growing shortage of mental health providers*. Chapter 2 provides data from the fields of both psychiatry and psychology to support the need for innovative solutions to the workforce shortage in mental health care. Using data from organizations that monitor supply and demand of professional services, this chapter demonstrates both the current and anticipated severe shortage of mental health professionals. It also discusses how TMH can address many, but not all, aspects of this crisis.

The shortage of mental health resources in socioeconomically disadvantaged areas such as inner-cities and correctional facilities is less recognized. Videoconferencing now allows hospital-based specialists to provide consultations to urban nursing homes, prisons, primary care offices, schools, and even day care centers that have difficulty obtaining needed on-site care. TMH allows for the sharing of this scarce valuable resource across geographic and socioeconomic boundaries. In particular, TMH has been used successfully to provide needed services to children, the elderly, rural veterans, and correctional populations and holds promise for reaching the larger population that relies on primary care for their mental health treatment (see Section IV). Cultural and community aspects of care are a crucial component of developing services for these populations. TMH allows patients to be treated within their own communities, whether inner city or rural reservation, accompanied by their families and other supports, if desired. Several chapters provide insights and advice gleaned from clinical practice on how the cultural context must be considered in TMH, particularly when making decisions about how to use TMH technology to provide culturally competent care (in particular see Chapter 4).

The second of the critical developments listed above, *advances in the quality and availability of desktop and internet videoconferencing solutions*, has greatly increased the feasibility of conducting TMH in multiple, diverse settings. These technological options and their relevance for practice are covered in Section III. The advent of videoconferencing technology that can be conducted on desktop computers and the use of secure Internet transmission of videoconferencing data obviates the need for a separate space dedicated to videoconferencing and large, high-definition and costly units. A desktop, computer-based, system allows the clinicians to alternate between usual same-room and TMH care within the standard workflow of clinical practice. In addition, the widespread increase in the recreational use of desktop videoconferencing, such as SKYPE and Google Talk, has familiarized clinicians with videoconferencing which may reduce their resistance to using TMH. The ease of desktop videoconferencing has also promoted the adoption of TMH from private practitioners' offices, or even their homes—which allows a unique option when balancing the demands of family and career. This is one of the first developments in TMH that has improved access and opportunities for the provider, rather than the patient. As provider acceptance is necessary for widespread adoption, this is no small benefit.

The relevance of these newer desktop videoconferencing systems, of course, is their ability to provide care comparable to that provided through traditional, more expensive, high-definition systems—and to same-room care. In Section II, clinical technique, therapeutic alliance, and efficient workflow are addressed to help potential TMH providers glean the relevant issues in selecting equipment. This section also addresses the ethical, privacy, and regulatory requirements of clinical practice that must be considered in choosing technology and establishing a practice.

The third critical area influencing the adoption of TMH is *reimbursement.* Medicare reimbursement for TMH has made great strides since the year 2000 and now includes coverage for psychiatric diagnostic interviews, pharmacologic management, and individual psychotherapy (Centers for Medicare and Medicaid Services, 2009). Further, reimbursement is the same as the current fee schedule for same-room care, and the facility where the patient is treated can also submit a "facility fee" (approximately $30–35 per visit). As Medicare guidelines in these areas are dynamic and influence regulations by private payers, potential TMH providers should consult the web site for the Centers for Medicare and Medicaid for further and up-to-date information (*www.cms.gov/Manuals/ downloads/bp102c15.pdf*).

As of 2011, 39 states have some form of reimbursement for telemedicine within their Medicaid population (Center for Telehealth and eHealth Law, 2011). In addition, state governments faced with large mental health provider shortages and geographic access issues are now passing legislation requiring private insurers within their states to reimburse for telemedicine, including TMH (American Psychological Association Practice Central, 2012). Reimbursement by private insurers opens many opportunities for private practitioners who typically are not eligible for Medicare or Medicaid payments. Further information can be obtained at http://www.apapracticecentral.org/update/2011/03-31/reimbursement.aspx.

Issues related to the fourth critical development, *the establishment of an evidence base*, is addressed in Chapter 19 (see Section VI). This candid look at the strengths and weaknesses of the current research allows potential providers to assess the quality of psychiatric assessment, psychiatric follow-up, and psychotherapy provided through TMH. In the past 10 years, well-designed randomized controlled trials have not only demonstrated that TMH is comparable to same-room care, it has also demonstrated that TMH is effective in treating mental illness. However, the importance of an evidence base underlies all of the chapters in this text, particularly the chapters addressing the treatment of special populations (see Section IV) and those addressing specific interventions (see Section V).

Finally, the fifth critical development, *a national mandate for health reform*, is evidenced by the active debate within the United States on the need for and nature of health care reform. On March 23, 2010, President Obama signed the Affordable Care Act enacting comprehensive health insurance reforms to expand the provision of health care to uninsured and underinsured Americans. At the time that this book goes to press, the constitutionality of this act will be determined by the US Supreme Court making some skeptical about whether the reform will actually occur. The decision of the Supreme Court is unknown, as is its impact. However, the open national debate has led to widespread acknowledgment that health care reform, in some version, is imperative given the inequities and spiraling costs of health care in the United States. In April 2012, the Centers for Medicare and Medicaid Services issued a report stating that the Affordable Care Act will save over $200 billion for taxpayers through 2016 (Centers for Medicare and Medicaid Services, 2012). This suggests that even if the Affordable Care Act is struck down, the imperative for health care reform lies within the larger federal structures responsible for providing health care for millions of Americans and is not tied solely to a single presidential administration.

Organization of This Book

This book was inspired by the converging evidence that the time for TMH has come. The book seeks to stimulate conversation and action among health providers and those interested in health innovation. Though innovations in TMH span video-conferencing, online therapy, eHealth, mobile technology, and health information technology, this book, with some exceptions, is primarily concerned with the provision of mental health care through real-time videoconferencing. This platform is most consistent with current approaches to mental health care, has the strongest evidence base supporting its feasibility, acceptability, and effectiveness, and is increasingly being accepted and reimbursed by both public and private payers. Other exciting platforms for providing TMH care have the potential to augment videoconferencing as well as to eventually stand on their own as service delivery models. Hopefully, their applications will soon be explored in other texts.

Each chapter presents new approaches for understanding and solving the disparities in mental health care by providing hands-on guidance on how to start and maintain a TMH practice including clinical, administrative, ethical, and financial guidance. The evidence base for this guidance is provided throughout the book.

The aims for this text are ambitious and comprehensive. There are six sections. Section I provides the context for the remaining sections by describing major demographic and professional changes that underlie the problem TMH seeks to remedy that of poor access to mental health services. Though Chapter 2 focuses on the declining psychiatry workforce, data on the declining psychology workforce and urban/rural differences in access to any form of mental health care are also discussed. The other sections describe potential solutions to this problem. Section II provides guidance on how to conduct clinical sessions through TMH while optimizing ethical and culturally competent care and minimizing risk. Clinicians and investigators with many years of experience in the use of videoconferencing to provide TMH services offer insights and advice to optimize TMH practice.

Section III follows with some "nuts-and-bolts" discussion of both the business and technical infrastructure needed to provide TMH. These chapters include discussions of the newer business models that are emerging in TMH care. Together, Sections II and III provide a tutorial on how to develop a TMH practice that meets all of the clinical and regulatory requirements found in same-room care.

TMH has arisen in response to provider shortages, most often in populations faced with multiple barriers to care, and TMH has the goal of redistributing the provider workforce. Section IV describes the research supporting TMH and offers guidelines for clinical practice with special populations. Children, the elderly, incarcerated, and geographically remote patients all suffer poor access to care so it is not surprising that the early development of TMH has focused on these populations. Section V complements Section IV with discussions of assessment and treatment provided through TMH.

Section VI focuses on future applications of TMH. There is growing excitement about the potential of TMH to address much needed mental health care in disaster relief. Chapter 17 discusses the challenges of such care as well as the cause for growing optimism. It also sets the agenda for what needs to be accomplished so the potential of TMH in this context can be realized. Like disaster relief, the potential of social networking in TMH care is just starting to be realized. Chapter 18 discusses the few case studies of how videoconferencing has entered the sphere of mental health care. The chapter also provides hands-on guidance for clinicians to consider before "friending" their professional relationships. As already stated, the aim of this text is to provide the evidence base for the topic addressed in each chapter. Therefore, Chapter 19 serves as an editorial review of the strengths and weaknesses of the current evidence base and indicates directions for future work. It also addresses the newer developments in TMH such as mobile applications and eHealth.

Telemedicine has been "just around the corner" for decades. How do we know that its time has truly come? The chapters in this book illustrate again and again that the convergence of unmet mental health need, technologic advances, changes in health care structure, a growing evidence base and clinical practice history make the time now. This book aims to facilitate the process by convincing readers interested in health innovation that a powerful solution is at our fingertips, and concerted efforts to promote TMH will benefit all.

References

American Psychological Association Practice Central (2012). *Reimbursement for telehealth services*. Legal and Regulatory Affairs Staff. <http://www.apapracticecentral.org/update/2011/03-31/reimbursement.aspx> Accessed 25.05.12.

Center for Telehealth and eHealth Law (2011). *Medicaid reimbursement*. <http://ctel.org/expertise/reimbursement/medicaid-reimbursement/> Accessed 25.05.12.

Centers for Medicare and Medicaid Services. (2009). *The Medicare benefit policy manual* (Chapter 15). <http://www.cms.gov/Regulations-and-Guidance/Guidance/Manuals/downloads/bp102c15.pdf> Accessed 25.05.12.

Centers for Medicare and Medicaid Services (2012). *The affordable care act: Lowering medicare costs by improving care.* <http://www.cms.gov/apps/files/ACA-savings-report-2012.pdf> Accessed 25.05.12.

Demyttenaere, K., Bruffaerts, R., Posada-Villa, J., Gasquet, I., Kovess, V., & Lepine, J. P., et al. (2004). Prevalence, severity, and unmet need for treatment of mental disorders in the World Health Organization world mental health surveys. *Journal of the American Medical Association, 291,* 2581−2590.

Kessler, R. C., Berglund, P. A., Bruce, M. L., Koch, J. R., Laska, E. M., Leaf, P. J., et al. (2001). The prevalence and correlates of untreated serious mental illness. *Health Services Research, 36,* 987−1007.

Kessler, R. C., Demler, O., Frank, R. G., Olfson, M., Pincus, H. A., Walters, E. E., et al. (2005). Prevalence and treatment of mental disorders 1990 to 2003. *New England Journal of Medicine, 352,* 2515−2523.

Lewis, R. B., Martin, G. L., Over, C. H., & Tucker, H. (1957). Television therapy: Effectiveness of closed-circuit television as a medium for therapy in treatment of the mentally ill. *A.M.A. Archives of Neurology and Psychiatry, 77,* 57−69.

Nelson, E. L., Barnard, M., & Cain, S. (2003). Treating childhood depression over videoconferencing. *Telemedicine Journal and E-health, 9,* 49−55.

Thomas, C. R., & Holzer, C. E., III (2006). The continuing shortage of child and adolescent psychiatrists. *Journal of the American Academy of Child and Adolescent Psychiatry, 45,* 1023−1031.

United States Public Health Service Office of the Surgeon General (1999). *Mental health: A report of the surgeon general,* United States Public Health Service Office of the Surgeon General, Rockville, MD.

World Health Organization (2001). *The world health report 2001—Mental health: New understanding, new hope.* Geneva, Switzerland: World Health Organization Press. <http://www.who.int/whr/2001/en/> Accessed 29.05.12.

2 Telemental Health as a Solution to the Widening Gap Between Supply and Demand for Mental Health Services

*Michael Flaum**

Department of Psychiatry, University of Iowa Carver College of Medicine, Iowa City, IA

Workforce Shortages in Mental Health: The Example of Psychiatry

What Is the Current Supply of Psychiatrists in the United States?

As of 2010, there were just under 50,000 psychiatrists practicing in the United States. (*Note*: source of all data in Figures 2.1–2.5 is from American Medical Association (2010).) This makes psychiatry the sixth most common specialty in medicine (behind internal medicine, pediatrics, family practice, obstetrics/gynecology, and anesthesia). Figure 2.1 shows how psychiatrists are distributed in terms of specialty and practice setting. Approximately 18% of US psychiatrists are certified in Child and Adolescent Psychiatry. More than 11% of all psychiatrists are currently in residency or fellowship training. About three-quarters (78%) are primarily in office-based outpatient settings.

In order to put these numbers into a meaningful context, it is necessary to look at trends over time, how these trends compare to the numbers of other physicians, and most importantly, how the trends over time correspond with trends in utilization of services.

Rate of Growth in Psychiatrists and All Physicians Over Time

Figure 2.2 shows the numbers of general and child psychiatrists over the past 40 years and Figure 2.3 shows the number of all physicians in the United States over

* Corresponding author: Michael Flaum, Department of Psychiatry, University of Iowa Carver College of Medicine, 1-400 Medical Education Building, Iowa City, IA 52242. Tel.: +1-319-353-4340, Fax: +1-319-353-3003, E-mail: michael-flaum@uiowa.edu

Telemental Health. DOI: http://dx.doi.org/10.1016/B978-0-12-416048-4.00002-6

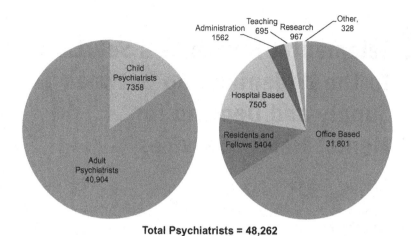

Total Psychiatrists = 48,262

Figure 2.1 Specialty and Treatment Setting for Psychiatrists in the United States, 2010.

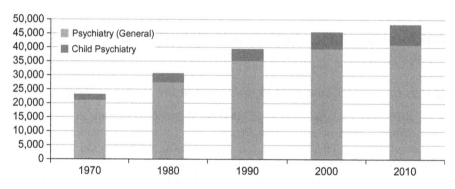

Figure 2.2 Number of General and Child Psychiatrists in the United States, 1970–2010.

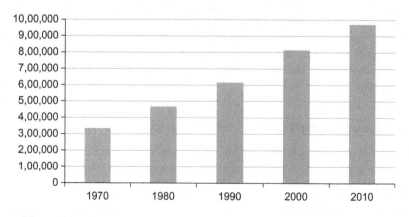

Figure 2.3 Total Number of Physicians in the United States, 1970–2010.

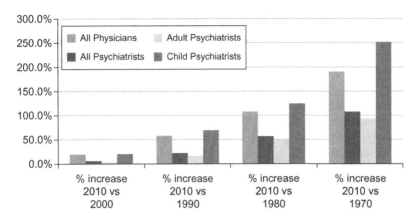

Figure 2.4 Percent Increase in General and Child Psychiatrists and All Physicians over the Past four Decades (2010 versus 2000, 1990, 1980, and 1970).

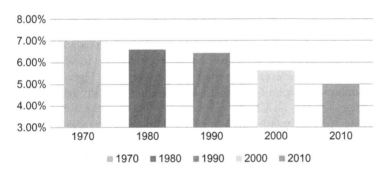

Figure 2.5 Percent of Psychiatrists of all US Physicians, 1970–2010.

the same time period. Several points are worth noting. First, while the increase in all physicians has been relatively constant over this time, the increase in numbers of psychiatrists has flattened out over the past two decades. Second, the rate of growth is substantially lower for psychiatrists than for all physicians (Figure 2.4). For example, while there has been a nearly 20% increase in the number of US physicians in the past decade, there has been less than a 6% increase in the number of psychiatrists during the same period. Third, growth in child psychiatry has substantially outpaced that of general psychiatry. Specifically, there has been a 20.2% and 69.4% increase in the numbers of child psychiatrists over the past 10 and 20 years, respectively, versus 3.6% and 16.3% for general psychiatrists over those two decades. Finally, as the increase in the numbers of psychiatrists has not kept pace with that of the increase in the numbers of physicians, the percentage of psychiatrists among physicians continues to fall (Figure 2.5).

The Psychiatry Pipeline: Trends in Residency Training

As can be seen in Figure 2.6, the number of psychiatry residents in the United States has been essentially flat over the past two decades (American Psychiatric Association Resident Census, Characteristics, and Distribution of Psychiatry Residents in the U.S., 2010–2011). The numbers of medical students nationally have increased steadily (American Medical Association, 2001), and this reflects an ongoing proportional decrease in the numbers of medical students choosing careers in psychiatry. There has been much discussion, concern, and debate about reasons for this, including financial concerns (psychiatry is consistently among the lowest paid of the medical specialties). What is clear from these data is that the number of psychiatrists entering the field, at least those trained in US programs, will not be expected to increase in the foreseeable future.

The Aging-Out Effect

Perhaps of greatest concern in predicting the future supply of psychiatrists comes from an analysis of the age distribution of the current psychiatric workforce (American Association of Medical Colleges, 2008). Psychiatrists as a group are older than their counterparts in almost every other field. Here is a sobering statistic that is easy to remember: *Fifty-five percent of all currently practicing psychiatrists in the United States are over the age of 55.* As shown in Figure 2.7, the corresponding numbers for each of the other most common specialty areas are all in the 30–40% range. (Across all US physicians, 37.6% are over the age of 55). Indeed, when looking at this metric across all 35 subspecialties categorized by the American Medical Association, psychiatry was second only to preventive medicine in the percentage aged 55 or older. Thus, the majority of current psychiatrists in the United States will enter retirement age within the next decade.

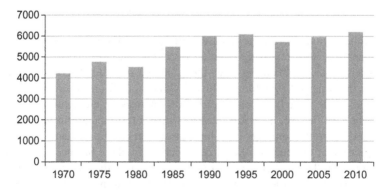

Figure 2.6 Number of Psychiatry Residents and Fellows in US programs, 1970–2010. *Source*: http://psych.org/MainMenu/EducationCareerDevelopment/EducationalInitiatives/ residentcensus./1011census.aspx?FT = .pdf.

What Is the Current Need or Demand for Psychiatrists in the United States?

Estimating the need or demand for psychiatrists and/or psychiatric services requires the modeling of a combination of epidemiological and health services utilization data.

Methodologically sound prevalence estimates of mental illness began in earnest in the early 1980s with the Epidemiological Catchment Area (ECA) study (Robins & Regier, 1991). The main finding was that of over 20,000 adults surveyed across five US sites, the estimated annual prevalence rate of having any of the psychiatric disorders included in the study was 28.1% (Regier et al., 1993). A second key finding was that a minority (28.5%) of those who met study criteria for a mental disorder accessed any kind of treatment.

In the early 1990s, the National Comorbidity Study (NCS) (Kessler et al., 1994) documented findings that were similar to the ECA study regarding both prevalence and treatment for mental disorders, despite some significant methodological differences. In the NCS of a nationally representative sample of over 8000 respondents, 29.4% of adults (ages 15−54) met criteria for a mental disorder within the previous 1 year. As with the ECA study, a minority (in this case about 20%) received some sort of treatment for the disorder. The methodological differences between the ECA and NCS studies did not allow for a clear comparison of any changes in either prevalence or utilization of services over time.

To do so, the methods utilized in the NCS were replicated in a larger sample in the early 2000s (2001−2003). That study, known as the NCS-R (NCS-Replication (Kessler, Berglund et al., 2005)), remains at the time of this writing the "gold standard" on prevalence of mental disorders and utilization of mental health services nationally. The study involved almost 10,000 completed interviews of a representative nationwide sample of adults ages 18 or older and included data on illness characteristics such as age of onset, severity, and comorbidity, as well as service

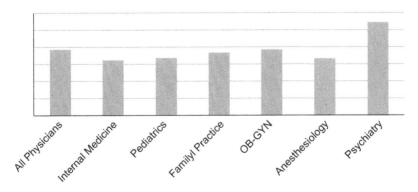

Figure 2.7 Percent of Active Physicians over the age of 55 by Specialty (top six specialties).
Source: https://www.aamc.org/download/47352/data/specialtydata.pdf.

utilization data including provider types and frequency (Kessler, Berglund et al., 2005; Kessler, Demler et al., 2005).

Two key findings emerged from the comparison of the NCS and NCS-R results and are as follows:

1. Prevalence of mental illness did not appear to change over time, with no evidence of an increase. The NCS-R overall prevalence rate was 30.5% versus 29.4% 10 years previously ($P = 0.52$).
2. Rates of treatment increased significantly from 12.2% of the total population in the 1990s to 20.1% a decade later ($P < 0.001$).

Thus, despite no evidence of a change in the underlying rate of mental illness, almost twice as many people were seeking some kind of treatment. There has been much speculation and study as to reasons for this trend which is often attributed to progress in the destigmatization of mental illness.

The NCS-R also detailed the type of providers accessed over the prior year by those individuals diagnosed with mental illness. Strikingly, as shown in Figure 2.8, less than half of those identified as having a mental illness in that sample accessed any kind of mental health treatment (broadly defined, including both medical and nonmedical services) (Kessler, Demler et al., 2005). An even smaller proportion accessed medical services, and of those who did, primary care physicians provided more psychiatric services than psychiatrists across all levels of severity of mental illness. This low penetration rate suggests that the actual demand for services may not yet be nearly commensurate with the underlying need.

Quantifying the need for different kinds of providers of mental health services

In the mid-2000s, the Health Resources and Services Administration (HRSA) commissioned a series of studies to further clarify the need for mental health professionals nationally. The series of resulting studies (Ellis, Konrad, Thomas, &

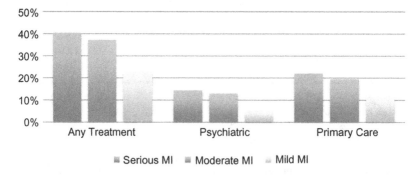

Figure 2.8 Percent of those identified in the NCR-S Sample with Mental Illness Accessing Mental Health Services over the Prior Year by Severity and Provider Type.

Morrissey, 2009; Konrad, Ellis, Thomas, Holzer, & Morrissey, 2009; Thomas, Ellis, Konrad, Holzer, & Morrissey, 2009) built on the NCS-R prevalence data and combined this with county-level population and workforce data nationally. Using licensure data, they compiled county-level estimates of six types of mental health professionals: psychiatrists, advanced practice psychiatric nurses, psychologists, social workers, marriage and family counselors, and licensed professional counselors. They categorized the first two as "mental health prescribers" and the others as "nonprescriber mental health professionals." A variety of data sources were used to examine utilization patterns, including different contributions of primary care physicians as mental health prescribers, allowing for estimates of the amount of time over a given year a person would be likely to spend with both prescribers and nonprescribing mental health professionals. They estimated the utilization of, and need for, mental health services separately for those with and without a "serious" mental illness.

Konrad et al. (2009) found that about half of those with serious mental illness accessed at least one kind of mental health service in the reference year studied. Specifically, those with serious mental illness spent about 10.5 h/year with a "nonprescriber" mental health professional and about 4.4 h/year with a prescriber, who might have been a psychiatrist, a psychiatric nurse practitioner, or a primary care physician. As expected, those without serious mental illness spent much less time, but nevertheless some time, on mental health needs—specifically, 7.8 and 12.6 min/year with nonprescribers and prescribers, respectively.

From these data, and taking into account different levels of contributions of primary care physicians, these investigators estimated the overall need for 25.9 psychiatrists/100,000 adult population. Based on 2010 census data, that translates into a need for over 60,000 psychiatrists, to care only for adults (ages 18 or over). If a similar level of needs is extrapolated to include children, then the corresponding number is just under 80,000.[1]

It is noteworthy that these estimates far exceed those developed over 30 years ago by the Graduate Medical Education National Advisory Committee, which was 15.4/100,000. Interestingly, our current supply of 48,000 fits the 30-year-old estimate but is far short of current estimates.

The HRSA-commissioned studies supplied further evidence and quantification of the supply and demand mismatch on a county level. Defining "severe shortage" as over half the estimated need unmet, they reported that over three-quarters of all counties in the United States (77%) met criteria for a "severe shortage" of psychiatric prescribers. Of those remaining, only 4% of all US counties appeared to have a supply of psychiatric prescribers equal to the demand. Finally, it is important to recognize that the data summarized above likely represent an underestimate of prevalence in light of several methodological limitations. Most notably, persons who are homeless or institutionalized (either in nursing, psychiatric, or correctional

---

[1] http://www.census.gov/compendia/statab/2012/tables/12s0007.pdf.
Calculations: $25.9/100,000 = x/234,564,000$ (2010 US population age 18); $x = 60$,
$75225.9/100,000 = x/308,746,000$ (total US population in 2010) $x = 79,965$.

facilities), as well as those in the military, tended to be excluded from most of the prevalence estimates.

Also, these studies do not tend to take into account trends in utilization that have occurred more recently than the early 2000s. However, there is certainly reason to suspect that utilization patterns are indeed continuing to grow. Pharmaceutical data show that Americans are utilizing psychoactive medications at markedly increased rates (Wang et al., 2005). For example, as of 2005, nearly one out of every ten Americans was taking an antidepressant medication (27 million people), more than double the number taking them a decade earlier. Stimulant medications are being prescribed to adults in rates that were unheard of a decade ago, and antipsychotics are being used as widely beyond psychotic disorders. The more common use of polypharmacy in psychiatry (e.g., augmentation of antipsychotics for mood disorders) and black box warnings on antidepressants in children and adolescents, or higher doses of commonly prescribed selective serotonin reuptake inhibitors (SSRIs) are likely to cause reluctance among primary care physicians to continue to take responsibility for mental health prescribing.

These factors, along with the implementation of federal and state parity mental health parity laws, increasingly aggressive direct marketing of psychoactive medications to consumers, economic hardships, and the toll of two long wars will likely result in an ongoing increase in the demand for psychiatric services in the foreseeable future.

The Distribution of Psychiatrists: The Iowa Example

The final, and perhaps most critical, piece of the supply and demand gap has to do with the geographic distribution of existing psychiatric resources. The author of this chapter has spent his career as a psychiatrist in the state of Iowa which provides the opportunity to describe trends in the psychiatric services gap that appears to be representative of the pattern throughout the country.

As shown in Figure 2.9, as of 2011, Iowa has 238 actively practicing psychiatrists (Kelly, 2006). With a population of about 3 million, this translates to a rate of about 8 psychiatrists/100,000, ranking it in the bottom 5 of states in terms of psychiatrists per capita (American Medical Association, 2010). But an even greater practical problem is that almost a quarter of all of the state's psychiatrists work in the same building, i.e., a large academic medical center. More than half of these are located in just two of Iowa's 99 counties. More than two-thirds of Iowa's counties have no psychiatrists at all, at least at their primary practice locations.

While "circuit riding,", i.e., spending time in many locations is common and an important contribution to solving this problem, it is still the case that the majority of the state does not have easy access to psychiatrists. Waiting lists are long and growing longer. There is widespread recognition that the situation has reached crisis proportion and stakeholders are coming together to seek alternatives.

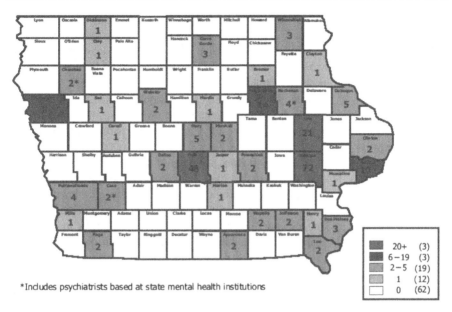

*Includes psychiatrists based at state mental health institutions

■ 20+	(3)
■ 6–19	(3)
▨ 2–5	(19)
▨ 1	(12)
□ 0	(62)

Figure 2.9 Geographic Distribution of Iowa Psychiatrists as of 2011.
Source: Iowa Health Professions Tracking Center, University of Iowa Carver College of Medicine, February 2011.

Telepsychiatry as a Key Strategy for Closing the Gap

Among the many strategies that have been discussed to address the state's marked maldistribution of psychiatric services, telepsychiatry has been the obvious front-runner, and its use is growing daily. There has been a significant investment in a telepsychiatry infrastructure, much of it funded through Magellan Health Services which manages behavioral health for Iowa's Medicaid population. Telepsychiatry suites are now available in a majority of the state's community mental health centers, with access points in more than two-thirds of all counties. Reimbursement policies have also been implemented allowing for equivalent fee-for-service payments for telepsychiatry visits as for same-room care, in addition to a small care coordination fee paid to the local site on a per patient per month basis. This is consistent with a national trend in which states are passing legislation mandating that private insurance policies must reimburse telepsychiatry visits at the same rate as same-room care.

Telepsychiatry has also been widely and successfully used for many years in Iowa's prison system and throughout the Veterans Administration Hospitals in the region. At least one rural hospital in Iowa is using telepsychiatry for its inpatient psychiatric services. A pilot program is under way using telepsychiatry services in several rural community hospital emergency rooms. A psychiatric physician's assistant (PA) has become one of the primary providers of child and adolescent psychiatric services in a rural corner of the state, with supervision being provided through videoconferencing by University of Iowa faculty.

Yet, despite all of this activity, telepsychiatry has not yet reached the "tipping point," at least not in Iowa where it is arguably needed more than in most places in the country. The use of telepsychiatry to meet service needs is still by far the exception rather than the rule. The numerous telepsychiatry suites sit empty most of the time. Less than 10% of the state's psychiatric workforce has had any telepsychiatry experience whatsoever, and it is not yet a routine part of our residency training programs.

Why not? Some of this can be explained in terms of system inertia. Systems, as well as individuals, tend to do what they have always done despite evidence that the world is changing rapidly. It is possible that most of the inertia in this particular area can be best understood as a direct result of the existing supply versus demand gap described above. That is, most currently practicing psychiatrists in Iowa, no matter what setting they are in, already have more business than they can handle. As such, finding ways to enhance access tends to be low on their priority lists. If, as the evidence presented above would suggest, the need has already outstretched supply, telepsychiatry alone will not substantially change that imbalance. Efficiencies that may be gained with the use of telepsychiatry are likely to be outpaced by the widening supply and demand gap.

That is, of the various efforts currently under way to address the psychiatric workforce shortage in Iowa, two small pilot projects are of particular interest. Both happen to require telehealth:

1. In one small effort to address the psychiatric workforce issue, the Iowa legislature in 2005 provided funding to develop and maintain an 1-year fellowship program in psychiatry for PAs. It is one of two or three programs of its type nationally, and thus far, it has been successful in that each of the PAs who have matriculated through it have gone on to focus in psychiatry. Recently, the program recruited what appeared to be its poster-child candidate: A PA who had been doing family practice in one of the most underserved areas of the state for 10 years, and who recognized the acute need for psychiatric services, wanted to obtain training in psychiatry to bring back to his hometown. His local health system was highly supportive and eager to hold his job for him through his training year. The problem, however, was that there was no psychiatrist in the area to supervise him once he completed training. With the endorsement of the state's PA licensure board, a model of distance supervision was developed in which the psychiatrists with whom he had trained provided his psychiatric supervision via telehealth. For better or worse (work is under way to look at various quality indicators), that PA-psychiatrist team is now the primary provider of psychiatric services in the area.

2. A child psychiatrist based at the University of Iowa has established service agreements with multiple rural pediatric practices to provide psychiatric consultative services to the primary care team. The model is based on the consultation service established at the University of Massachusetts to provide telephone consultation statewide to primary care physicians and expanded by the University of Washington to supplement telephone consultation with TMH consultation as needed (Hilt, McDonell, Rockhill, Golombek, & Thompson, 2009; Sarvet, Gold, & Straus, 2011). In the University of Iowa service, patients and families are evaluated directly when necessary, but much of the

communication is limited to consultation between the psychiatrist and the pediatrician or, in some cases, between the psychiatrist and a care coordinator. There is also a didactic educational element with "lunch and learn" sessions monthly. All of the interactions, the direct patient care, the supervision, and the educational sessions are conducted via telehealth.

These are two examples that illustrate how telepsychiatry is most likely to be able to address the supply and demand gap. The simple algebra presented in this chapter (and illustrated below) is that the substantial gap which already exists between the need and workforce capacity for psychiatric services is predicted to widen over time.

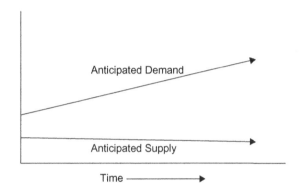

If psychiatrists continue to spend most of their time providing direct care to patients on a one-to-one basis, whether that is via telepsychiatry or same-room care, the visits will be even shorter than they already are, and fewer and farther between. Collaborative, team-based approaches will be necessary in which psychiatrists interact efficiently and effectively with other providers of psychiatric services, including primary care physicians, nurse practitioners, and PAs, as well as more innovative members of an expanding mental health workforce (e.g., allied health, consumers, and family members). Telepsychiatry can play a critical role in facilitating these approaches, and the degree to which it is successfully exploited to do so may allow for an optimal balance between supply and demand for psychiatric services.

Workforce Issues of Psychology Health Service Providers

Most of this chapter has focused on psychiatry which, as part of the medical profession, has several sources for data pertaining to workforce issues. It is not clear whether these issues also pertain to mental health professionals in general. Some comparable data are available for psychologist providers and suggest that the issues described above apply to the broader mental health workforce.

U.S. Department of Labor, 2011 estimates that in 2011 there were approximately 100,850 clinical, counseling, and school psychologists. Comparable to the trend in psychiatry, a 2008 American Psychological Association (APA) report reveals that 48% of its members were aged 55 and older. A survey of health service providers conducted by the APA reported a mean age of 52. Though the response rate for this survey was low, it should be noted that it was not restricted to APA members. Therefore, the "aging-out" phenomenon in psychiatry will also occur in psychology.

Fortunately, this 2008 APA survey included questions about telepsychology. Using a broad definition of telepsychology which included phone contact, the survey asked providers to report whether and how they used communication technology in their clinical practice. The respondents were prompted to respond "yes" only if they used the technology for actual communications about therapeutic issues which included appointment scheduling. Of 1226 survey respondents, 87.3% reported using telepsychology to deliver health services. As shown in Figure 2.10, the predominant media used was the telephone, with 85% reporting use. In total, 45.4% used e-mail. Far smaller percentages used listserves (12.6%), Internet videoconference (6.7%), non-Internet videoconference (6.3%), podcast (2.8%), and Internet chat room (2.3%).

Therefore, the predominant use of communication technology was the phone, with far fewer using videoconferencing. The most common types of services provided were appointment scheduling (71.8%), communication between sessions (64.7%), providing resources (63.2%), and referrals (62.4%). Actual provision of psychotherapy (33.5%) or counseling (20.6%) were far less frequently endorsed.

More recent American Psychological Association Center for Workforce Studies data also indicates disparities in availability of psychological services related to urban/rural status (American Psychological Association, 2011). A 2011 report based on data collected in 2008 estimates that approximately 85% of licensed psychologists are located in designated metropolitan areas, whereas 60% of the US population lives in metropolitan areas.

Data from Iowa regarding its licensed psychologist workforce confirms this finding (Kelly, 2006). Iowa has 19.1 licensed psychologists per 100,000 population which gives it a rank of 46th nationwide on this metric. It is far lower than neighboring states such as Minnesota (59.8/100,000) or Missouri (27.5/100,000). However, it is not lower than South Dakota (14.6/100,000), which is Iowa's

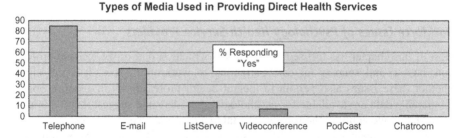

Figure 2.10 Survey of Psychologists Regarding their use of Electronic Media in Patient Care.

neighbor in national ranking, 47th. Among Iowa's psychiatrists, advanced registered nurse practitioners, social workers, and marital and family therapists, psychology has the highest percentage of practitioners aged 55 and older at 47%.

Efforts to relieve this shortage have focused on attracting and retaining providers in the state through support of psychology doctoral training programs and establishment of attractive internship opportunities. TMH solutions are currently being explored to address this shortage and the primary insurer for Medicaid, Magellan Behavioral Health, currently supports TMH throughout the state.

Conclusions: The Optimal Use of Telemental Health to Address Workforce Shortages

Remedying the workforce shortages in mental health care will require multiple new approaches. TMH is one approach to overcome the geographic disparity in the distribution of mental health providers, but TMH is not a stand-alone solution. It should be incorporated into evolving models of multidisciplinary collaboration.

Collaborative care models in which mental health specialists provide consultation and guidance to other professionals, or even to lay providers, is one of the most well-documented means of multiplying workforce capacity (Bauer et al., 2011; Richardson, McCauley, & Katon, 2009). These models could be readily adapted to TMH. In one of the most interesting demonstrations of this process, Hilty, Yellowlees, and Nesbitt (2006) demonstrated that consultation through TMH to rural primary care providers was associated with an increase over time in accuracy of diagnosis and medication dosing. Medication dosing adequacy, as defined by national guidelines, increased from 47.4% to 63.6% ($P = 0.001$) over a period of 6 years. Rural primary care providers' perceptions of being able to treat more patients for psychiatric problems also increased over time. Though many TMH consultants have noted such change over time in the knowledge base developed by their consultees, this is one of the first studies to document such success. Perhaps making such skill acquisition an explicit goal of TMH consultation, in addition to improved patient outcomes, would accelerate and increase the degree to which rural primary care providers can independently treat mental health problems.

Another way TMH can expand the mental health workforce is through online interventions that require minimal or no therapist contact (Andersson, 2009). This research is reviewed in Chapter 19. The research supporting online cognitive behavioral therapy indicates moderate effect sizes on average. Attrition from treatment remains a major issue but one that can be addressed in future research. Perhaps a combination of online therapy sites with a tethered social networking site will provide the needed interpersonal benefits of psychotherapy without using professional resources.

In short, TMH can improve access and increase efficiency in the distribution of mental health resources. However, the field must "think outside the box" to harness communication technology in ways that meaningfully expand and/or reallocate mental health resources in light of the inevitable growing need.

References

American Association of Medical Colleges. (2008). *Physician specialty data.* <https://www.aamc.org/download/47352/data/specialtydata.pdf> Accessed 25.05.12.

American Medical Association. (2001). *Graduate medical education database—AMA physician masterfile.* <http://www.ama-assn.org/ama/pub/about-ama/physician-data-resources/phsician-masterfile.page> Accessed 25.05.12.

American Medical Association. (2010). *Physician characteristics and distribution in the U.S.* Washington, DC: American Medical Association Press.

American Psychiatric Association Resident Census, Characteristics, and Distribution of Psychiatry Residents in the U.S. (2010−2011). <http://www.psychiatry.org/learn/research–training/resident-census> Accessed 25.05.12.

American Psychological Association. (2008). *2008 APA survey of psychology health service providers.* <http://www.apa.org/workforce/publications/08-hsp/index.aspx> Accessed 25.05.12.

American Psychological Association. (2011). *Underserved populations: Practice setting matters.* <http://www.apa.org/workforce/snapshots/2011/underserved-population.pdf> Accessed 25.05.12.

Andersson, G. (2009). Using the Internet to provide cognitive behaviour therapy. *Behaviour Research and Therapy, 47,* 175−180.

Bauer, A. M., Azzone, V., Goldman, H. H., Alexander, L., Unutzer, J., Coleman-Beattie, B., et al. (2011). Implementation of collaborative depression management at community-based primary care clinics: An evaluation. *Psychiatric Services, 62,* 1047−1053.

Ellis, A. R., Konrad, T. R., Thomas, K. C., & Morrissey, J. P. (2009). County-level estimates of mental health professional supply in the United States. *Psychiatric Services, 60,* 1315−1322.

Hilt, R., McDonell, M. G., Rockhill, C., Golombek, A., & Thompson, J. (2009). The partnership access line: Establishing an empirically-based child psychiatry consultation program for Washington State. *Report on Emotional and Behavioral Disorders in Youth, 9,* 9−12.

Hilty, D. M., Yellowlees, P. M., & Nesbitt, T. S. (2006). Evolution of telepsychiatry to rural sites: Changes over time in types of referral and in primary care providers' knowledge, skills and satisfaction. *General Hospital Psychiatry, 28,* 367−373.

Kelly, M. (2006). *Iowa's mental health workforce.* Iowa Department of Public Health. <www.idph.state.ia/hpcdp/health_care_access.asp> Accessed 25.05.12.

Kessler, R. C., Berglund, P., Demler, O., Jin, R., Merikangas, K. R., & Walters, E. E. (2005). Lifetime prevalence and age-of-onset distributions of DSM-IV disorders in the national comorbidity survey replication. *Archives of General Psychiatry, 62,* 593−602.

Kessler, R. C., Demler, O., Frank, R. G., Olfson, M., Pincus, H. A., Walters, E. E., et al. (2005). Prevalence and treatment of mental disorders, 1990 to 2003. *The New England Journal of Medicine, 352,* 2515−2523.

Kessler, R. C., McGonagle, K. A., Zhao, S., Nelson, C. B., Hughes, M., Eshleman, S., et al. (1994). Lifetime and 12-month prevalence of DSM-III-R psychiatric disorders in the U.S. Results from the national comorbidity survey. *Archives of General Psychiatry, 51*, 8−19.

Konrad, T. R., Ellis, A. R., Thomas, K. C., Holzer, C. E., & Morrissey, J. P. (2009). County-level estimates of need for mental health professionals in the United States. *Psychiatric Services, 60*, 1307−1314.

Regier, D. A., Narrow, W. E., Rae, D. S., Manderscheid, R. W., Locke, B. Z., & Goodwin, F. K. (1993). The de facto US mental and addictive disorders service system. Epidemiologic catchment area prospective 1-year prevalence rates of disorders and services. *Archives of General Psychiatry, 50*, 85−94.

Richardson, L., McCauley, E., & Katon, W. (2009). Collaborative care for adolescent depression: A pilot study. *General Hospital Psychiatry, 31*, 36−45.

Robins, L. N., & Regier, D. A. (1991). *Psychiatric disorders in America: The epidemiologic catchment area study*. New York, Toronto: Free Press, Collier Macmillan Canada, Maxwell Macmillan International.

Sarvet, B., Gold, J., & Straus, J. H. (2011). Bridging the divide between child psychiatry and primary care: The use of telephone consultation within a population-based collaborative system. *Child and Adolescent Psychiatric Clinics of North America, 20*, 41−53.

Thomas, K. C., Ellis, A. R., Konrad, T. R., Holzer, C. E., & Morrissey, J. P. (2009). County-level estimates of mental health professional shortage in the United States. *Psychiatric Services, 60*, 1323−1328.

U.S. Department of Labor. (2011). *Occupational employment and wages, May 2011*. <http://www.bls.gov/oes/current/oes193031.htm#nat> Accessed 25.05.12.

Wang, P. S., Lane, M., Olfson, M., Pincus, H. A., Wells, K. B., & Kessler, R. C. (2005). Twelve-month use of mental health services in the United States: Results from the national comorbidity survey replication. *Archives of General Psychiatry, 62*, 629−640.

Section Two

Developing a Therapeutic Space During Telemental Health

3 Establishing Therapeutic Rapport in Telemental Health

*Dehra Glueck**

Department of Psychiatry, Washington University School of Medicine, Washington University, St. Louis, MO

Introduction

Many clinicians who are considering a telemental health practice have questions about the impact videoconferencing technology (VTC) will have on their ability to establish rapport with their patients. Kaplan and Sadock define rapport as "the spontaneous, conscious feeling of harmonious responsiveness that promotes the development of a constructive therapeutic alliance" (Sadock, Sadock, Ruiz, & Kaplan, 2009). While the term rapport can be used across many settings, the related concept of therapeutic alliance has been well researched and found to a robust predictor of treatment response in mental health settings. For example, in a meta-analysis of 24 studies, Horvath and Symonds (1991) found that therapeutic alliance moderately accounted for treatment response per patients' perspective. Therapeutic alliance appears to be one of the most robust predictors of positive outcome in mental health treatment and does not appear to be a function of type of therapy or length of treatment. Understanding rapport in telemental health has additional nuance given the potentially negative impact of technology on the ability to develop an alliance, especially when the distant patient's community differs culturally and demographically from the clinician's own community. Nonetheless, experienced teleclinicians and preliminary research suggest that clinicians and patients can, and do, establish a solid rapport, therapeutic alliance, and satisfaction during telemental health treatment that equals face-to-face treatment (Bishop, O'Reilly, Maddox, & Hutchinson, 2002; Cook & Doyle, 2002; De Las Cuevas, Arredondo, Cabrera, Sulzenbacher, & Meise, 2006; Ghosh, McLaren, & Watson, 1997; Knaevelsrud & Maercker, 2006; Modai et al. 2006). Rather than seeing rapport as a fixed dimension, definitions focus on the "responsiveness" and bidirectional nature of this construct. Rapport is a concept that can be better understood by

* Corresponding author: Dehra Glueck, Department of Psychiatry, Washington University School of Medicine, 660 South Euclid, Campus Box 8134, St. Louis, MO 63110. Tel.: +1-314-286-1754, Fax: +1-314-286-1730, E-mail: glueckd@psychiatry.wustl.edu

Telemental Health. DOI: http://dx.doi.org/10.1016/B978-0-12-416048-4.00003-8

deconstructing how various clinicians establish rapport within the telemental health setting and understanding their techniques for addressing technical limitations. Thus, the goal of this chapter is to help clinicians to optimize rapport, and working alliance, during telemental health practice.

Review of the Literature on Rapport and Alliance

In light of the impact therapeutic alliance has as one of the strongest predictors of outcome in psychotherapy research, it has become an important developing area in telemental health research. Studies regarding rapport and therapeutic alliance join an emerging evidence base that includes studies that have more broadly examined patient's satisfaction, including a randomized clinical trial of 495 patients in Ontario, Canada, who received evaluations through either traditional face-to-face care or VTC care and subsequent follow-up. Patients in the VTC group demonstrated similar levels of satisfaction with their care as well as comparable clinical outcomes (O'Reilly et al., 2007). To date, several studies with small samples and a handful of larger studies have examined the relationship between alliance and the mode of service delivery. The most commonly used measure to assess alliance has been the Working Alliance Inventory (WAI; Andrusyna, Tang, DeRubeis, & Luborsky, 2001; Horvath & Greenberg, 1989). The WAI is a 36-item self-report measure with three main subscales: Task, Bond, and Goal. The Task subscale relates to therapeutic techniques used during the treatment, the Bond subscale assesses trust, empathy, and attachment to the therapist, and the Goal subscale assesses the degree to which the clinician and patient agree on treatment goals and work together toward these goals.

Most studies, both large and small, have not found major differences in the therapeutic alliance when comparing care that is delivered face-to-face with care through VTC (Bouchard et al., 2004; Ertlelt et al., 2010; Himle et al., 2006; Knaevelsrud & Maercker, 2006; Morgan, Patrick, & Magaletta, 2008). A solid alliance may be established with a typically difficult-to-treat groups such as those struggling with bulimia nervosa (Ertlelt et al., 2010) or obsessive compulsive disorder (Himle et al., 2006). In a study using the WAI with a sample of 100 incarcerated patients who were receiving mental health care, neither the WAI subscales nor the inmates' overall satisfaction with care varied according to the modality of service delivery (Morgan et al., 2008). Similarly, in a smaller sample of 21 patients with eating disorders, Bouchard et al. (2004) found no difference for patients' WAI scores for VTC versus face-to-face modalities.

Overall, the available literature on rapport and therapeutic alliance has supported the capability of clinicians and patients to develop a therapeutic alliance through VTC. However, the number of studies and subjects is not large, methodologies have differed across studies, and most have focused on patient ratings. Only occasionally do patients rate alliance, or rapport, as significantly lower for the VTC versus the face-to-face modality. Recently, Morland et al. (2010) found that patients rated leader alliance as lower in the VTC condition. This was associated with individual patient's outcomes but was not significant in contributing to group-level outcomes. These latter studies demonstrate the importance of continuing to refine the information gathered from studies in this emerging field in a way that reflects the diversity of settings in which telemental health is being used and its wide variety of applications.

Some studies have looked at rapport and therapeutic alliance as dyadic constructs that need input from both the patient and the treating clinician. For example, Ertlelt et al., (2010) used the WAI to assess therapeutic factors affecting the delivery of cognitive behavioral therapy through VTC versus face-to-face care for 116 patients with bulimia nervosa. They found that patients reported no overall differences according to treatment modality in the key components of Goals and Bond subscales including the dimensions of empathy and trust. However, the clinicians rated alliance on the Task, Bond, and Goal subscales as significantly lower for the group receiving care through VTC. Clearly, both patients' and clinicians' perspectives are important, particularly in efforts to expand the telemental health workforce. Additional questions remain regarding how clinicians can understand and positively impact therapeutic relationships within "virtual" settings.

Related studies that used online interventions, but not VTC, have also been used to shed light on the concepts of rapport and therapeutic alliance within therapeutic settings that use new or emerging technology. In a convenience sample of patients suffering posttraumatic stress, those who received an online intervention endorsed a better working alliance with their therapist than did patients receiving face-to-face care (Knaevelsrud & Maercker, 2006). However, the association between therapeutic alliance and positive outcomes was not as strong as found in the usual mental health intervention studies. Similarly, Cook and Doyle (2002) found no differences on the WAI in an online therapy treatment that included intensive writing exercises that were then submitted to a clinician. These investigators asked open-ended questions about patients' experiences and reported that a major theme in these comments was patients' sense of freedom to express themselves online without embarrassment. Even without real-time clinician contact, patients experienced the presence of the clinician. Extrapolation to VTC suggests that the interpersonal distance, or virtual relationship, that technology imposes might have benefits for patients. It also raises interesting questions as to how rapport and therapeutic alliances develop. As with any area of innovation, research has shown there are additional nuances to understand and indications that more work needs to be done to explore rapport and alliance when using telemental health. These studies begin to demonstrate the ability of telemental health clinicians and patients to establish therapeutic rapport sufficient to effect clinical improvements and to engage in evidence-based care and suggest avenues for further research.

Experience with health-care innovations across a broad array of settings suggests that there may be a wide range of factors, such as risk tolerance, comfort with change, and interest in innovation that impact an individual provider's willingness to adopt new technologies. It is also likely that these factors affect patients in significantly different ways. Consistent with this is the finding across a number of studies that patients are often more comfortable with receiving care through telemental health than clinicians are at providing it. One reason for this is thought to be patients' recognition of the ability of technology to deliver care that is not otherwise available in their area. It is also noted that there are certain convenience effects for patients such as not needing to travel long distances to obtain care and decreased stigma when care is provided by clinicians that patients do not have to encounter in their communities. Consistent with this split between patient and provider factors, Ertlelt et al. (2010) found that teleclinicians generally endorsed a higher working alliance in face-to-face care over telemental health care, although their patients did not. Rather than interpreting this finding as a fixed aspect of telemental health, Ertlet et al. suggested that clinicians will need additional training to increase their comfort with this method of service delivery. This conclusion is commensurate with the author's experience. In addition to encouraging clinicians to gain experience with telemedicine, it is often helpful to deconstruct complex concepts such as rapport into concrete techniques and suggestions that can be implemented and adapted by teleclinicians. Rapport is not a black or white concept, which develops, or not. It can be cultivated and more discussion and empirical investigation are needed to determine the best strategies for developing rapport and therapist competence in delivering VTC in general (Andersson & Cuipers, 2009). The remainder of this chapter aims to describe such strategies and to begin an ongoing discussion of how to best optimize patient's response to telemental health in light of how it impacts patients and clinicians.

Technological Considerations Impacting Rapport

Clinicians often rely on subtle observations of patient's affect and body movements to make diagnoses and convey nuances in meaning and emotional context. The ability to observe these subtleties is highly related to having sufficient bandwidth to allow fast transmission. When there is adequate bandwidth, the video images have very high resolution, so that even small movements are appreciated. There is also no time lapse in verbal transmission such that the patient and the teleclinician can freely converse including speaking at the same time. This need to approximate in-person communication is one of the most important indications for high bandwidth (>384 kbits/s), i.e., to ensure as fast and reliable a connection and as fast a frame rate (>30 frames/s) as possible. If the transmission has fluid motion and good resolution, then subtle changes in facial expression can be detected, such as tearfulness or even the blunting and quivering that precedes tearfulness. Affective withdrawal due to internal stimuli and oddities in prosody can also be readily appreciated. By contrast, at low bandwidth, these features may be difficult to pick up, and the desynchronization of verbal and visual input can make it difficult to assess such aspects of the mental status examination as latency of speech. It may also interfere with rapport due to the difficulties in communication.

High-speed transmissions are also important for detecting abnormal movements such as tremor in a patient with anxiety or in a patient suspected of having Parkinsonism. With fluid transmission, patients can be observed informally for movements such as tics as well as more formal assessments such as the Abnormal Involuntary Movement Scale (AIMS) when monitoring for side effects of antipsychotic medication. A study by Amerendran (2011) showed that administration of the AIMS by telemental health was as reliable as direct in person observation. Demonstration of conducting the AIMS through VTC can be viewed at http://www.rbha.net/presentations/RealWorldTelepsychRev/player.html (Gibson, 2012).

In addition to direct observation, staff at the remote site can be trained to administer the AIMS and provide reliable observations of patients.

In addition to bandwidth considerations, rapport may be impacted by camera placement and use. Advances in camera technology now provide excellent ability to detect subtle motions, interactions, and other factors that affect rapport. Adequate lighting in the room is critical. Cameras should be placed to allow easy observation of the room and of the patient's full body. It is important to avoid convenience placement in large multipurpose, sterile conference rooms or in small rooms with major obstacles to full visualization. For example, when working with hyperactive children, it is important to have adequate space to observe the child's gross motor, organizational, and play skills as well to follow the child's actions by controlling the distant camera. However, too large a room may be overstimulating and may interfere with the parent's ability to control the child. As another example, elderly or physically challenged patients will likely be accompanied by a caregiver and thus adequate space and camera movement will be needed to relate to both individuals and capture their interactions. On the other hand, when working with a patient suffering from depression or anxiety, a large conference room may feel too impersonal. The room should be sufficiently large to capture tremors in the lower extremities but small enough to convey confidentiality and "connectedness" with the teleclinician. The ability to zoom the camera in and out at the patient's site helps the telemental health clinician to assess dysmorphia, affective shifts, and relatedness. Often finding a balance of correct camera placement and utilization will enhance the teleclinicians' comfort and ability to establish both rapport and excellent observational skills.

It is also important to make sure that the microphones have sufficient sensitivity and placement to clearly detect the patient's speech. When the microphone is separate from the camera, placing the microphone close to the patient and on a table rather than on the ceiling is recommended. This allows the patient to move the microphone closer if there are difficulties in communicating. In contrast, ceiling placement often results in diminished quality and increased interference from echoes or background noises. Similar to concerns about camera use, it is best to avoid placement of the microphone in a conference room as it can be difficult to pick up speech, especially if the patient whispers, or the room causes an echo, or the microphone is placed too far from the patient. Some rooms benefit from carpeting or a large area rug on the floor or draperies on the windows so that there is less ambient noise. Similarly, carpeting in hallways outside the interview room can further decrease interference from outside noise. Some practitioners have used sound machines in the hallway outside the telemental health room both to decrease interference from outside noise as well as to increase auditory privacy for patients, especially if elderly patients require higher volume on the monitor to adequately hear the telemental health clinician. Finally, the telemental health room should not be near a window that opens onto a major roadway or walkway as the microphone will be affected by these outside noises. Sometimes detection of such noise can provide some comic relief. For example, during a session in a clinician's well positioned and appointed office at a major medical center, a "code purple" was called indicating possible fire. The soft alarm was detected at the patient's site by an elderly patient with hearing difficulties. He asked the calm clinician whether she wanted to check to see whether someone was trying to break into her office.

Like all modern technology, including popular cell phones, there can be disruptions in telemental health sessions when there are unavoidable technology failures, such as lost Internet connection, camera malfunctions, or changes in Internet usage that affect bandwidth. These impacts can be minimized by establishing backup systems, such as a telephone, to complete the session. This possibility should be discussed with patients at the beginning of telemental health care. Patients generally tolerate these vicissitudes fine. But it also highlights the importance of having good technical support so disruptions are minimized. It is recommended that the telemental health clinician maintains the contact numbers for remote sites and also for the direct contact of the patients in the event of a technical disruption.

Establishing Therapeutic Rapport with the Patient

One key element of establishing rapport is the ability to fluidly respond to the emotions of the other person. This is essential for conveying empathy and for discussing a patient's responses to the session. It is also important that patients feel that they can "read" the responses and emotional tone of the clinician and know that they are understood. As previously discussed, one important aspect of this exchange is having adequate bandwidth to ensure high-resolution video so that teleclinicians can use real-time changes in visual cues to determine the affective state of another person. Often, clinicians who are new to telemental health are surprised, and pleased, to note that patients cry and laugh in their sessions just as patients do in face-to-face care. When clinicians are experiencing lower resolution or are unsure of the patient's response, based on visual cues, they can seek verbal confirmation of their observation and interpretation. This adaptation can provide additional opportunities to positively impact rapport as patients have the opportunity to confirm or clarify the teleclinician's understanding of their response. For instance, asking a patient "Is something we are talking about making you sad?" is an opportunity both to inquire about the relationship between therapeutic content and affect and to clarify the clinician's read of the patient's emotional response through VTC.

Telemental health allows the opportunity to not only observe but also mirror patients' emotions and expressions. Studies of embodied emotions indicate that emotional information is processed, in part, through visual cues such as facial expression and postural movements (Niedenthal, 2007). Not only do individuals notice the emotions of others, but also they often mimic them, subconsciously or intentionally, as part of establishing rapport. This mirroring is readily accomplished in videoconferencing. Perhaps telemental health is uniquely suited to this task because of the teleclinician's ability to make detailed visual observations and to monitor their own body language by using the picture-in-picture (PIP) function on their monitor. The PIP function displays in a corner of the teleclinician's monitor the same image of themselves that the patient sees. One humorous example of this related to a teleclinician who felt as if all of his patients that day were "watching a tennis match" as their eyes were going from one side of the screen to the other. When the teleclinician switched on the PIP function, he realized his cat was walking back and forth on a cabinet behind him. Clinicians are encouraged to use the PIP function to monitor not only their environment but also their responses and facial expressions with patients. Some teleclinicians note that seeing the sad expression on their own face makes them aware of an empathic dimension they might not have previously detected. New telemental health clinicians often report feeling self-conscious when they first see themselves on their monitor. This is a normal part of adapting to the telemental health practice and can, in fact, become an important area of feedback and self-monitoring. Experienced teleclinicians will often discuss this aspect of telemental health openly with patients when they are showing some self-consciousness. Discussing the clinicians' own experience of first seeing themselves on the monitor can be another way to emphasize a common experience and respect for the novelty of the situation for the patient.

In addition to observation of facial expressions, eye contact is always important to the clinical interview and may take on increased importance in a telemental health encounter if there is decreased access to other nonverbal means of communication. The literature has discussed the maintenance of eye contact during the encounter as essential for building rapport. This is more a technical than a clinical issue. Patients and clinicians naturally communicate by looking at one another on the monitor. To obtain direct eye contact, the camera would have to be placed in the middle of the monitor, which is not technically possible. The camera is usually above, below, or to the side of the monitor, and the monitor is typically mounted relatively high on the wall. Eye contact then appears averted down, up, or sideways, respectively, as participants look at the monitor and not at the camera. The approximation of eye contact can be enhanced by optimizing camera placement directly in front of the patient at eye level for a seated person. This minimizes eye-gaze distortions. The monitor is then set higher or lower on the wall and not at eye level. Telemental health clinicians can also alternate their gaze from the monitor to the camera as the patient speaks, thereby providing the patient better eye contact. To help patients know where the clinician's eye gaze is directed, it is frequently helpful to have a written list of the participants' names in the room, so that questions can be directed by first saying the name of the person with whom the clinician wants to speak.

Desktop systems can also cause eye-gaze distortion based on camera placement, especially when using a built-in camera function. It is important to experiment prior to a session with determining the optimal distance from the camera in order to approximate normal eye gaze. Use of the PIP function can help with determining placement. Staff at the patient's site might also provide relevant information. Some teleclinicians like the relative mobility of desktop systems. It is important to make note of the eye contact prior to each session if the desktop system is routinely moved. If there is a small screen size, it is also recommended that clinicians provide regular feedback to the distant site regarding placement of patients in relation to the camera. They may also consider discussing placement directly with patients in order to improve the encounter and optimize rapport. Some clinicians note that built-in cameras can significantly change the "shape of the face." This distortion may impact comfort with using such a system. Overall, larger, high-definition screens provide optimal resolution, full viewing of the patient's site, and best approximate in person encounters. If such systems are not available, then clinicians are encouraged to manipulate the distant camera to obtain needed information and/or to discuss with patients how to optimize images and communication.

Some telemental health clinicians also avoid taking notes or using the electronic medical record during the encounter in order to maintain eye contact. If the camera is zoomed above the mid chest, some basic notes may be taken without disrupting eye contact, providing the clinician can write or type without looking away. Patient notes can be completed at the end of the session if the change in eye contact is negatively impacting the session. A potential downside of camera focus on such a small area of the teleclinician's physical image is that it does not convey the entire person as well and may not adequately approximate an in-person session. More research is needed on how clinician image affects rapport.

Explaining Telemental Health to Patients

One of the quickest ways to increase patients' comfort with telemental health is to explain what to expect and to demonstrate its use early in the process. This succinct explanation of telemental health has been referred to as "the pitch." A good pitch contains a basic explanation of the process, confidentiality and the equipment. The essential components of a sample pitch are as follows:

1. It is helpful to ask whether the patient has ever seen a doctor through television (TV) and, if not, whether he/she has used any VTC. If the patient has not seen a doctor through VTC, it is helpful to make references to common lay technology, such as Facetime or Skype and explain key differences.
2. It is helpful to let patients know why telemental health is being used in their community. For example, mental health clinicians are using technology to bring the patient expert care without burden to the patient of travel or missing work.
3. Patients can then be told that the session is happening in "real time." This can be nicely demonstrated by commenting on what the patient is wearing and his/her current gestures saying that "everything you can see about me, I can see about you. For instance, you are

wearing. . ." and "you just. . ." Children in particular seem to really like this exercise and proof that they too are being seen by the clinician.

4. The next step is to discuss security, such as encrypted technology, which is the HIPAA (Health Information Portability and Accountability Act) standard and can be described as having an "electronic tunnel from the camera where the clinician is sitting to the one where the patient is sitting." Additional information regarding technological specifications should be available if requested.

5. It is important to inform patients as to whether or not a session is being recorded. If the clinician wants to record a session, then the clinician must obtain explicit consent from the patient. Many patients appreciate being reassured that the session is not "on the Internet" in the sense that it can neither be openly viewed nor will it be placed on TV.

6. An important next step is to establish a visual context of where the clinician is sitting. Patients can be asked if they would like to see the clinician's office. Using the camera's zoom and pan features, clinicians can give patients a virtual tour of their offices so as to assure them that no one else is present and/or give some context to the clinical setting. In some settings it may be possible, or even desirable, to allow patients to manipulate the remote control at their end to conduct their own tour of the clinician's office and/or to give the clinician a tour of their clinic room. After the tour, it is helpful to let the patient know that most of the time the camera will be zoomed in sufficiently so that the patient can see the clinician's facial expressions.

7. Clinicians are then encouraged to discuss any technical difficulties noticed during the introduction. For instance, if there is a slight lag in audio that makes it seem as if the clinician and patient are talking over each other, the clinician can suggest adding a small pause after each statement. Clinicians can also take this opportunity to discuss any video lag or distortions. After such discussion by the clinician, patients are then free to bring up their concerns.

8. The final portion of "the pitch" is to give patients an opportunity to ask questions before starting the session. This may be especially helpful to younger and older patients who are not as comfortable with electronic media.

At the end of the pitch, it is common for patients to ask a few questions about the clinician personally or professionally and say something about telemental health being "different, but neat." At this time, patients can be asked whether they are comfortable proceeding with the session. The majority of patients will readily proceed; however, some may remain uncomfortable and convey this directly or indirectly by having reserved body language or looking to other people in the room for confirmation to proceed. Commonly their discomfort is shown by increased self-grooming or nervousness that they express by looking at others in the room or avoiding direct eye contact with the clinician. If additional reservations are expressed, clinicians are encouraged to ask patients to talk more about their concerns in case there are specific adaptations that may increase their comfort. For example, one way to minimize patients' discomfort is to take away the option many cameras have for displaying the PIP features, i.e., the ability for patients to see themselves in a corner of their screen. Though this view may be helpful when initially demonstrating the technology, it may increase some patient's self-consciousness and can be very distracting to children with high levels of distractibility who can spend the entire session making faces at themselves. Elderly patients with dementia or developmentally delayed adults may be confused about this feature of seeing themselves on the monitor. Many teleclinicians report that patients' nervousness disappears as they engage in conversation.

If the patient continues to express discomfort, referral to a clinician for traditional face-to-face care should be considered, either in the patient's community or at a metropolitan site. Patient's choice should be honored especially if adaptations to the telemental health encounter are not deemed to be adequate to address concerns. Having said this, telemental health has been used for patients with the most serious illnesses such as schizophrenia, substance abuse, posttraumatic stress disorders, cognitive impairment, personality disorders, and autism (De Las Cuevas et al., 2006; Elford et al., 2000; Jones & Ruskin, 2001; Kopel, Nunn, & Dossetor, 2001; O'Reilly et al., 2007; Ruskin et al., 2004). Clinical experience has shown that even patients with the most severe illnesses generally agree to telemental health care and there are no specific contraindications to its use for any disorder or age range.

It is recommended that discussions of rapport and assessments of patient's satisfaction with telemental health care continue to be openly discussed over time. In addition, when the clinician is not present, clinic staff are encouraged to routinely ask patients whether they are comfortable with the care they are receiving. This allows the patient to discuss telemental health, without concerns about how the telemental health clinician might respond. If the patient indicates that he or she is not comfortable, then standard risk management procedures should be followed regarding terminating the doctor−patient relationship and making appropriate referrals to another clinician.

Many patients find the experience of telemental health to be enjoyable once they gain experience, especially children. One patient diagnosed with autism was so excited about his monthly appointments that he told everyone at school about it. He told his teachers that he was going to see the "TV doctor." The patient's teacher was unaware of his receiving care through telemental health and asked the patient's grandfather "why are the TV sets in the house always broken." She assumed the TVs were in need of repair, i.e., it was the TVs that needed a doctor. For the elderly who have seen the coming of the "TV age" up to interactive videoconferencing, it might provide an opportunity to engage them in some discussion of their overall life experience with technology.

Developing Rapport with Special Populations

One of the best ways to develop rapport is to have fun with the patients, and telemental health presents the opportunity to explore the virtual world together. For instance, young children who are initially uncomfortable can be allowed to play "hide and seek." This can be accomplished by moving the distant camera to face the back wall while the clinician counts out loud. The child hides. Then the clinician uses the camera to search the room for the child's hiding place. Children also like to draw pictures and then hold them up to the camera or to have the staff send them to the clinician via fax or e-mail. Then the clinician can display the pictures at their site and ask the child to discuss them. The teleMental health uide web site, www.tmhguide.org, developed by the University of Colorado in collaboration with SAMHSA (Substance Abuse and Mental Health Services Administration) has coloring pages that show telemental health encounters with "doctors in the TV". This web site has been developed with robust content regarding starting telemental health programs and includes helpful links such as the coloring pages that can increase patient comfort with technology. These coloring pages can be printed at the patient's site and given to children to be colored during the session. Some teleclinicians arrange to have toys present at the patient's site and use these to talk about and engage caretakers in play. There is also an option to have a staff person on-site with the patient who can help engage young children in play.

A frequent question of clinicians is how to handle emotional outbursts at the patient's site. There are three broad options. The first, for patients who are accompanied by a caregiver, is to use the opportunity to coach caregivers on how to respond to negative or difficult behaviors. Additionally, if there is good rapport with the telemental health clinician, the clinician can directly intervene by speaking to the patient and getting his/her attention or distracting the patient. For more severe situations, such as an elderly patient who becomes disoriented, or a traumatized individual who experiences a flashback, or a suicidal patient, likely staff at the distant site will need to be involved to ensure safety. Indeed, protocols for such situations should be in place prior to starting a telemental health service.

Adolescent patients generally have greater comfort with technology than earlier generations, including their parents. It is important to discuss their experiences of commercially available videoconferencing, such as Facetime or Skype, and elicit specific feedback or questions in light of their knowledge and experience. This can also provide a natural bridge to discussing confidentiality. Similar to a face-to-face session, rules of confidentiality apply such that concerns expressed by the adolescent are kept confidential unless there are specific concerns about safety. Potentially unique to the telemental health setting are adolescent concerns about the security and privacy of the teleclinician's videoconferencing system and the inability for others to enter the session or observe without their knowing. Adolescents may need to be assured that their sessions will not be recorded and "shared on the Internet" or shown to their parents. Clinicians are encouraged to discuss this directly with patients and ensure confidentiality comparable to what they uphold in a face-to-face encounter.

There are several rapport-building options that stem from adolescents' frequent use of technology. If computers are available at both the teleclinician's and patient's site, clinicians are able to look at the same web site as a patient. This can allow them to look at social networking sites, such as Facebook, at the same time. Another example is to have the clinician ask adolescents about their favorite musical artist. Then, the teleclinician can search free musical sites, such as Youtube, on their computer and play the teen's favorite music through their computer's speakers while the adolescent listens at the remote site. The excellent sensitivity of the microphones provides a reasonable listening experience. Alternatively, adolescents can bring an MP3 player and place it near the microphone of the videoconferencing equipment in order to play music for the clinician. Adolescents can also be given opportunities to move the camera or explore the clinician's office. Some clinicians will put objects in their office such as landscape photographs or small sculptures that can be shared with adolescents and discussed as they tour the office.

Many clinicians express concern about how their elderly patients will respond to the technology. Clinical experience has shown that there can be elements of initial skepticism about care, but these are often overcome with experience. There are options of adjusting the volume of the monitor if there are concerns about hearing impairment as well as offering written materials or repeating explanations. In addition, age-appropriate attempts to communicate a shared world can be attempted. For instance, if there is significant distance between the sites, discussing the weather at each site or local events can be helpful. In the author's experience, elderly people often have increased comfort when other family members accompany them to the telemental health session. Also, for some racial or ethnic groups, several extended family members, or unrelated kin, may attend the session in order to be involved in the patient's care. Involving these folks is part of rendering culturally competent care. It is recommended that teleclinicians spend time understanding the cultural context of the community in which they practice. Accommodations may have to be made with the room, equipment, time of session or other factors in order to practice competently in selected situations or communities. For example, the use of telemental health is being examined with depressed Chinese Americans (Yeung, Hails, Chang, Trinh, & Fava, 2011).

Establishing Therapeutic Rapport with the Referring Clinic

Staff at the patient's site are an important ally of, and advocate for, telemental health. They can assist the telehealth clinician by providing cultural and ecological context regarding patients and the community. This is especially important if the patient lives in a community that differs ethnically and/or racially from the telehealth clinician's community. But, it is also important for community differences such as rural versus urban environments. Staff also often know how difficult it is to get specialty mental health services for individuals in their community. It is important to discuss the national shortages of specialty mental health care available in nonmetropolitan communities, particularly the shortages of psychiatrists, and the ability of telemental health to provide this expertise and access to evidence-based mental health care in their area. It is often helpful to also discuss the difficulties most families outside of metropolitan areas have faced in accessing expert mental health care such as long travel times, delays in referrals, underuse of specialty care, and lack of follow-up care. Telemental health can then be discussed as a "value added" service for patients as well as for their primary care physicians who struggle with caring for patients with mental health disorders and with navigating the barriers to finding adequate services for them. Some sites that provide telemental health services will also provide specialty telemedicine services such as cardiovascular treatment, diabetes management, or neurodevelopmental assessments. It can be helpful to discuss telemental health in the context of a spectrum of specialty health services for patients who lack access to such care. Teleclinicians can also build liaisons in the community by calling local primary care clinicians to discuss telemental health and referral to specialty care.

How the staff perceives telemental health is a primary determinant for how patients will perceive telemental health. Therefore, therapeutic rapport starts with the teleclinician establishing rapport with the clinic staff at the patient's site. One critical early factor in building this rapport is to designate a liaison with patients, such as a staff at the patient's site with good credibility in both the clinic and the larger community, who recognizes the value of telemental health and who likes or appreciates the telemental health clinician. As with any endeavor, and especially those involving technology, there will be problems and it also helps to have someone who is not afraid of the technology. This staff could be a clinician such as a nurse practitioner with whom the teleclinician might also serve a supervisory role or a therapist who refers to the telemental health program or even a clinic manager who has responsibility for the quality of patient's care. At some sites, this technology liaison might even be a medical assistant or supportive staff. The goal is an advocate for the service and someone who can troubleshoot simple problems.

As mentioned, the clinic's buy-in for telemental health is essential for the patient's buy-in. It helps if clinics discuss during, or before, scheduling that the visit will be via videoconferencing—that way there are no "surprises." This should be reiterated in any letter sent to families reminding them of their upcoming appointment. It can again be addressed when patients register in the clinic and sign forms to consent to treatment. Staff at the clinic can show patients the videoconferencing equipment before their first visit and begin an introduction to the process. This also gives patients a chance to ask questions in a setting where they do not have to worry about "offending" the telemental health clinician who will not be present and do not have to worry about looking uninformed. It is important to have clear protocols for staff's handling simpler technical problems as well as guidelines for contacting official audiovisual staff for major technical problems.

Finally, freedom of choice is often a key element of the telemental health buy-in. It is helpful in contracting with an agency to request that the agency establishes a referral line for face-to-face clinicians in case patients do not feel comfortable with telemental health (Quill & Brody, 1996). Although this may represent additional travel or expense for patients, it is important that they have options. Most agencies and clinicians attest that it is unusual for patients to refuse telemental health. If patients are hesitant, it is often helpful to have them experience a first session and then encourage them to complete two to three sessions before making a decision, unless there are urgent concerns that would prompt a more immediate face-to-face referral. Telemental health clinicians may also feel uncomfortable treating certain patients, and it is important that they also have the option for referral to other clinicians. There is not yet any definitive work on matching telemental health interventions to specific patients or diagnoses but, the American Telemedicine Association has published practice guidelines for telemental health (Grady, Myers, & Nelson, 2009a). There is also information regarding the provision of evidence-based care through telemental health that may aid in determining a patient's suitability for telemental health (Grady, Myers, & Nelson, 2009b). These guidelines also provide some information regarding the minimal technological specifications for a particular application of telemental health, although clearly this topic needs further investigation and is evolving rapidly. For example, most work on rapport building in telemental health has used higher bandwidth systems, but increasingly desktop and mobile devices are being considered and there are not data on their effects on rapport building.

Building Rapport with Staff: An Open-Door Policy

One thing clinicians fear about telemental health is the loss of informal time spent with other clinicians such as the old "lunchroom or water cooler talk" or the building of general rapport with coworkers which affects the work milieu and collegiality. One effective modification is to have an "open-door policy" that is a combination of dedicated staffing time and open availability to talk with staff via VTC. Depending on the patient volume for each clinic, the telemental health clinician can meet with the staff on a weekly or monthly basis via videoconferencing. During this staffing time, clinicians at the patient's site can be invited to come into the telemental health suite to discuss about the patients with the teleclinician. This allows clinicians at the patient's site to experience the technology first hand, which may be helpful in later describing the experience to their patients, and to discuss shared patients' needs. This time can be used for direct supervision or informal support as local clinicians share their difficult cases. Some patients also appreciate having their therapists or support staff attend the telemental health visits and this should be encouraged when appropriate. Inclusion of referring therapists or other clinicians also serves the purpose of providing consultee-centered consultation.

Open availability can be greatly enhanced by letting the clinic know by email or instant messaging any time the telemental health clinician has a cancelation, so that local clinicians can stop by the telemental health suite to discuss issues of concern or interest. After a while, clinicians learn that they are welcomed to drop by for unscheduled discussions. This kind of informal accessibility goes a long way toward establishing a sense of community and obtaining insights about patients and their lives as well as insights about clinical staff's needs in caring for complex patients.

Another rapport-building technique is letting the referring clinicians know that they can reach the telemental health clinician whenever needed. In addition to a formal on-call system, encouraging clinicians to call on the telephone whenever they have questions will build a sense of shared mission in patient's care. However, since telephone contact is not always possible, secure email and instant messaging can provide a useful alternative for ready access to the telemental health clinician. A 24-h turn around for email responses during the week is reasonable. It is also helpful to identify a dedicated staff member who is in contact with the teleclinician throughout the day and week and who can use instant messaging or email to serve as a liaison between the telemental health clinician and the clinical staff.

The Importance of a Clinical Coordinator in Facilitating Rapport at the Patient Site

One useful model is to have a dedicated contact person as a telemental health coordinator within the clinic. This coordinator is a tool of the telemental health service and extends the reach of the teleclinician. The coordinator handles schedules, ensures implementation of the teleclinician's treatment plan, functions as the contact person for patients and clinic staff, and may even track patients' appointments or adherence to treatment. It is not necessary for this individual to be an employee of the telemental health clinician; in fact, it is often helpful if he/she is integrated into the clinic's care model, such as being a care coordinator or behavioral health technician. There are several important characteristics desired in a telemental health coordinator, such as likability, organization skills, and flexibility. The coordinator will often be the patient's first point of contact with telemental health, similar to the office staff of a traditional practice. Thus, it is very important that this individual is respectful and has good communication skills.

Many telemental health clinicians find it helpful if the coordinator is present during the clinical session. This takes a special kind of person, one who can be present, but not intervene in the interaction with the telemental health clinician. Sometimes, experienced coordinators can help facilitate clinical care by sharing observations, such as the recognition that a patient or family member is crying off camera. Also, patients often talk with the coordinator before the connection is made and again this can be a valuable source of information and patients should be informed ahead of time that this will be shared with the clinician. The coordinator may also help with disruptive children, disabled adults, or folks who are new to the process.

On a practical level, when working with a telepsychiatrist, the telemental health coordinator can be responsible for handling requests for laboratory tests and prescriptions, and liaise with other professionals in the community. This can be as simple as handing a laboratory slip to the patient that the coordinator fills out with the help of the telepsychiatrist or arranging a referral for an electrocardiogram or magnetic resonance imaging. Additional roles can include helping patients to receive appropriate handouts on their diagnosis and treatment. With sufficient training, coordinators can also be tasked with obtaining vital signs and can be used to facilitate administration of certain instruments, such as the AIMS. The coordinator can also be trained to conduct basic troubleshooting for the videoconferencing equipment, and when there is a technical disruption, the coordinator serves as an on-site contact for technical help. Telemental health coordinators often assist with triage when there is an emergent or urgent situation involving the patient. Thus, comfort with the vicissitudes of clinical care is another desirable characteristic. The coordinator's overall likability, respect in the community, and availability to explain recommendations by the clinician can also enhance rapport. The coordinator is often the "glue" that makes various members of the telemental health group a true team.

Establishing Rapport with the Broader Community

One of the challenges to distance medicine is obtaining an accurate sense of the community in which patients live. There are several practical strategies for building relationships with the community. The first is getting to know staff and querying them about community events. In addition, many local papers are now available online and some telemental health clinicians review them or have relevant articles sent to them by clinic coordinators. For example, a coordinator can send World Wide Web links about major town events such as crimes that may impact patients and their families or new transportation services that may help patients. Sometimes it amounts to knowing that a new "family fun center" opened and is now available to families or that a senior center is planning to offer free lunches.

It can be helpful in building rapport to occasionally visit the partner community. During such visits, the telemental health clinician may host an open house to meet patients and other community members, such as child protective service workers, judges, and probation officers. The teleclinician may also coordinate or participate in health-promoting events such as a depression screening day. Local newspapers might be interested in interviewing the visiting teleclinician, which helps not only to advertise the service but also to demystify it, and educate the community about mental illness and its treatment. Equally important is spending informal time with staff and visiting a local "hot spot." Interestingly, clinical experience suggests that these visits may be more helpful to the teleclinician than to the patients themselves and there is no requirement for such on-site visits. Similar to the overall discussion of rapport, it is often felt to be the clinician's interest in the community rather than their direct presence, which is felt to be the key element of developing broader relationships in telemental health.

Conclusion

Clinical reports, existing research, and patient's personal attestations support the use of VTC and show the ability to establish rapport, a therapeutic alliance, and emotional connection through telemental health. Telemental health clinicians note that establishing rapport through VTC is not a unique endeavor but represents the adaptation of existing rapport-building techniques to a virtual environment. There are also practical considerations such as technology that allows sufficient bandwidth for fluid transmissions and detailed observations of patients. Additional studies are needed to continue to delineate specific aspects of clinical care that aid in rapport development in this setting as well as continuing collaboration on best practices. As increased emphasis is placed on the implementation of evidence-based care across the nation, telemental health is uniquely situated to disseminate such care to distant areas and help to rectify the disparities in access to specialty mental health care. Careful consideration of rapport within the context of individual interactions, relationships with local clinicians, and communities at large will greatly facilitate the success of telemental health in underserved communities.

References

Amerendran, V. (2011). The reliability of telepsychiatry for neuropsychiatric assessment. *Telemedicine Journal and e-Health, 17*(3), 223–225.

Andersson, G., & Cuipers, P. (2009). Internet-based and other computerized psychological treatments for adult depression: A meta-analysis. *Cognitive Behaviour Therapy, 38*, 196–205.

Andrusyna, T. P., Tang, T. Z., DeRubeis, R. J., & Luborsky, L. (2001). The factor structure of the working alliance inventory in cognitive-behavioral therapy. *Journal of Psychotherapy Practice and Research, 10*, 173–178.

Bishop, J., O'Reilly, R., Maddox, K., & Hutchinson, L. (2002). Client satisfaction in a feasibility study comparing face-to-face interviews with telepsychiatry. *Journal of Telemedicine and Telecare, 8*, 217–221.

Bouchard, S., Paquin, B., Payeur, R., Allard, M., Rivard, V., Fournier, T., et al. (2004). Delivering cognitive-behavior therapy for panic disorder with agoraphobia in videoconference. *Telemedicine Journal and e-Health, 10*, 13–25.

Cook, J., & Doyle, C. (2002). Working alliance in online therapy as compared to face-to-face therapy: Preliminary results. *Cyberpsychological Behavior, 5*, 95–105.

De Las Cuevas, C., Arredondo, M., Cabrera, M., Sulzenbacher, M., & Meise, U. (2006). Randomized clinical trial of telepsychiatry through videoconference versus face-to-face conventional psychiatric treatment. *Telemedicine Journal and e-Health, 12*, 341–350.

Elford, R., White, H., Bowering, R., Ghandi, A., Maddiggan, B., St John, K., et al. (2000). A randomized, controlled trial of child psychiatric assessments conducted using videoconferencing. *Journal of Telemedicine and Telecare, 6*(2), 73–82.

Ertlelt, T., Crosby, R., Marino, J., Mitchell, J., Lancaster, K., & Crow, S. (2010). Therapeutic factors affecting the cognitive behavioral treatment of bulimia nervosa via telemedicine versus face-to-face delivery. *International Journal of Eating Disorders, 44*, 687–691.

Ghosh, G., McLaren, P., & Watson, J. (1997). Evaluating the alliance in videolink teletherapy. *Journal of Telemedicine and Telecare, 3S*, 33–35.

Gibson, S. (2012). *Real world telepsychiatry provision*. Northern Arizona Regional Behavioral Health Association. <http://www.rbha.net/presentations/RealWorldTelepsychRev/player.html> Accessed 16.08.12.

Grady, B., Myers, K., & Nelson, E. L. (2009a). *Telemental health standards and guidelines working group. Practice guidelines for videoconferencing-based telemental health.* American Telemedicine Association. <http://www.americantelemed.org/files/public/standards/PracticeGuidelinesforVideoconferencing-Based TeleMentalHealth.pdf> Accessed 16.08.12.

Grady, B., Myers, K., & Nelson, E. L. (2009b). *Telemental health standards and guidelines working group. Evidence-based practice for telemental health.* American

Telemedicine Association. <http://www.americantelemed.org/files/public/standards/EvidenceBasedTelementalHealth_WithCover.pdf> Accessed 16.08.12.

Himle, J. A., Fischer, D. J., Muroff, J. R., VanEtten, M. L., Loker, L. M., Abelson, J. L., et al. (2006). Videoconference-based cognitive behavior therapy for obsessive compulsive disorder. *Behaviour Research and Therapy, 44*, 1821−1829.

Horvath, A. O., & Greenberg, L. S. (1989). Development and validation of the working alliance inventory. *Journal of Counseling Psychology, 36*, 223−233.

Horvath, A. O., & Symonds, D. B. (1991). Relation between working alliance and outcome in psychotherapy: A meta-analysis. *Journal of Counseling Psychology, 38*, 139−149.

Jones, B., III, & Ruskin, P. (2001). Telemedicine and geriatric psychiatry: Directions for future research and policy. *Journal of Geriatric Psychiatry and Neurology, 14*(2), 59−62.

Knaevelsrud, C., & Maercker, A. (2006). Does the quality of the working alliance predict treatment outcome in online psychotherapy for traumatized patients? *Medical Internet Research, 8*, 31.

Kopel, H., Nunn, K., & Dossetor, D. (2001). Evaluating satisfaction with a child and adolescent psychological telemedicine outreach service. *Journal of Telemedicine and Telecare, 7*(Suppl. 2), 35−40.

Modai, I., Jabarin, M., Kurs, R., Barak, P., Hannan, I., & Kitain, L. (2006). Cost effectiveness, safety, and satisfaction with video telepsychiatry versus face-to-face care in ambulatory settings. *Telemedicine Journal and e-Health, 12*, 515−520.

Morgan, R., Patrick, A., & Magaletta, P. (2008). Does the use of telemental health alter the treatment experience? Inmates' perceptions of telemental health versus face-to-face treatment modalities. *Journal of Consulting and Clinical Psychology, 76*, 158−162.

Morland, L. A., Greene, C. J., Rosen, C. S., Foy, D., Reilly, P., Shore, J., et al. (2010). Telemedicine for anger management therapy in a rural population of combat veterans with posttraumatic stress disorder: A randomized noninferiority trial. *Journal of Clinical Psychiatry, 71*, 855−861.

Niedenthal, P. (2007). Embodying emotion. *Science, 316*, 1002−1005.

O'Reilly, R., Bishop, J., Maddox, K., Hutchison, L., Fisman, M., & Takhar, J. (2007). Is telepsychiatry equivalent to face-to-face psychiatry? Results from a randomized controlled equivalency trial. *Psychiatric Services, 58*, 836−843.

Quill, T., & Brody, H. (1996). Physician recommendations and patient autonomy: Finding a balance between physician power and patient choice. *Annals of Internal Medicine, 125*, 763−769.

Ruskin, P., Silver-Aylaian, M., Kling, M., Reed, S., Bradham, D., Hebel, J., et al. (2004). Treatment outcomes in depression: Comparison of remote treatment through telepsychiatry to in-person treatment. *American Journal of Psychiatry, 161*(**8**), 1471−1476.

Sadock, B., Sadock, V., Ruiz, P., & Kaplan, H. (2009). *Kaplan and Sadock's comprehensive textbook of psychiatry*. Philadelphia, PA: Wolters Kluwer Health and Lippincott Williams & Wilkins.

The telemental health guide. University of Colorado Denver. <www.tmhguide.org> Accessed 01.09.12.

Yeung, A., Hails, K., Chang, T., Trinh, N., & Fava, M. (2011). A study of the effectiveness of telepsychiatry-based culturally sensitive collaborative treatment of Chinese Americans. *BMC Psychiatry, 11*, 154−161.

4 Ethical Considerations in Providing Mental Health Services Over Videoteleconferencing

Eve-Lynn Nelson[a,b,]*, Kathy Davis[a] and Sarah E. Velasquez[b]

[a]Pediatrics Department, University of Kansas Medical Center, Kansas City, KS, [b]KU Center for Telemedicine and Telehealth, University of Kansas Medical Center, Kansas City, KS

Introduction

Technology brings many new opportunities for mental health services, but with these opportunities come new ethical considerations and dilemmas. Similar to traditional face-to-face clinical settings, the core ethical concern to protect the client remains paramount in the telemental health setting. The American Psychological Association (APA) Code of Ethics (American Psychological Association, 2002) posits five general principles to guide discussion about how to best protect the client: (1) beneficence and nonmaleficence, (2) fidelity and responsibility, (3) integrity, (4) justice, and (5) respect for people's rights and dignity. The principles encompass broad ethical concepts across mental health professions (American Psychological Association, 2002; Gunter, Srinivasaraghavan, & Terry, 2003; Kaplan & Litewka, 2008) and common ethical issues such as informed consent, privacy, conflict of interest, and access. Leading telehealth and mental health associations strongly emphasize the ethical–legal importance of translating onsite ethical best practice to the telehealth setting (Grady et al., 2011; Merrell & Doarn, 2009). With newer practices such as telemental health, the American Psychological Association (2002) advises that telemental health professionals "... take reasonable steps to ensure the competence of their work and to protect clients/clients, students, supervisees, research participants, organizational clients, and others from harm." This is particularly true as the purpose of telemental health is often to extend services to vulnerable populations who otherwise do not have access to specialists.

* Corresponding Author: Eve-Lynn Nelson, PhD, 2012 Wahl Annex, MS 1048, 3901 Rainbow Blvd., Kansas City, KS 66160, Tel.: (913)588-2413, Fax: (913)588-2227, E-mail: enelson2@kumc.edu

Telemental Health. DOI: http://dx.doi.org/10.1016/B978-0-12-416048-4.00004-X

This chapter will focus on ethical mental health practice with interactive videoteleconferencing (VTC), as well as address ethical considerations with emerging video-based technologies, including home telehealth and mobile devices. Additionally, this chapter will address "reasonable steps" to promote ethical telemental health practice. Nonvideo and nonclinical technologies, including social media, are also important areas for ethical review but are beyond the scope of the chapter.

To illustrate each ethical principle reviewed, each section includes a case description that builds on the following example: *Don is an elderly man living in a rural community and suffering from low mood since his wife died 1 year ago. He has a local primary care professional who wants to help Don, but has had little training in treating elder clients with low mood due to widowhood. Don is not able to travel 6 h to the academic health center where one of the few geriatric mental health specialists in his state practices (note for the example the specialist could be any mental health professional). However, the mental health specialist provides monthly services over VTC.*

Applying Ethical Principles in Telemental Health

The authors will first briefly describe the ethical principles delineated above and discuss how each principle can be applied in a telemental health setting. While the VTC modality is highlighted, the ethical questions raised are intended to generalize to other telemental health technologies.

Principle A: Beneficence and Nonmaleficence

Broadly, beneficence refers to acts that benefit clients by relieving distress or illness, or by preventing harm. Nonmaleficence, which is often coupled with beneficence, literally means to "do no harm." Not only do mental health professionals ensure that they do not engage in harmful practices, but they also strive to provide treatments known to be effective. The rationale for telemental health practice underscores benefits that are anticipated for clients, including increased access to care, decreased client costs, and increased communication between specialists and local professionals. High client satisfaction with telemental health services is often used as a measure of these anticipated benefits, and high satisfaction is reported across telemental health settings (Bishop, O'Reilly, Maddox, & Hutchinson, 2002; Myers, Valentine, & Melzer, 2007; Wagnild, Leenknecht, & Zauher, 2006). However, there are potential risks with technology-delivered services, including an altered client—patient relationship and potential decreased feelings of autonomy and connectedness (see Glueck, this volume).

Telemental health professionals strive to benefit their clients and take care to do no harm (van Wysberghe & Gastmans, 2009). To maximize beneficence, telemental health generally offers to approximate the same in-person assessment and treatment procedures, not "half" of the services or lower quality services. Accepted standards for ethical practice may include the use of a comprehensive informed consent procedure, guidance on how to handle emergency situations, documentation procedures, and the specifics of fees and financial arrangements (Barnett & Scheetz, 2003).

The professional and the patient talk together about the purpose of the telemental health clinic and there is an ongoing discussion to confirm telemental health is meeting the patient's needs over time. As in the face-to-face setting, the consent process includes both verbal and written components and focuses on ensuring patient safety. Following best practices in risk management, the informed consent procedure addresses the relative risks and benefits associated with telemental health, taking into consideration the current empirical evidence and consensus guidelines. The professional's role in the telemental health session is defined, noting his/her role as a one-time consultant, an ongoing care provider, a coach, or another role. The professional notes his/her completion of any licensing requirements as well as training related to telemental health service delivery. The professional works with distant sites to understand community standards of care as well as reasonable alternatives that are available for patients and their families. The professional describes how confidentiality is preserved, noting technology-related issues such as encryption, as well as measures taken to maintain privacy in the clinic room and in transmitting written information. The professional addresses the legal limits to confidentiality that exist in the client's state of residence, including procedures in the event of clinical emergencies (described below). As in the face-to-face setting, the professional discusses standard procedures around vacation, cancellations, and similar issues, as well as approaches specific to the technology setting, such as the steps to be taken should the VTC equipment stop working during the session. When groups are conducted over VTC, group members are socialized to the same ground rules of group participation and respect of confidentiality as in the onsite setting.

Prior to the initiation of clinics, the professional establishes procedures related to patients presenting in crisis. Professionals determine criteria for which patients will be seen remotely and may decide to refer patients at higher risk for crisis, dysfunction, or noncompliance to onsite treatment. As in traditional mental health services, the professional takes care to check that the patient can see and hear using the VTC unit and is comfortable within the room setting. The professional assesses whether there are any needs for medical interpreting, addressing concerns around stigma, or concerns specific to the individual patient.

Emergency procedures for telemental health practice approximate face-to-face procedures. Protocols specify whom the patient contacts in the event of a crisis situation—often a local crisis management option—and acknowledge limits to the telemental health professional's management due to geographic distance. In addition, the patient site personnel complete initial and ongoing training concerning the management of patients who present with safety and other crisis concerns.

Standards of practicing within one's scope of clinical competence are all the more important when delivering service over VTC. Professionals may feel compelled to practice outside of their area of competence by rationalizing that the client will not get care otherwise, thus compromising ethical practice. However, telemental health professionals must first follow the same competence standards applied in face-to-face practice, including professional standards for assessment and treatment across age groups. A variety of professional and legal mechanisms function to assure professional competence is met. Licensure requirements are particularly important, both for interstate (see www.ctel.org) and for international practice. In addition to their own standards of competence, mental health professionals must also consider the competence required of possible telemental health presenters assisting on the distant side of the telemental health encounter (American Telemental Health Association, 2011). The telemental health presenter, also referred to as telemental health coordinator, is usually a nurse or other healthcare staff specially trained in assisting the professional and patient at the patient site during the VTC visit. The mental health professional is responsible for addressing both the clinical competence and knowledge of standard ethical practice in order to support telehealth presenters in providing high-quality, compassionate care using VTC technology.

Due to the newness of the field, there are no established performance competences specific to technology, but telehealth guidelines provide recommendations and direction (American Telemental Health Association, 2009; Grady et al., 2011; Myers & Cain, 2008). Technology competence includes how to select equipment that will meet specific clinical purpose, how to use the equipment appropriately, and how to seek mentoring and supervision from established telemental health professionals. Professionals are encouraged to observe other telemental health professionals and to complete "test runs" in order to build confidence with the technology (Nelson, Bui, & Sharp, 2011; Yellowlees et al., 2010). Professionals must consult their own institution, as well as the distant hospitals served, regarding credentialing requirements. Some, but not all, institutions will accept credentialing completed at another major telemedicine site.

In addition to beneficence, telemental health professionals must consider professional obligations to do no harm and avoid maleficence. Forethought through detailed and continuously updated telehealth protocols help to reduce such potential harm. This includes backup plans with the telemental health coordinator in the event the client reports suicidal, homicidal, abusive, or other safety concerns. As in traditional settings, expectations concerning professional coverage are outlined within the informed consent. In addition to the safety plans, the informed consent should outline who the client would to contact with crisis needs, and what the expectations are when the patient site is unavailable, such as when school is not in session.

One of the most common ethical dilemmas occurs is the attempt to balance beneficence and nonmaleficence. Since most therapies have both benefits and risks, this concept is applied accurately when professionals thoughtfully evaluate the risk—benefit ratio of their practice and conduct only those treatments that clearly benefit the client. As a new science, the evidence base in telemental health is growing. There is strong evidence for feasibility and satisfaction, but the outcome literature is minimal and there are only a handful of well-controlled randomized trials to date (Grady et al., 2011; Hyler & Gangure, 2004). While informative, the pilot trials common in the literature have not had sufficient power to assess equivalence across presenting concerns, although the emerging results across equivalence trials are promising. Thus, telemental health professionals must weigh the anticipated benefits of the VTC service with the remaining questions concerning VTC equivalence across the diverse clients seen over VTC and the range of interventions delivered. To address this ethical concern, more research is needed to understand the unique benefits that telehealth provides as well as the unique drawbacks.

Recall the case study example of Don. *Don's primary care provider asks if he would be interested in undergoing an evaluation from the mental health professional. The mental health professional is practicing within his area of competence based on the professional board and licensing requirements related to geriatric psychiatry, and he has sought out additional mentoring from long-standing telemental health professionals. What must the geriatric specialist consider before conducting the assessment that ensures he is practicing beneficence and nonmaleficence? What is the evidence base for services for elders with depression? Although there is not a large quantity of literature, there are some studies demonstrating acceptance and efficacy of telemental health with elders for a range of psychiatric disorders (Holden & Dew, 2008). The mental health professional is also experienced in conducting mental health evaluations and has standard protocols for client education, confidentiality, data security, and emergency management based on guidelines presented by telemental health professional organizations. What harms are there in the VTC encounter over harms related to a traditional onsite consultation?*

Principle B: Fidelity and Responsibility

Fidelity and responsibility refer to establishing the trust of clients, colleagues, and the public at large in the practice of telemental health. It is closely tied to concerns of competence, in that a telemental health professional promotes fidelity and responsibility by conducting evidence-supported, and guideline concordant, mental health care. However, the concept of responsibility also refers to the importance of addressing other professionals' practices if there is evidence of misconduct or betrayal of trust.

Confidentiality is a key concern in telemental health. There is frequently tension between the benefits of telemental health and the loss of direct control over the clinical environment and the ability to ensure confidential therapeutic encounters. To ensure confidentiality, best practices must be used in technology selection. The American Telemental Health Association's (2009) *Practice Guidelines for Videoconferencing-Based Telemental Health* recommends the use of encrypted, point-to-point technologies to make certain that videoconferencing has an additional level of security to ensure privacy. The recommendation is to employ a dedicated network with high bandwidth to not only ensure privacy but also to allow for the greatest possible detail during the video conference (van Wysberghe & Gastmans, 2009). The dedicated network with sufficient, stable bandwidth maintains the continuous high-quality connection encouraged for clinical communication without dropped calls, audio-visual interruptions, or a choppy onscreen image.

The professional takes into consideration VTC monitors with sufficient detail and good lighting in order to create a user-friendly VTC environment that supports rapport building and interactive patient–professional communication.

Staff often assume new or expanded roles when assisting with telemental health and therefore need support in building a trusted environment at the patient site. Training should be provided in expectations around maintaining confidentiality, especially when coordinators are likely to be working with their neighbors in small communities. This includes approximately all the safeguards and paperwork of the face-to-face setting, including a comprehensive informed consent and the Health Information Portability and Accountability Act (HIPAA)-compliant Notice of Privacy Plan (NPP) (Stanberry, 2006). Maheu, Pulier, Wilhelm, McMenamin, and Brown-Connolly (2004) give detailed examples of considerations for model consents for mental health services over VTC. Training at both the mental health professional and the patient site is also needed to treat the telemental health space as secure clinical space, and to ensure conversations are not inadvertently overheard or that no one (parent, child, other) eavesdrops at the door. Prior to the session, the professional should scan the patient site room with the camera to make sure clients know who, if anyone else, is in the professional's room. The telemental health consultant is also responsible for confidential transport of client documentation between the consulting and the patient site, both in electronic and in paper versions.

Technology decisions around privacy and security are rarely clear-cut and usually involve weighing the advantages and disadvantages for the specific telemental health purpose. When selecting the technology, it is important to understand not only the labeling of encryption, but the publically available information about the encryption process and who could potentially access the information. If there are potential risks, the therapist is encouraged to be transparent with the client about limitations with the particular technology. In addition, the professional follows best practices in health information exchange between the professional site and the patient site, and maintains the secure designated medical record. To date, telemental health protocols most often address the secure transfer of patient written information by fax and/or secure e-mail. Protocols should detail procedures for shared information between institutions for both paper and electronic health records associated with telemental health care.

Fidelity and responsibility also refers to engendering trust in colleagues and the public at large. This relies on the professional's responsibility to correct unethical practice when it arises. For example, if a professional conducting telemental health as part of a large health care system learns that the system's administrators chose to discontinue using encryption software but they have not informed the clients, he should tell the administrators that this is not ethical practice. The organization is not adequately protecting client confidentiality and practicing informed consent. Such a breach should be taken as seriously as systematic breaches of confidentiality for clients receiving face-to-face care.

Returning to the case study of Don, *the mental health professional begins work with Don by describing what to expect with the telemental health sessions and continuously checks in with Don about his understanding and comfort level with the technology. He reassures that only Don can see him and vice versa, the information is neither viewable by other sites nor is it taped. The psychiatrist asks Don if he is alone in the room and Don's daughter comes on camera to let the psychiatrist know she is there to support her father. Don confirms what he has previously conveyed to his team that he consents to his daughter's participation and prefers that she attend the appointment with him. Don says that he doesn't have concerns about the technology but worries about what people at church, some of whom work at the clinic, will think about him "seeing a shrink." Don's mental health professional normalizes his worry, addresses concerns about stigma, and explains that the role of mental health professional in supporting Don. He also discussed the clinic staff's responsibility to follow the same high standards of confidentiality in the local community.*

Principle C: Integrity

Integrity refers to the accurate, honest, and truthful clinical and scientific practice of mental health care. Mental health professionals need to honestly describe the risks and benefits of telemental health care to the client. During the informed consent process, professionals should acknowledge the early state of the science and research gaps concerning rigorous telemental health evaluation. Although professionals may be caught up in the excitement of the technology delivery, a candid discussion of its limitations, as well as alternatives to care, is warranted. Optimally, face-to-face options are available and the client is able to make the choice of being seen over VTC. Realistically, this choice may mean the client would need to drive some distance to treatment. Moreover, professionals should avoid conflicts of interest through financial relationships with videoconferencing technology companies or, at the very least, these conflicts of interest should be disclosed to the client and to the referring clinic. In addition, professionals must review Fraud and Abuse regulations (e.g., Stark Laws) in relation to their proposed telehealth service.

Integrity also relates to the mental health professionals to accurately describe the scope of telemental health services. For example, cross-state licensure requires considerable professional resources when delivering direct clinical services over VTC. Some professionals have focused on coaching services over VTC to address these legal complexities. Harris and Younggren (2011) advise that to avoid allegations of unlicensed practice, coaches often provide written disclaimers "to alert the client to the differences between the services they regulate and health care."

In the ongoing example, let us add that *the mental health professional has just started consulting with the company that makes the videoconferencing equipment he uses. He receives a stipend from the company but pays full price for his equipment. He consults because he wants to influence the types of improvements the company makes on its equipment and he is not dependent on the stipend in any way. He does not realize this is a conflict of interest, comparable to the relationship some psychiatrists have with a pharmaceutical company. Thus, he does not disclose this information to his client or to the referring clinic. The technical*

support person at the clinic learns that the mental health professional has this rela-
tionship. He discusses it with the mental health professional directly. Although
what the professional is doing is not illegal, it would be more ethical to be open
with both the client and the referring clinic about his relationship with the com-
pany. The referring clinic asks the professional to disclose this information at the
beginning of each consultation in case the patient will have any problems with this
relationship. In addition, all clients are provided the option of face-to-face care,
though it will require travel by the client.

Principle D: Justice

Justice in the APA's guidelines refers to entitling all persons access to, and benefit
from, care. Telemental health has much potential to support access and equity in
health care because it extends the ability of mental health professionals to provide
services. The reach of telemental health has extended state borders, and now even
national borders, and may literally link clients and professionals worldwide. This
leads to new questions of justice, or who is served, as well as professional competence with the population served. The issue of equality of care is raised when
deciding who will have access to telemental health services and who will make
such decisions. Telemental health professionals strive to approximate or exceed the
quality of face-to-face care and make sure telemental health is not misused to
deliver inferior services to underserved populations.

For example, telemental health professionals have delivered services to underserved urban populations, including urban schools, daycares, and other settings
(Spaulding, Cain, & Sonnenschein, 2011). The rationale for such services is that
using the technology to link health care with other systems of care trusted by the
client, such as the school, will improve the health of this underserved population.
Questions of justice relate to site selection: Are sites selected based on highest
need or based on ability to buy equipment? In addition, which clients at the site are
selected to be seen in the telemental health clinic? Does the client have a choice
between face-to-face and telemental health care? Is there equivalent buy-in from
parents or do they feel pressured by the school to initiate services?

Another issue to consider is that access issues remain even with telemental
health availability, particularly with tight budgetary times purchasing, maintaining,
and supporting the telemental health clinic. This may limit both the expansion and
the sustainability of telemental health services. Some individuals do not have
access to transportation for travel to the patient site, making emerging home telehealth and mobile options appealing from a justice perspective (Demiris, Oliver, &
Courtney, 2006). Luxton, McCann, Bush, Mishkind, and Reger (2011) summarize
potential uses of mHealth (mobile health) in behavioral health care, including psychoeducational, monitoring, support, coaching, and clinical purposes. They emphasize that to date, data is scant and professionals should acknowledge limitations
with patients. In addition to the same ethical considerations discussed in relation to
nonmobile videoconferencing, they outline mHealth ethical considerations including usability/acceptance issues, quality standards and safety, and data security/

privacy concerns. Professionals have less control of the client environment with home and mobile devices and this leads to different risks related to privacy/confidentiality and managing crises as well as very limited information to inform behavioral health outcomes.

Continuing with our case study, *the mental health professional originally agreed to do telemental health consultations to rural clinics, but only those with high-resolution technology that allows for better video and audio transmission. In this particular state, money to purchase equipment is tied closely to the taxable income of the local population. Therefore, only the wealthier counties were able to afford such equipment. The end result is raises ethical concerns as only elders in wealthy rural counties had access to the geriatric specialist. To remedy this, the mental health professional assisted poor rural clinics in applying for funds to purchase equipment from both national and state organizations concerned about health disparities.*

Principle E: Respect for People's Rights and Dignity

This principle means that professionals respect the dignity and worth of all people, and the rights of individuals to privacy, confidentiality, and self-determination. Self-determination includes autonomy and a person's right to make informed choices. Informed choices can only be made after a client has been provided comprehensive information about all possible choices for the full complement of treatment options, as well as the choice to refuse treatment. The mental health professional carefully informs the client, and then assesses for client understanding, before making treatment plans and decisions with the client. Careful attention to the holistic view of the client is important in guiding the professional in identifying the form of care that is the most appropriate and beneficial to the individual (van Wysberghe & Gastmans, 2009).

Just as in the face-to-face setting, mental health professionals refrain from providing interventions if there are concerns about whether or not a client is able to make autonomous decisions. Special consideration must be taken with telemental health as telehealth increases services to vulnerable populations who may have limited access otherwise, including diverse populations that have little experience with mental health services. For example, what special precautions would be needed over VTC if Don was cognitively impaired by dementia? Or what if Don was incarcerated, how would standard onsite safeguards be translated for the VTC setting?

The same expectations for professionalism and cultural competence are paramount in the telemental health setting across differences based on age, gender, gender identity, race, ethnicity, culture, national origin, religion, sexual orientation, disability, language, or socioeconomic status, as well as perceived differences that are important to the client. The key point is that telemental health is not just dependent on a technical fix. It also requires a comprehensive understanding of the cultural and legal differences in the communities served across the nation or the globe. Along these lines, providing culturally competent care over VTC is just as important as providing culturally competent care in face-to-face settings. Some examples of ways to provide this care over VTC would be to inquire about the client's level of comfort with technology and be mindful of how culturally specific nonverbal communication styles might be affected by the VTC technology (Savin, Glueck, Chardavoyne, Yager, & Novins, 2011).

One challenge in telemental health is to ensure that distant staff has training in these same expectations across clients with mental health concerns. Cultural competence is expected in the broadest sense as VTC opens the door to see almost any client at any time, regardless of one's training or experience working with the population. In addition to cultural competence across ethnicities, competence also refers to proficiency with rural culture. Linguistic competence is equally important and the same expectations for quality medical interpreting are required over VTC. Knowledge of resources in the client's local area is critical should an emergency arise or the need for a referral. When clients or families speak a different language than the professional, all standards of medical interpreting should be followed.

How would the situation be different *if Don was Mexican-American and was predominantly Spanish-speaking? What interpreting services are adequate to support the health care interaction over VTC? Aging and treatment of the elderly have strong cultural determinants, so the mental health professional seeks consultation about mental health care for Mexican-American elders from an expert in the state as well as through secondary reading. Don is also experiencing significant stress due a severe drought impacting their family farm. The professional seeks out local resources to understand the drought's impact on the community and potential sources of support for Don.*

Concerns Specific to Research

There is a significant and strong need for research to further telemental health practice (Merrell & Doarn, 2009). Standard ethical research practices apply in the context of telemental health research, including those regarding informed consent, confidentiality, voluntary participation, and commitment to participant safety. However, there are additional challenges specific to conducting research where collaborators and participants are located at a patient site.

The informed consent and witness of consent process may sometimes occur without the presence of the investigator from the research site. The investigator must ensure the full formal consent process is followed at the patient site by trained staff. This includes an explanation of the nature of telemental health and a discussion of how telemental health is at an early stage of development so the participant fully understands the research prior to consent. As telemental health is often used with underserved populations who may lack experience with medical research, a discussion of voluntary participation and of the risks and benefits of the research is critical.

One challenge of telemental health research is selecting sites that are willing to commit to the staff time that is needed to collaborate in ethical research. Such collaboration often requires staff training at the patient site, including formal human subject research training. The availability of online human subject training provided by either the research site or the National Institutes of Health can facilitate remote ethics training, but these courses can last several hours. The investigator at the research site is then responsible for ongoing supervision to ensure the patient sites are compliant with ethical standards.

Concerns about HIPAA must also be addressed, as the researcher cannot have access to clinical information at patient sites until the study participant consents to join the study. This can influence recruitment as staff at patient sites may not make study recruitment a priority. Similarly, patient sites participating in quality improvement efforts using telemental health must make sure that their organization's HIPAA language covers these efforts. In addition, data collection and storage at the patient site must follow ethical guidelines about privacy and, when indicated, delete information that personally identifies a participant. All of these concerns make considerable demands on the patient collaborating site and underscore why selection of collaborators must be well investigated.

Finally, the client's right to refuse, or to discontinue, participation needs to be explained clearly from the outset. Optimally, participants can seek care comparable to that offered in the research study so that treatment options are not linked to study participation. Clients should be informed of treatment alternatives including those that may require travel. Then, the clients themselves can evaluate the risks and benefits of participation.

In the example with the client Don, *assume that the mental health professional is able to provide a consult as part of research project funded by the National Institute of Health. Both he and the referring staff are required to complete human subject research training. The referring professional is trained to provide informed consent and does a full explanation of the study before arranging for the initial consultation. In his explanation, he states that the client can receive a consultation without participating, but the client would have to travel to the hospital. As part of the consent procedure, the referring clinic staff member acknowledges that formal investigation about the efficacy of VTC services is still in its early stages, though the work to date is promising.*

Don agrees to participate. However, after three meetings with the mental health professional, Don decides that he is uncomfortable with VTC services. He feels he cannot "express himself to a television set." Both the mental health professional and referring clinic accept this decision and arrange for Don to have follow-up care onsite. This is ethical practice of telemental health research where protecting the client's rights and dignity is the first priority.

Emerging VTC-Related Technologies

Technology options abound for VTC services. Two particularly relevant areas for telemental health practice over VTC are home telehealth and mobile technologies.

Each brings additional ethical considerations related to the five ethical principles highlighted above. While not the focus of this chapter, nonvideotelemental health practice can inform VTC practice, including delivery by telephone, computer-aided therapy, e-mail, and virtual worlds (Anthony, Nagel, & Goss, 2010; Hsiung, 2001).

Home Telehealth and VTC

Home telehealth has been utilized for chronic disease management and data collection for some time and some mental health purposes (Demiris et al., 2006). VTC has recently expanded in-home telehealth, further expanding mental health possibilities to the home setting. Early work used videophones to deliver home-based VTC for depressed elderly veterans (Egede et al., 2009), and some of the same lessons apply to the emerging home-based videoconferencing. They note the benefits of the service with utility to address challenges to access for rural residents, capacity to reduce stigma associated with traditional mental health care, and utility to overcome significant age-related problems in ambulation and transportation. New concerns arise related to client safety in clinically unsupervised settings when the client is alone without a telemental health presenter. How will the telemental health professional address potential safety concerns in the event the client discloses a suicidal plan? How will the telemental health professional work with the client to create a shared environment to translate evidence-supported strategies with the potential changes in the environment and with perceived boundaries? Pilot projects from the Veteran's Administration, military, and other settings are beginning to inform these important questions with emerging telemental health technologies and settings. Such approaches generally rely on detailed consents and written patient agreements to contact named local providers in the event a crisis or safety concern arises. The Veteran's Administration and military home-based telemental health also asks patients to provide the contact information for a patient support person who will assist in emergency management when needed. The patient support person is contacted before the start of treatment and informed about their potential role in managing the patient's safety. Sometimes, the professional may ask for the patient support person to be present in the household during each session. Though this increases the amount of preparatory work when compared to in-person therapy, it addresses the concerns of managing emergencies in clinically unsupervised settings.

Mobile Devices and VTC

Mobile phones offer appeal to continue to expand access to telemental health services (Anthony et al., 2010). Cell phones have become "a near-ubiquitous tool for information seeking and communicating—83% of American adults own some kind of cell phone," and one-third of these users possess smartphones (Pew Research Center, 2011). This is relevant to the current chapter as there are an ever-expanding number of downloadable applications to deliver secure videoconferencing to smartphone and tablet devices. There is limited information about mobile texting and written communication for mental health (Anthony et al., 2010; Clough & Casey, 2011); however, information on mobile VTC for mental health services is emerging. There is a strong need for research to inform professionals and patients about the unique benefits and risks with mobile devices. Research is needed to understand how VTC services over mobile devices compare to both face-to-face consultations and nonmobile VTC services. This raises new ethical concerns. For example, will there be equal access to mobile services given the lower mobile adoption rates among Don's age group? What expectations will be set around where the VTC consult occurs given the increased ability to connect at almost any location? What happens if the mobile device used to connect is lost or stolen? What will be the quality of video transmission with the mobile devices and will it be sufficient to meet the clinical purpose?

Integration of Technologies

The next horizon is balancing the ethical and clinical considerations of the advantages and disadvantages of the full complement of technologies for the individual client. We are coming closer to the ability to tailor the particular set of therapeutic strategies and technologies to best fit the needs of the individual patient (Mohr, 2009). For example, some electronic health record companies are developing videoconferencing capabilities. Therefore, the teleconference can be integrated immediately into the patient's electronic health record and may even be accessible for review by the patient through his or her own patient portal to the electronic health record. The Department of Veterans Affairs has a personal health record called My HealtheVet which is developing a format for integrating My Recovery Plan software. Mental health patients and their professionals can develop a recovery plan, store it on the patient's personal health record, and review progress through My HealtheVet during either in-person or teleconferencing visits. However, these new possibilities bring new and continued ethical dilemmas, including verifying the identity of the client and considering ways to train mental health professionals in this very broad technology skill set.

Conclusion

Ethical practice in telemental health is within the context of the mental health professional's overall personal commitment to act ethically across practice settings. The authors present the APA ethical framework to illustrate ethical principles in the VTC context, but many other mental health professional organizations have related guidance and the reader is encouraged to review practices specific to their practice (see resources lists at www.ohpsych.org/telepsychologystandards.aspx and http://kspope.com/ethics/email.php).

Regulatory entities have not widely addressed telemental health practices, but some states have begun to address best practices for telemental health (Ohio

Psychological Board, 2009). Reed, McLaughlin, and Millholland (2000) provide interdisciplinary guidance in practicing ethical telemental health, emphasizing that each telemental health professional's ethical and professional requirements do not change with the introduction of the new technologies. The core principles they present focus on protecting clients, providing common ground for different health care professions and providing a basis for additional development of professional and clinical guidelines for telemental health practice. Just as with face-to-face mental health services, telemental health professionals are encouraged to follow best practices in risk management, including careful documentation of anticipated advantages and disadvantages of telemental health practice and use of comprehensive informed consent (Maheu et al., 2004). As with other new areas of practice, it is recommended that telemental health professionals frequently consult with peers and specialists as they work with new populations and encounter unique ethical challenges. In addition, ethicists may utilize the very technologies described to extend their consultation reach in complex ethical cases involving technologies (Kon, Rich, Sadorra, & Marcin, 2009).

Telemental health is rapidly changing with new technologies, new sites of service, and other innovations. These new opportunities bring new ethical dilemmas. Moreover, there is likely to be greater integration across technologies including video applications and data applications, such as electronic health records, and ethical considerations related to each will need exploration. In the future, mental health services over VTC offer tremendous promise to benefit clients just like Don and clients across the world. However, the ethical guidelines presented must be kept in mind in order to guarantee technology delivers our best possible clinical services to underserved clients and their families.

References

American Psychological Association (2002). Ethical principles of psychologists and code of conduct. *American Psychologist, 57,* 1060–1073.

American Telemental Health Association (2009). *Practice guidelines for videoconferencing-based telemental health.* ATA. <http://www.americantelemed.org/files/public/standards/PracticeGuidelinesforVideoconferencing-Based%20TelementalHealth.pdf> Accessed 26.01.12.

American Telemental Health Association (2011). *Expert consensus recommendations for videoconferencing-based telepresenting.* ATA. <http://www.americantelemed.org/i4a/pages/index.cfm?pageid=3311> Accessed 26.01.12.

Anthony, K., Nagel, D. M., & Goss, S. (2010). *The use of technology in mental health: Applications, ethics, and practice.* Springfield, IL: Thomas.

Barnett, J., & Scheetz, K. (2003). Technology advances and telehealth: Ethics, law, and the practice of psychotherapy. *Psychotherapy: Theory, Research, 1 Practice, and Training, 40,* 86–93.

Bishop, J. E., O'Reilly, R. L., Maddox, K., & Hutchinson, L. J. (2002). Client satisfaction in a feasibility study comparing face-to-face interviews with telepsychiatry. *Journal of Telemental Health and Telecare, 8,* 217–221.

Clough, B. A., & Casey, L. M. (2011). Technological adjuncts to enhance current psychotherapy practices: A review. *Clinical Psychology Review*, *31*, 279—292.

Demiris, G., Oliver, D. P., & Courtney, K. L. (2006). Ethical considerations for the utilization of tele-health technologies in home and hospice care by the nursing profession. *Nursing Administration Quarterly*, *30*, 56—66.

Egede, L. E., Frueh, C. B., Richardson, L. K., Acierno, R., Mauldin, P. D., & Knapp, R. G., et al. (2009). Rationale and design: Telepsychology service delivery for depressed elderly veterans. *Trials*, *10*, 22.

Grady, B., Myers, K. M., Nelson, E. L., Belz, N., Bennett, L., & Carnahan, L., et al. (2011). Evidence-based practice for telemental health. *Telemental Health Journal of E-Health*, *17*, 131—148.

Gunter, T. D., Srinivasaraghavan, J., & Terry, N. P. (2003). Misinformed regulation of electronic medicine is unfair to responsible telepsychiatry. *Journal of the American Academy of Psychiatry Law*, *31*, 10—14.

Harris, E., & Younggren, J. N. (2011). Risk management in the digital world. *Professional Psychology: Research and Practice*, *42*, 412—418.

Holden, D., & Dew, E. (2008). Telemental health in a rural gero-psychiatric inpatient unit: Comparison of perception/satisfaction to onsite psychiatric care. *Telemental Health Journal of E-Health*, *14*, 381—384.

Hsiung, R. C. (2001). Suggested principles of professional ethics for the online provision of mental health services. *Telemental Health Journal of E-Health*, *84*, 1296—1300.

Hyler, S. E., & Gangure, D. P. (2004). Legal and ethical challenges in telepsychiatry. *Journal of Psychiatric Practice*, *10*, 272—276.

Kaplan, B., & Litewka, S. (2008). Ethical challenges of telemental health and telehealth. *Cambraige Quarterly of Healthcare Ethics*, *17*, 401—416.

Kon, A. A., Rich, B., Sadorra, C., & Marcin, J. P. (2009). Complex bioethics consultation in rural hospitals: Using telemental health to bring academic bioethicists into outlying communities. *Journal of Telemental Health and Telecare*, *15*, 264—267.

Luxton, D. D., McCann, R. A., Bush, N. E., Mishkind, M. C., & Reger, G. M. (2011). mHealth for mental health: Integrating smartphone technology in behavioral healthcare. *Professional Psychology: Research and Practice*, *42*, 505—512.

Maheu, M., Pulier, M., Wilhelm, F. H., McMenamin, J. P., & Brown-Connolly, N. (2004). *The mental health professional and the new technologies: A handbook for practice today*. Mahwah, NJ: Erlbaum.

Merrell, R. C., & Doarn, C. R. (2009). Ethics in telemental health research. *Telemental Health Journal of E-Health*, *15*, 123—124.

Mohr, D. C. (2009). Telemental health: Reflections on how to move the field forward. *Clinical Psychology Science and Practice*, *16*, 343—347.

Myers, K., & Cain, S. (2008). Telepsychiatry. In M. Dulcan (Ed.), *Dulcan's textbook of child and adolescent psychiatry* (pp. 649—665). Arlington, VA: American Psychiatric Publishing.

Myers, K. M., Valentine, J. M., & Melzer, S. M. (2007). Feasibility, acceptability, and sustainability of telepsychiatry for children and adolescents. *Psychiatric Services*, *58*, 1493—1496.

Nelson, E., Bui, T., & Sharp, S. (2011). Telemental health competencies: Training examples from a youth depression VTC clinic. In M. Gregerson (Ed.), *Technology innovations for behavioral education* (pp. 41—48). New York, NY: Springer.

Ohio Psychological Association. (2009). *Telepsychology: Guidelines for Ohio psychologists*. Retrieved on February 2, 2011 from http://www.ohpsych.org/psychologists/files/2011/06/OPATelepsychologyGuidelines41710.pdf.

Pew Research Center (2011). *Americans and their cell phones report.* PRC. <www. pewinternet.org/~/media/Files/Reports/2011/Cell%20Phones%202011.pdf> Accessed 26.01.12.

Reed, G. M., McLaughlin, C. J., & Millholland, K. (2000). Ten interdisciplinary principles for professional practice in telehealth. *Professional Psychology Research and Practice,* *31,* 170−178.

Savin, D., Glueck, D. A., Chardavoyne, J., Yager, J., & Novins, D. K. (2011). Bridging cultures: Child psychiatry via videoconferencing. *Child Adolescent Psychiatrics Clinics of North America, 20,* 125−134.

Spaulding, R., Cain, S., & Sonnenschein, K. (2011). Urban telepsychiatry: Uncommon service for a common need. *Child Adolescent Psychiatrics Clinics of North America, 20,* 29−39.

Stanberry, B. (2006). Legal and ethical aspects of telemental health. *Journal of Telemental Health and Telecare, 12,* 166−175.

Wagnild, G., Leenknecht, C., & Zauher, J. (2006). Psychiatrists' satisfaction with telepsychiatry. *Telemental Health Journal of E-Health, 12,* 546−551.

van Wysberghe, A., & Gastmans, C. (2009). Telepsychiatry and the meaning of in-person contact: A preliminary ethical appraisal. *Medicine, Health Care and Philosophy, 12,* 469−476.

Yellowlees, P. M., Odor, A., Parish, M. B., Iosif, A. M., Haught, K., & Hilty, D. (2010). A feasibility study of the use of asynchronous telepsychiatry for psychiatric consultations. *Psychiatric Services, 61,* 838−840.

5 Integrating Culturally Appropriate Care into Telemental Health Practice

Elizabeth Brooks[a], Garret Spargo[b], Peter Yellowlees[c], Patrick O'Neill[d] and Jay H. Shore[a]

[a]Centers for American Indian and Alaska Native Health, University of Colorado Denver, Aurora, CO, [b]ANTHC—AFHCAN, [c]UC Davis, [d]Tulane University School of Medicine

Culturally Appropriate Care and Telemental Health: An Introduction

What Is Culturally Appropriate Care?

Individual culture often defines how patients express and interpret their personal health symptoms and, ultimately, the health care choices they make. For example, some traditional Chinese American and American Indian cultures rely on the healing powers of traditional medicines, herbs, and rituals instead of, or as an adjunct to, the use of modern Westernized medicine. Because of this, there has been a growing awareness of the interplay of culture and healing among many service providers who wish to practice culturally appropriate care. While there is not a universal definition for what constitutes such treatment, telemental health experts have identified culturally appropriate care as "the delivery of mental health services that are guided by the cultural concerns of all racial or ethnic groups, including psychosocial background, typical styles of symptom presentation, immigration histories, and other cultural traditions, beliefs, and values" (Yellowlees, Marks, Hilty, & Shore, 2008). This particular definition is used because of its focus on mental health and its reflection of the different ways that culture can vary between individuals. Yet, the definition is limited in that it restricts culture to race and ethnicity lines only. Important to this discussion is the understanding that cultural differences can exist among many different groups—such as the urban-based provider who sees a primarily rural patient population. Accordingly, the aforementioned definition of culturally appropriate care is expanded to include the care of *any* group of individuals who have distinct customs, beliefs, values, histories, and

Telemental Health. DOI: http://dx.doi.org/10.1016/B978-0-12-416048-4.00005-1

communication styles. This chapter illustrates many different examples in which cultural differences may present in the clinical setting and relate to telemental health practice.

To facilitate the understanding and clinical practice of culturally appropriate care, several organizations and entities have developed practice guidelines and recommendations. One of the most commonly referred to set of cultural guidelines was issued by the American Psychological Association (APA) (Task Force on the Delivery of Services to Ethnic Minority Populations, 2011). These recommendations stress that providers should actively learn about the cultural practices and beliefs among members of the patient population while also being aware of their own limited knowledge and competency in this area. The guidelines further stress the importance that providers reflect on their own cultural identity and acknowledge their individual attitudes and stereotypes toward their patients' culture. Another set of popular practice recommendations stem from the *Diagnostic and Statistical Manual*, 4th Edition (DSM-IV-TR), *Outline for Cultural Formulation* (American Psychiatric Association, 2000). The formulation offers a systematic method of incorporating cultural issues into the clinical evaluation. Similar to APA guidelines, the need to understand a patient's cultural identity is stressed and physicians are encouraged to explore the role of the cultural in the expression and evaluation of symptoms and dysfunction. The cultural formulation also advises providers to consider ways in which culture influences the therapeutic relationship. When providers practice culturally appropriate care, they are better able to understand, communicate with, and effectively relate to patients across diverse backgrounds and dissimilar experiences.

The Use of Telemental Health with Rural, Distant, and Underserved Populations

The expansion of high-speed Internet and wireless networks, videoconferencing, and other personal communication devices offers new opportunities to meet the health needs of many patient groups (Alverson et al., 2008). Perhaps the utmost hallmark of telehealth-based care lies in its ability to bridge large geographical distances between the patient and the provider. Because of this, telemental health is frequently used in rural and distant areas. Rural and distant populations are often distinct given their tendency for strong kinship ties and shared local community and economic concerns (Dwyer, Lee, & Coward, 1990; Phillips & McLeroy, 2004). Ample research has documented the existence of health disparities in rural areas, which frequently exist because of the long distances required to access care, as well as a shortage of local qualified providers (Agency for Healthcare Research and Quality, 2009). Oftentimes, health disparities are compounded for large factions of diverse patient populations who live in rural areas. For example, many American Indian and Alaska Natives reside in distant tribal reservation communities where access to specialized health care is difficult to obtain, often hundreds of miles away from one's home (Baldwin et al., 2008; Government Accountability Office, 2005). Many rural areas suffer from elevated rates of post-traumatic stress disorder (PTSD), depression, and other mental health disorders and help seeking for these conditions is much lower than expected (Beals, Manson, Shore et al., 2002; Beals, Manson, Whitesell et al., 2005).

Telemental health is also used in many medically underserved areas (MUAs) or with medically underserved populations (MUPs). MUAs and MUPs are defined as having a relative or absolute shortage of medical personnel or resources. While MUAs and MUPs are not necessarily located in rural communities, they include groups of people who often face economic, cultural, or linguistic barriers to health care. Oftentimes, the medically underserved include a high percentage of patients who are elderly, who suffer from chronic conditions, and who are enrolled Medicaid programs (Coburn, Lundblad, MacKinney, McBride, & Mueller, 2010).

The Interplay Between Culture and Telemental Health

While the patients using telemental health services are frequently located in rural, distant, and underserved areas, the providers often reside in large urban centers and their backgrounds may be distinctly different from the population that they serve. There are many ways in which backgrounds may differ. For example, the provider may encounter patients who do not speak the same language or share the same social history and values. Because the general demographic and diversity of the United States are quickly changing and health care needs are growing, the likelihood that providers will encounter larger groups of diverse patient populations when using telemental health is expected to increase. In fact, many times telehealth clinics are established specifically to address the needs of traditionally underserved communities. It is increasingly important that such providers are aware of and are trained in culturally appropriate care practices.

A further consideration regarding the interplay of telemental health and culture is that individual background has a strong contextual influence on whether and how technology is used. Studies demonstrate that the acceptance and diffusion of technology differs across cultures (Brooks, Manson, Bair, Dailey, & Shore, 2012; Nwabueze et al., 2009) and that different groups tend to use technologies differently. For example, some research shows that men's decisions to use technology may be more influenced by its perceived usefulness while women's decisions may be based more on usability aspects (Gefen & Straub, 1997). Accordingly, the successful implementation of telemental health may not be universally implemented across groups of individuals, despite concerted efforts to make technology customizable to the patient. Moreover, when using telemental health with specific populations, the telehealth delivery mechanism should be suited to the needs, resources, and technological infrastructure (e.g., availability of high-speed/high-definition dedicated T1 lines vs desktop systems) of the local community.

Prior Research Examining Telehealth with Cultural Subgroups

While research specifically examining the interplay of culture and telehealth is still sparse (Yellowlees, Marks et al., 2008), a growing number of investigators have published reports discussing changes that occur when telehealth is used with populations that differ from the provider. This has largely been achieved by publishing case illustrations or sharing reports of successful clinic models. There is little in the way of quantitative reports. Several other publications highlight the successful implementation of telehealth demonstration projects with MUPs, minority groups, or disadvantaged populations, although the study aims or findings did not expressly address cultural considerations. The following section reviews a few of the more salient publications concerning telehealth and culture issues. Due the present lack of available literature, this section encompasses the practice of telemental health in particular but also includes other medical specialties as well.

American Indian Veteran Telemental Health Clinics

A series of papers have been published describing the cultural issues that surround a telemental health program which addresses the needs of American Indian veterans. (In disclosure, the administration of these clinics and subsequent clinic reports are largely the work of two of the chapter authors.) The clinics, which offer individual and group therapy, diagnostic evaluation and medication management, have demonstrated positive study findings for diagnostic reliability, patient and clinician acceptability, economic indicators, and the feasibility of videoconferencing with a specific subgroup (Shore, Brooks, Savin, Manson, & Libby, 2007; Shore, Brooks, Savin, Orton, et al., 2008; Shore & Manson, 2005; Shore, Savin, Orton, Beals, & Manson, 2007). Researchers working with these clinics documented ways in which the treatment process was altered given the interplay of cultural factors and the use of videoconferencing technology. For example, rapport building and general communication between the patient and the provider occasionally needed to be adjusted to accommodate for background differences as well as nuances imposed by the network transmission delay (Shore, Savin, Novins, & Manson, 2006). The researchers also documented that the diffusion and acceptance of telemental health services within the patient community was impacted, in part, by the cultural understanding and sensitivity displayed by key stakeholders (Brooks, Manson et al., 2012). Based on their several years of providing telehealth-based care to American Indian patients, the authors developed a model for adapting remote monitoring to specific populations which focused on (a) information gathering, (b) process and dialogue changes, (c) testing, and (d) patient and administrative feedback (Brooks, Novins et al., in press). Researchers suggested that input should be gathered from a variety of individuals who understand area needs and can speak about local technological and resource capabilities. Adaptation changes included the incorporation of patient-specific information into telehealth care. This might include acknowledging historical discrimination faced by community members and educating patients about the relationship of such inequities to current health concerns. The use of this model serves as one example by which other clinicians and investigators may incorporate telehealth technologies into successful, culturally appropriate care.

Telehealth Treatment with the Elderly, Child, and Adolescent Populations

Other authors have discussed the ability of telehealth to be successfully utilized with differing age groups. The elderly are some of the highest consumers of health care and providing specialized services to this population can be difficult. However, failure to do so may result in significant stress, impairment, or death. Consequently, the rendering of telehealth services to the elderly population can provide a much needed avenue for care. While some may question the ability of older adults to effectively use or accept telehealth-based medical care given their relative lack of technological exposure, studies have demonstrated that telehealth with the elderly can be successfully provided in both residential settings and at home (Barlow, Singh, Bayer, & Curry, 2007; Sheeran et al., 2011; Wakefield et al., 2008; Yeung, Johnson, Trinh, Weng, Kvedar, & Fava, 2009). Moreover, research has shown that the provision of telemental health services has resulted in significant cost savings in nursing homes (Rabinowitz et al., 2010) and may prevent or reduce subsequent hospitalizations (Jerant, Azari, & Nesbitt, 2001). Conversely, telehealth services have been shown to be effectively used with children and adolescents (Marcin et al., 2004; Myers, Valentine, & Melzer, 2007; Nelson, Barnard, & Cain, 2003). This area of research is particularly important as many rural areas lack access to psychiatrists and other mental health specialists trained to provide care to children and adolescents. Investigations show that younger patients tend to be very enthusiastic about technology-based care and the care modality is beneficial and well accepted by this age group (Myers et al., 2007; Myers, Valentine, & Melzer, 2008; Pesamaa et al., 2004).

Treatment with Linguistically Diverse Populations

Earlier, it was discussed how the US population demographic is rapidly shifting. As a result, providers are encountering a rising number of patients who have limited, or no, English proficiency (Ku & Flores, 2005). A growing number of individuals and organizations have developed guidelines and best practices to use when working with non-English-speaking populations. The US Office of Minority Health developed the *Culturally and Linguistically Appropriate Services (CLAS)* standards in 2001 in an effort to supersede the previous patchwork of recommendations in this area. Although none of the 14 standards mentions the use of telehealth-based care specifically, 6 standards greatly lend themselves to the provision of telehealth by addressing issues largely focused on language barriers (Table 5.1). In particular, these guidelines stress the importance of delivering care and information in the patient's native or preferred language. In an effort to provide more effective, appropriate care in this manner, providers have begun using telehealth in novel ways with non-English-speaking patients. For example, Yellowlees, Hilty et al. (in press) tested the feasibility and reliability of asynchronous psychiatric consultations demonstrating the successful use of store-and-forward-based Spanish to English translations. Real-time interpreter services have been used as well, with the researchers citing either equivalent or better satisfaction ratings for telehealth-based interpreter

Table 5.1 CLAS Standards Lending Themselves to the Provision of Telehealth[1]

- *Standard*: Health care organizations should ensure that patients receive *effective, understandable, and respectful care that is provided in a manner compatible with their cultural health beliefs and practices and preferred language.*

- *Standard*: Health care organizations should ensure that *staff receives education and training in culturally and linguistically appropriate service delivery.*

- *Standard*: Health care organizations must *provide language assistance services*, including bilingual staff and interpreter services, at no cost to each patient/consumer with limited English proficiency.

- *Standard*: Health care organizations must *provide to patients both verbal offers and written notices in their preferred language* which inform them of their right to receive language assistance services.

- *Standard*: Health care organizations must *assure the competence of language assistance provided to limited English proficient patients* by interpreters and bilingual staff. *Family and friends should not be used to provide interpretation service* (expect on request by the patient).

- *Standard*: Health care organizations must *make available patient-related materials and post signage in the language of the commonly encountered groups* in the service area.

[1]Modified from the US Department of Health and Human Services Office of Minority Health, http://minorityhealth .hhs.gov/templates/browse.aspx?lvl = 2&lvlID = 15.

services (Hornberger et al., 1996; Jones, Gill, Harrison, Meakin, & Wallace, 2003). Researchers have also found better accuracy of telehealth-based interpretation services compared to in-person care. Other researchers have found that prerecorded clinical reminders in the patients' native tongue increased appointment attendance (Tanke & Leirer, 1994), while another study found that handheld personal digital assistants were helpful in assisting Spanish-speaking mothers learn problem-solving skills to care for their children with cancer (Askins et al., 2009).

Treatment with Other Cultural Subgroups

In addition to these specific areas of cultural research, various journal articles and briefs have outlined considerations and lessons learned when using telemental health with African-American populations (Bondmass, Bolger, Castro, & Avitall, 2000). For example, a recent diabetes self-care management program was implemented with an urban African-American population who had very few health care resources (Carter, Nunlee-Bland, & Callender, 2011). Patients effectively learned to take and transmit their own medical information using a personal laptop computer equipped with peripheral devices

Despite these advances, there has been a limited effort to create national policies concerning the practice of culturally appropriate care via telemental health although a number of authors have called for the development of policy recommendations in this area (Shore, Savin, Novins, & Manson 2006; Tirado, 2011; Yellowlees, Marks et al., 2008).

The Appropriateness of Telemedicine

Only a limited number of studies have been conducted regarding the appropriateness of telemental health services with special populations. Even fewer studies exist that look at how to assess whether the technology and services are appropriate for a specific group. Given the dearth of data, a level of inference is required to assess how special populations may respond to issues around technology and human interaction during the use of telemental health.

There is some concern about telemental health services that are heavily dependent upon reading and comprehension of textual and verbal materials among those who have limited fluency in English (Campbell-Grossman, Hudson, Keating-Lefler, Yank, & Obafunwa, 2009; Markstrom, Stamm, Stamm, Berthold, & Running Wolf, 2003; Tirado, 2011; Viruell-Fuentes, Morenoff, Williams, & House, 2011). This may be particularly detrimental for text-based telehealth tools such as remote monitoring dialogues. Other studies report concerns about compliance and timely completion of Internet-based therapies that rely heavily on written cognitive-behavioral homework assignments. Concerns surround cultural differences for populations whose sense of time may be less stringent or whose compliance rates may be below that of other populations (Andersson, Carlbring, Berger, Almlov, & Cuijpers, 2009). Note, however, that these issues may be mitigated by changing the frequency, duration, or method of communication and interaction between the patient and the provider.

Understanding the Patient Culture and Community

Throughout this chapter it has been important to stress the need for providers to understand the local culture and community which they serve. Many cultural subgroups have wide ranging concerns about accessing behavioral health services. Moreover, because different groups vary in their personal histories and experiences with governmental, medical, and other institutions, the scope and degree of their concerns may also vary widely. Within immigrant populations, seeking behavioral health treatment may be avoided due to fears about deportation or the affordability of care (Campbell-Grossman et al., 2009; Markstrom et al., 2003). Alaska Native, American Indian, and African-American populations—who have experienced various levels of abuse or apathy in governmental programs—report feeling disenfranchised or disinterested in pursuing treatment from outside sources (Briggs, Briggs, Miller, & Paulson, 2011; Champion & Collins, 2010; Goodkind et al., 2011; Walters & Simoni, 2009). Rural communities also have witnessed the "revolving door" of short-term medical practitioners in their area, and, consequently, some are hesitant to engage in services that they fear will not be available in the long term (Goodkind et al., 2011). Additionally, populations may possess stigmas around mental health care (Briggs et al., 2011) or have beliefs that their condition is somehow fated or a part of "God's will" (Becker, Affonso, & Beard, 2006; Markstrom et al., 2003; Natale-Pereira et al., 2008). The following section addresses some ways that providers and clinic administrators can gain a better understanding of the local community.

Community Leaders and Key Informants

Local leadership enables providers to better understand the concerns and specific needs of the community. The exact structure of local leadership can vary widely between regions and cultures, ranging from respected individuals, to existing programs and service providers, to community organizations, to sovereign tribal entities and tribal councils. Other key informants include network engineers who understand the local technological infrastructure, capabilities, and limitations. Health care providers or other individuals who know the medical needs of the area are also helpful to talk to. A single community may contain a diverse mix of these formally and informally recognized leaders.

During conversations with community leaders, the information gathered not only helps to understand the area needs but also allows the ability to gauge the telemental health program's potential impact, suitably, and appropriateness. It is often important to offer community leaders a forum for voicing concerns, to provide an avenue to incorporate them in future decisions, progress updates, and planning efforts, and to clearly identify how their participation can help with the development of behavioral health services. For example, the development of an emergency protocol is necessary in most telehealth programs. Area leaders can help to foster relationships and facilitate communication or collaboration between the telehealth clinic administrators and local emergency services. Community relationships may also be enhanced by the use of technology. For example, some meetings can be held by videoconferencing, allowing participants a more similar experience to in-person meetings when traveling to distant sites is not an option.

A benefit of engaging in the discussion with the local community is that efforts to engage in program development may be more thoroughly understood by local leaders, who may in turn work with their community members to educate them on how and why to participate in new programs. Additional benefits can arise from the leaders' connections to the community, resulting in an increase in outreach opportunities as they interact with their constituents and other community members. Furthermore, these individuals may also be able to address fears, uncertainty, and doubts about the nature of the clinical services.

Local Outreach Workers

One of the most effective ways to learn about the patient community is to hire an outreach worker to help with the telemental health clinic. Although there are many models for outreach workers (Brooks, Manson et al., 2012), these critical staff are often situated at the patient site and are members of the local community. The importance of the outreach worker cannot be undervalued. In many programs, the outreach worker will assist with patient scheduling, orient new patients to the telehealth equipment, and be on hand to assist with technological problems that arise during the clinical encounter.

However, perhaps the most important role of the outreach worker is to serve as a "cultural bridge" or liaison between the clinic and the patients and community. When initially orienting new patients to telehealth services, the presence of an outreach worker who is of a similar cultural background can increase patients' comfort and trust. By hiring a respected member of the community, that individual is able to promote the services, recruit patients, and gain local acceptance for the use of technology-based medical services. The outreach worker position can also provide an avenue for the public to voice concerns about the clinic and offer ideas about ways to improve or expand services to the area.

Often, outreach workers provide valuable cultural information to the providers. For example, they may share information about local customs or holidays, or they may provide updates about particularly important issues affecting the community. In many rural areas, accidents or local deaths can affect a large number of people and may impact the current focus of the telehealth clinic. The outreach worker is in a unique position to inform the provider about these issues in advance of seeing patients, allowing the provider to restructure individual sessions as appropriate.

Outreach workers can be especially useful in areas for which seeking mental health care still holds a negative stigma. In some rural areas, outreach workers might be patients of the clinic themselves. While there are certainly issues of dual relationships to consider, the ability of an outreach worker to publicly identify as both a patient and a respected member of the community helps to encourage others to seek treatment.

Utilizing Local Information

Apart from community leaders and outreach workers, there are many other ways to stay abreast of local events. Clinicians can visit community web sites, read local papers, and learn about local organizations. It may also be important to hold occasional site visits in the patient community. Site visits offer patients the opportunity to meet their providers face to face and may strengthen the clinical relationship. They also lend a sense of credibility and commitment by the provider. This can be extremely important in areas where most new clinicians leave once their education commitments and debt repayment obligations are fulfilled. Thus, telemental health may offer a level of continuity of care that may not be possible in other models that seek to rectify disparities in access to mental health care.

Incorporating the Community for Effective Telemental Health Services

Oftentimes, the success of a distant telemental health clinic requires establishing local collaborations. This section reviews why community members are important partners and how their assistance might be resourced. Challenges that arise from such collaborations, such as dual relationships, are also discussed.

Establishing Local Partnerships and Collaborations

Earlier in the chapter it was discussed how local leadership can help providers to understand the cultural concerns of the community. It was also stressed that these individuals are valuable assets when planning services and establishing collaborative partners. Partnering with community leaders can provide access to additional resources such as office space, local pharmaceutical care, and nearby emergency services. Local leaders may also help with overcoming jurisdictional or legal obstacles. It is important to partner with these local groups and individuals in the early planning stages so that their regional and cultural expertise can be utilized, and so that their concerns and input can be addressed as the program grows.

Community leaders' participation can take different forms, depending, in part, on their individual cultures and roles within the community. It is best to identify and involve leaders early in the process of planning services. Formal involvement early in the process can help provide guidance on the scope and goals of the program, and may also provide introductions to other key community members and organizations. More formal methods of involvement may include requesting their participation in a steering committee or other position. Less formal involvement may include the use of talking circles, public forums, or town-hall style meetings to gather community feedback.

Another way to increase community collaboration is to establish ways in which the telemental health resources might be leveraged to provide additional services to meet local needs. Examples of this include providing access to videoconferencing equipment or allowing the use of bandwidth to other groups for clinical and administrative purposes. It may also consist of providing training opportunities for local health care practitioners and community members.

Collaborations with local partners may be a onetime occurrence, but often, longer relationships are beneficial. Maintaining community members' involvement in continued discussions and steering committees can ensure that their role in the development of the program continues. Consider developing methods for communicating program information with the community to assist in continued outreach and education regarding the availability of telemental health services. This should include a mechanism for feedback with the broader community as well as with the individuals utilizing the telemental health services. Both of these groups may provide valuable feedback regarding the struggles, successes, and ongoing concerns about treatment delivered through telemedicine.

Dual Relationships in Rural Areas

Dual relationships are an almost unavoidable reality of working in rural communities. Whereas these relationships have historically been considered unethical, some professional associations have updated their code of ethics to reflect the view that these relationships can be acceptable if properly and transparently handled. Given that the outreach coordinator or on-site clinician may have familial or professional relationships with the patients, the question is not whether dual relationships should be allowed, but how they will be handled. While the delivery of telemental health services reduces the risk of dual relationships between the patient and the provider, the clinician should still understand that many such relationships may still exist and special consideration should be given to understand how such relationships may impact the delivery of services. Patients may obtain prescriptions from a prescriber in the community or medical billing information may be handled by a neighbor. Clear policies should be in place to properly address how dual relationship issues will be addressed.

Neutral third-party interpreter services are not likely to be present within small communities. As such, the impact of the relationship between the patient and interpreter should be taken into consideration. Issues can arise if the interpreter censors, editorializes, or misinterprets pertinent information. Further, if using interpreter services during sessions conducted through videoconferencing, nuances of interpersonal relatedness might be missed that could help in detecting problems in interpretation. There may be issues beyond the scope of patient–provider interactions, as well. Concerns about the stigma attached to mental health treatment may cause patients to refrain from seeking services if their access to the facilities is clearly and publicly broadcast. Providing discrete entrances to the clinical setting can reduce the impact of this issue, as can siting telemental clinics within facilities that contain other, less stigmatized, organizations or services, such as colocating the telemental health clinic in a medical clinic.

Technological Considerations When Working with Diverse Populations

Here, the discussion focuses on the integration of culturally appropriate care into telemental health practice. In particular, specific factors that need to be considered when using technology with diverse populations—typically via videoconferencing—are provided. To better illustrate these issues, examples from a variety of patient backgrounds are provided. It is important to note, however, not every example applies to all members of the group.

Communication

Cultural differences often impact the communication between the clinician and the patient. Oftentimes, *how* a message is relayed may be a more accurate reflection of a message rather than what is actually said. Miscommunication is likely to affect the accuracy of diagnoses and effectiveness of the treatment (Savin, Glueck, Chardavoyne, Yager, & Novins, 2011). Because of this, clinicians must be familiar with the communication style of the patient population.

Verbal Communication

Cultures vary in their use of verbal communications in respect to the use of silence, the pace of the dialogue, and the tone of the conversation. Silence, for example, may be awkward and uncomfortable for some groups, while others tend to value quiet periods and intersperse them liberally into conversation. Silence is an especially important aspect to be aware of as it pertains to videoconferencing. Videoconferencing may alter the power of silence because the technology often creates unnatural pauses due to the mild delay in signal transmissions. Clinicians should be cautious not to overuse pauses or mistakenly attribute patients' silence to anything other than their reaction to the technology.

Many cultures have different communications styles; some speak very rapidly, others slowly. Cultural conventions determine when it is appropriate to speak and patients may need to be asked directly and specifically about a topic for which more information is needed. Further, many groups believe that it is extremely rude to interrupt people when they talk—especially an elder. Some cultures, such as several American Indian tribes, embrace a story-telling tradition. Consequently, responses to clinical questions may appear to be relatively long or off-topic in comparison with other groups. In instances in which the clinician determines that the client responses need to be refocused, redirection must be handled delicately and respectfully. Due to the wide variety of communication styles, clinicians may need to alter the way they address and respond to patients of differing backgrounds. Clinicians may find the need to be more direct when talking with a patient over telehealth, especially in a group setting. It is further important to note that rapport may take longer to establish both initially and at the beginning of each session. To overcome this, the clinician may use more initial small talk. When working with diverse populations, it can be particularly effective to raise issues about local community events which impact the patient. Toward the end of the chapter, a case study is presented to illustrate how one therapist incorporates a "talking circle" format in telehealth-based group therapy. Using this technique, many of the cultural considerations noted above can be effectively addressed.

Nonverbal Communication

Nonverbal cues vary widely in many cultures. For example, Hispanic cultures rely heavily on facial expressions such as frowning or tipping the head (Nieves & Stack, 2007). In some Asian and American Indian groups, direct eye contact is considered rude and disrespectful (Elliott, 1999). A provider needs to be careful not to misinterpret lack of eye contact in these patients as a clinical sign (e.g., depression). Some providers find it more difficult to establish eye contact while using telehealth technologies. Often, this is the result of the camera placement, which typically sits on top of the monitor. Clinicians should also be cognizant of how their own image is projected to the patient. A more distant image diminishes the appearance of eye contact. Personal space is another crucial element that can interact with culture and videoconferencing. Different groups vary widely in their comfort levels with interpersonal proximity. Many Caucasians or European-Americans prefer about 2−3 ft in distance from one another, or about arm's length (Fairlie, 2003). Videoconferencing has the ability to manipulate the proximity between the patient and the provider by use of the "zoom" function on the camera. For cultures that require more personal distance from one another, the camera's zoom lens should be set relatively far from the clinician; this will help to convey the feeling of physical distance. Providers may also allow patients to operate the camera on their end so they might adjust it to their personal comfort level.

Working with a diverse population often means that the clinician's characteristics have a greater impact on the patient's impression of the provider. The clinician should wear clothing that is appropriate to the population. "Overdressing" may create an unintentional impression of aloofness and be an unwelcome reminder of the unbalanced power dynamic in the patient−provider relationship. "Underdressing" for a particular patient population may create an impression of sloppiness and lack of professionalism. Speaking with other clinicians who work with the target population can help to understand the appropriate level of dress and expectations of attire for the group of interest.

Symbolism

Many cultures identify with specific symbols, objects, and designs, and the use of these items can help put patients at ease in a clinical setting. The use of culturally appropriate symbolism of the videoconferencing rooms can be an effective way to help bridge the distance between locations. It is often recommended that providers display objects that have some meaning to their patients, such as pictures, posters, and other wall hangings. For example, in a particular clinic that works with Northern Plains-based American Indians, the clinician hangs a star quilt on the wall during each encounter. The star quilt is frequently used to honor American Indians and their guests at traditional ceremonies and rites of passage. With the quilt hanging behind the clinician, the image is captured by the videoconferencing camera and provides cultural relevance to the clinical environment.

Technological Knowledge and Comfort

The patient's comfort with videoconferencing is critical to the success of treatment. Frequently, comfort is related to individuals past experience with technology. Not surprisingly, exposure to technology is often related to the patient's age and education; however, many older generations have used and expressed a high degree of satisfaction with videoconferencing. Rurality and ethnicity have also been found to be negative indicators of technology exposure (Fairlie, 2003; Lorence, Park, & Fox, 2006; Warren, 2007). In general, virtually no technical knowledge is necessary in order for patients to use most telemental health applications, which often do not require the use of peripheral medical equipment, and the initial introduction to telehealth can go a long way in making patients feel more comfortable. When orienting new patients to videoconferencing, clinicians should directly ask about the clients' prior experience with computers, videoconferencing, or other electronic instruments. During this session, it is often important to explain how the technology will be used and to assure patients of the privacy and confidentiality standards used in the clinic as many individuals are often wary about what will be seen by whom. For patients who have little prior experience with telehealth, their comfort level typically improves as they gain more exposure to the technology.

Conclusion

As emphasized throughout this chapter, cultural differences between the patient and the provider are an important consideration in the provision of mental health care. Culture can be expressed in a number of ways such as with language, social customs, and general attitudes about illness or disease management. When unrecognized differences exist in the clinical setting, the provider risks the delivery of substandard care. Cultural considerations are particularly salient when using telehealth technologies. Because telehealth is frequently used to bridge large geographic distances, the background, experiences, and concerns among patients and providers are more likely to differ. The technology, itself, may also make cultural differences more evident. Fortunately, variations between patients and providers do not have to impede the use of telemental health. Using technologies appropriately, as well as modifications to clinical care or processes, can help bridge cultural differences. This chapter concludes with three case studies to illustrate how culturally appropriate care can be integrated into the delivery of telemental health practice.

Case Studies

The Use of Talking Circles in Telemental Health Group Therapy

This case describes the cultural adaptation and modification of clinical processes for a working with specific population. One telemental health clinic serving a distant rural Northern Plains reservation offers ongoing supportive therapy group for chronic mental illnesses such as depression, anxiety, and substance use disorders using videoconferencing. The therapist is located in an urban center which is hundreds of miles away from the community. The group process is run along the line of a traditional talking circle. Talking circles are widespread Northern Plains' ceremonies in which participants gather in a circle and then pass ceremonial objects (e.g., talking stick, feather) around the circle in a systematic fashion. Members of the circle speak in turn when they are holding the object while other members listen. Modeling this in the telehealth group, the clinician in this case goes around the group inviting members to speak one at a time. The session often concludes with a larger group discussion that is guided by the therapist and follows on topics raised by the individual members. The adoption of this process has a number of clinical benefits which include presenting individual members with a format with which they are already familiar, as well as ensuring that all members have an opportunity to speak and are encouraged to participate in the group session. Using a talking circle further avoids the risk that a group could deteriorate into a "talking head" format with the therapist dominating the session in lecture-based style. It also allows the therapist to play an important role in managing and facilitating the group process while participating as an active member of the group remotely.

Using Telemental Health to Increase Access in a Medically Underserved Area

This example shows how telemental health has been used to bridge the high demand and low availability of mental health services in rural Louisiana, a setting that presents with difficulties similar to other MUAs. Throughout this chapter, the discussion has revolved around the ability of telemental health to meet the needs of geographically diverse, MUAs. The telehealth clinic extended to the community of Allen Parish is one such case. Allen Parish spans about 750 square miles and houses a population of about 25,000. Residents living in Allen Parish are located roughly 4 h away from the largest nearby cities of New Orleans and Houston. The population is 71% Caucasian, 25% African-American, and nearly 2% Native American with nearly 20% of residents living below the national poverty line. For the African-American population, residents are typically the fifth to sixth generation natives of the area, many are descendants of freed slaves and, economically, conditions are still very difficult for many of these families. Prior to the implementation of the telemental health program, the parish did not have regular behavioral health services, notwithstanding a general practitioner who would visit the clinic once a week to provide basic psychiatric medication management. The wait for a psychiatric evaluation was over a year in duration although there were counseling services provided. All emergent presentations were referred to a local emergency room.

Due to residents' difficulty of obtaining care, a telemental health clinic was established in 2009 connecting Allen Parish mental health clinic patients to psychiatric specialists at Tulane University. New telemental health services include adult and child psychiatric care via videoconferencing. The average wait for a psychiatric evaluation was drastically reduced from the previous delay of a year to 2–4 weeks through telehealth. The telehealth clinic also employs the use of a local, on-site nurse or social worker who remains with the patient during the medical appointment. As discussed in this chapter, the on-site clinical worker provides several benefits to the clinic. Not only does this person help to facilitate patient care but his/her presence also helps to bridge any cultural issues that might arise during the appointment. Additionally, the clinical worker serves as a liaison between the individual, the community, and the medical facility.

As an example of how the telemental health clinic has helped individuals in the community, the case of Mary C. is presented. Mary is a middle-aged, never married, African-American woman. She began receiving intermittent mental health care after battling depression which stemmed from the death of her infant daughter. Mary currently suffers from PTSD as a result of childhood, parental incest and struggles with obesity, hypertension, asthma, arthritis, chronic anemia, and hepatitis C. She frequently abuses alcohol and has a history of suicide attempts, drug overdose, and violent interpersonal relationships. Mary's housing situation is frequently uncertain with many long stays at shelters in the region. Similar to many local residents, Mary has no private insurance and is on Medicaid. Prior to receiving disability payments, Mary's income consisted of about $200/month. Since she began first seeking care for mental health problems, Mary visited over eight different outpatient programs and her compliance with treatment during this period was poor. She had been off all psychiatric medications for 3 years prior to telemental health treatment. However, since enrolling in the telemental health clinic, Mary is receiving evidenced-based medication management, nursing assessments of her physical condition, case management, housing assistance, and psychotherapy. Her condition has stabilized; she has an apartment and is becoming more involved in church and in the lives of her children.

The Use of Asynchronous Technology to Bridge Language Barriers

This case study describes how certain delivery mechanisms can advance health care quality and access among individuals who do not speak the community's dominant language. In this particular example, asynchronous telepsychiatric interpretive services are effectively used with a largely Spanish-speaking patient population.

As the US general demographic shifts, more regions have a growing patient population that is largely Hispanic, mainly of Mexican heritage. In the rural Northern California town featured here, many such patients are seen, several of whom are low-wage laborers and do not speak English. Access to and the quality of mental health services is limited not only by language barriers and geography but because many residents are undocumented citizens. As such, residents frequently do not seek care for fear that their immigration status will be discovered. Help seeking is also limited because local labor options—often farm work—do not include employee-supported health care coverage. Access to treatment is further hindered by one's ability to get time off work and arrange for, or pay for, daycare. Diminished care-seeking behavior has been a particular problem among the local Hispanic women, who—because of cultural norms—must often stay at home to tend to the house and children and, consequently, do not develop English-language skills as readily. When patients do present for health services, the language barrier quickly becomes a problem. In this clinic, as with many others, protocol dictates that non-English-speaking patients arrange for, and are accompanied by, an interpreter. lOftentimes, the interpreter is either related to the patient—a spouse or child—or a close friend. This poses serious concerns for patient privacy and often results in missing or inaccurate information in the medical history.

Store-and-forward videoconferencing is proving to be an effective mechanism to address these concerns and improve access. In this example, a program was created to test the feasibility and diagnostic validity of using asynchronous consultation services between the rural area and psychiatrists residing in a larger urban city (Yellowlees, Hilty et al., in press). In particular, patients in the rural area met with a bilingual provider who administered a standardized diagnostic interview and took the patient history. The patient's information was collected in Spanish with the entire interview recorded on video. The data were then translated to English and transferred to English-speaking psychiatrists via store-and-forward technology for evaluation. The demonstration project showed that the translation services and video could be implemented with accurate and reliable results. Further, it provides evidence that language barriers can be effectively removed in an assessment-type situation and may hasten enrollment in regular ongoing therapy.

References

Agency for Healthcare Research and Quality (2009). *National healthcare disparities report #09-0002*. Rockville, MD: US Department of Health and Human Services.

Alverson, D. C., Holtz, B., D'Iorio, J., DeVany, M., Simmons, S., & Poropatich, R. K. (2008). One size doesn't fit all: Bringing telehealth services to special populations. *Telemedicine and e-Health, 14*, 957–963.

American Psychiatric Association (2000). *Diagnostic and statistical manual of mental disorders* (4th ed., (text revision)). Washington, DC: American Psychiatric Association.

Andersson, G., Carlbring, P., Berger, T., Almlov, J., & Cuijpers, P. (2009). What makes internet therapy work? *Cognitive Behaviour Therapy, 38*, 1–6.

Askins, M. A., Sahler, O. J., Sherman, S. A., Fairclough, D. L., Butler, R. W., & Katz, E. R., et al. (2009). Report from a multi-institutional randomized clinical trial examining computer-assisted problem-solving skills training for English- and Spanish-speaking mothers of children with newly diagnosed cancer. *Journal of Pediatric Psychiatry, 34*, 551–563.

Baldwin, L. M., Hollow, W. B., Casey, S., Hart, L. G., Larson, E. H., & Moore, K., et al. (2008). Access to specialty health care for rural American Indians in two states. *The Journal of Rural Health, 24*, 269–278.

Barlow, J., Singh, D., Bayer, S., & Curry, R. (2007). A systematic review of the benefits of home telecare for frail elderly people and those with long-term conditions. *Journal of Telemedicine and Telecare, 13*, 172–179.

Beals, J., Manson, S. M., Shore, J. H., Friedman, M., Ashcraft, M., & Fairbank, J. A., et al. (2002). The prevalence of posttraumatic stress disorder among American Indian Vietnam veterans: Disparities and context. *Journal of Traumatic Stress, 15*, 89–97.

Beals, J., Manson, S. M., Whitesell, N. R., Mitchell, C. M., Novins, D. K., & Simpson, S., et al. (2005). Prevalence of major depressive episode in two American Indian reservation populations: Unexpected findings with a structured interview. *American Journal of Psychiatry, 162*, 1713–1722.

Becker, S. A., Affonso, D. D., & Beard, M. B. H. (2006). Talking circles: Northern plains tribes American Indian women's views of cancer as a health issue. *Public Health Nursing, 23*, 27–36.

Bondmass, M., Bolger, N., Castro, G., & Avitall, B. (2000). The effect of home monitoring and telemanagement on blood pressure control among African Americans. *Telemedicine Journal, 6*, 15−23.

Briggs, H. E., Briggs, A. C., Miller, K. M., & Paulson, R. I. (2011). Combating persistent cultural incompetence in mental health care systems serving African Americans. *Best Practice in Mental Health, 7*, 1−25.

Brooks, E., Manson, S., Bair, B., Dailey, N., & Shore, J. (2012). The diffusion of telehealth in rural American Indian communities: A retrospective survey of key stakeholders. *Telemedicine and e-Health, 18*, 60−66.

Brooks, E., Novins, D. K., Noe, T., Lowe, J., Richardson, W., Bair, B., et al. (in press). Reaching Rural Communities with Culturally-Appropriate Care: A Model for Adapting Remote Monitoring to American Indian Veterans with Post Traumatic Stress Disorder. *Journal of Telemedicine and e-Health.*

Campbell-Grossman, C., Hudson, D. B., Keating-Lefler, R., Yank, J. R., & Obafunwa, T. (2009). Community leaders' perceptions of Hispanic, single, low-income mothers' needs, concerns, social support, and interactions with health care services. *Issues in Comprehensive Pediatric Nursing, 32*, 31−46.

Carter, E. L., Nunlee-Bland, G., & Callender, C. (2011). A patient-centric, provider-assisted diabetes telehealth self-management intervention for urban minorities. *Perspectives in Health Information Management, 8*, 1−11.

Champion, J. D., & Collins, J. L. (2010). The path to intervention: Community partnerships and development of a cognitive behavioral intervention for ethnic minority adolescent females. *Issues in Mental Health Nursing, 31*, 739−747.

Coburn, A. F., Lundblad, J. P., MacKinney, A. C., McBride, T. D., & Mueller, P. K. J. (2010). *Designating health professional shortage areas and medically underserved populations and medically underserved areas: A primer on basic issues to resolve.* Rural Policy Research Institute, Columbia, MO.

Dwyer, J. W., Lee, G. R., & Coward, R. T. (1990). The health status, health services utilization, and support networks of the rural elderly: A decade review. *The Journal of Rural Health, 6*, 379−398.

Elliott, C. E. (1999). Communication patterns and assumptions of differing cultural groups in the United States. Pre-publication Master's Thesis.

Fairlie, R. W. (2003). Is there a digital divide? Ethnic and racial differences in access to technology and possible explanations. Report to the University of California, Latino Policy Institute and California Policy Research Center. Online publication <http://cjtc.ucsc.edu/docs/r_techreport5.pdf>.

Gefen, D., & Straub, D. W. (1997). Gender differences in the perception and use of e-mail: An extension to the technology acceptance model. *MIS Quarterly, 21*, 389−400.

Goodkind, J. R., Ross-Toledo, K., John, S., Hall, J. L., Ross, L., & Freeland, L., et al. (2011). Rebuilding trust: A community, multiagency, state, and university partnership to improve behavioral health care for American Indian youth, their families, and communities. *Journal of Community Psychology, 39*, 452−477.

Government Accountability Office (2005). *Health care services are not always available to native Americans.* Washington, DC: Indian Health Service.

Hornberger, J. C., Gibson, C. D., Jr., Wood, W., Dequeldre, C., Corso, I., & Palla, B., et al. (1996). Eliminating language barriers for non-English-speaking patients. *Medical Care, 34*, 845−856.

Jerant, A. F., Azari, R., & Nesbitt, T. S. (2001). Reducing the cost of frequent hospital admissions for congestive heart failure: A randomized trial of a home telecare intervention. *Medical Care, 39*, 1234–1245.

Jones, D., Gill, P., Harrison, R., Meakin, R., & Wallace, P. (2003). An exploratory study of language interpretation services provided by videoconferencing. *Journal of Telemedicine and Telecare, 9*, 51–56.

Ku, L., & Flores, G. (2005). Pay now or pay later: Providing interpreter services in health care. *Health Affairs, 24*, 435–444.

Lorence, D. P., Park, H., & Fox, S. (2006). Racial disparities in health information access: Resilience of the digital divide. *Journal of Medical Systems, 30*, 241–249.

Marcin, J. P., Ellis, J., Mawis, R., Nagrampa, E., Nesbitt, T. S., & Dimand, R. J. (2004). Using telemedicine to provide pediatric subspecialty care to children with special health care needs in an underserved rural community. *Pediatrics, 113*, 1–6.

Markstrom, C. A., Stamm, B. H., Stamm, H. E., Berthold, S. M., & Running Wolf, P. (2003). *Rural behavioral health care: An interdisciplinary guide*. Washington, DC: American Psychological Association.

Myers, K. M., Valentine, J. M., & Melzer, S. M. (2007). Feasibility, acceptability, and sustainability of telepsychiatry for children and adolescents. *Psychiatric Services, 58*, 1493–1496.

Myers, K. M., Valentine, J. M., & Melzer, S. M. (2008). Child and adolescent telepsychiatry: Utilization and satisfaction. *Telemedicine and e-Health, 14*, 131–137.

Natale-Pereira, A., Marks, J., Vega, M., Mouzon, D., Hudson, S. V., & Salas-Lopez, D. (2008). Barriers and facilitators for colorectal cancer screening practices in the Latino community: Perspectives from community leaders. *Cancer Control, 15*, 157–165.

Nelson, E. L., Barnard, M., & Cain, S. (2003). Treating childhood depression over videoconferencing. *Telemedicine and e-Health, 9*, 49–55.

Nieves, J. E., & Stack, K. M. (2007). Hispanics and telepsychiatry. *Psychiatric Services, 58*, 877–878.

Nwabueze, S. N., Meso, P. N., Mbarika, V. W., Kifle, M., Okoli, C., & Chustz, M. (2009). The effects of culture of adoption of telemedicine in medically underserved communities. *System Sciences*1–10.

Office of Minority Health (2012). National Standards on Culturally and Linguistically Appropriate Services (CLAS). U.S. Department of Health and Human Services. Retrieved Aug 9, 2012 from < http://minorityhealth.hhs.gov/templates/browse.aspx?lvl=2&lvlID=15 > .

Pesamaa, L., Ebeling, H., Kuusimaki, M. L., Winblad, I., Isohanni, M., & Moilanen, I. (2004). Videoconferencing in child and adolescent telepsychiatry: A systematic review of the literature. *Journal of Telemedicine and Telecare, 10*, 187–192.

Phillips, C. D., & McLeroy, K. R. (2004). Health in rural America: Remembering the importance of place. *American Journal of Public Health, 94*, 1661–1663.

Rabinowitz, T., Murphy, K. M., Amour, J. L., Ricci, M. A., Caputo, M. P., & Newhouse, P. A. (2010). Benefits of a telepsychiatry consultation service for rural nursing home residents. *Telemedicine and e-Health, 16*, 34–40.

Savin, D., Glueck, D. A., Chardavoyne, J., Yager, J., & Novins, D. K. (2011). Bridging cultures: Child psychiatry via videoconferencing. *Child and Adolescent Psychiatric Clinics of North America, 20*, 125–134.

Sheeran, T., Rabinowitz, T., Lotterman, J., Reilly, C. F., Brown, S., & Donehower, P., et al. (2011). Feasibility and impact of telemonitor-based depression care management for geriatric homecare patients. *Telemedicine and e-Health, 17*, 620–626.

Shore, J. H., Brooks, E., Savin, D. M., Manson, S. M., & Libby, A. M. (2007). An economic evaluation of telehealth data collection with rural populations. *Psychiatric Services, 58,* 830—835.

Shore, J. H., Brooks, E., Savin, D., Orton, H., Grigsby, J., & Manson, S. M. (2008). Acceptability of telepsychiatry in American Indians. *Telemedicine and e-Health, 14,* 461—466.

Shore, J. H., & Manson, S. M. (2005). A developmental model for rural telepsychiatry. *Psychiatric Services, 56,* 976—980.

Shore, J. H., Savin, D. M., Novins, D., & Manson, S. M. (2006). Cultural aspects of telepsychiatry. *Journal of Telemedicine and Telecare, 12,* 116—121.

Shore, J. H., Savin, D., Orton, H., Beals, J., & Manson, S. M. (2007). Diagnostic reliability of telepsychiatry in American Indian veterans. *American Journal of Psychiatry, 164,* 115—118.

Tanke, E. D., & Leirer, V. O. (1994). Automated telephone reminders in tuberculosis care. *Medical Care, 32,* 380—389.

Task Force on the Delivery of Services to Ethnic Minority Populations (2011). *Guidelines for providers of psychological services to ethnic, linguistic, and culturally diverse populations.* American Psychological Association. Retrieved June 12, 2011 from <http://www.apa.org/pi/oema/resources/policy/provider-guidelines.aspx>.

Tirado, M. (2011). Role of mobile health in the care of culturally and linguistically diverse US populations. *Perspectives in Health Information Management, 8,* 1e.

Viruell-Fuentes, E. A., Morenoff, J. D., Williams, D. R., & House, J. S. (2011). Language of interview, self-rated health, and the other Latino health puzzle. *American Journal of Public Health, 101,* 1306—1313.

Wakefield, B. J., Ward, M. M., Holman, J. E., Ray, A., Scherubel, M., & Burns, T. L., et al. (2008). Evaluation of home telehealth following hospitalization for heart failure: A randomized trial. *Telemedicine and e-Health, 14,* 753—761.

Walters, K. L., & Simoni, J. M. (2009). Decolonizing strategies for mentoring American Indians and Alaska Natives in HIV and mental health research. *American Journal of Public Health, 99,* S71—76.

Warren, M. (2007). The digital vicious cycle: Links between social disadvantage and digital exclusion in rural areas. *Telecommunications Policy, 31,* 374—388.

Yellowlees, P., Hilty, D., Odor, A., Losif, A., Parish, M. B., Nafiz, N., et al. (in press). Transcultural psychiatry made simple—Asynchronous telepsychiatry as a disruptive innovation. *Psychiatric Services.*

Yellowlees, P., Marks, S., Hilty, D., & Shore, J. H. (2008). Using e-health to enable culturally appropriate mental healthcare in rural areas. *Telemedicine and e-Health, 14,* 486—492.

Yeung, A., Johnson, D. P., Trinh, N. H., Weng, W. C., Kvedar, J., & Fava, M. (2009). Feasibility and effectiveness of telepsychiatry services for chinese immigrants in a nursing home. *Telemedicine and e-Health, 15,* 336—341.

6 Managing Risk and Protecting Privacy in Telemental Health: An Overview of Legal, Regulatory, and Risk-Management Issues [☆]

Greg M. Kramer[a,], Matt C. Mishkind[a], David D. Luxton[a] and Jay H. Shore[b]*

[a]National Center for Telehealth and Technology (T2), Tacoma, WA, [b]Centers for American Indian and Alaska Native Health, University of Colorado Denver, Aurora, CO

Introduction

Telemental health (TMH: the term "telehealth" is used in this chapter when referring to broader-level issues and throughout this chapter, the terms "telehealth" and "telemedicine" are used interchangeably) facilitates access to and defines psychological, psychiatric, and traumatic brain injury health care and other mental healthcare delivery between geographically distant sites. This health care access from a distance raises a number of legal and regulatory issues relevant for safe and effective practices. Some of these issues are related to concerns within the broader health-care community, while others are specific to or are uniquely modified for TMH. For example, how to manage patient's safety, protect patient's privacy, and protect oneself against licensure and malpractice claims are concerns for all healthcare providers. However, for potential or new TMH practitioners, these concerns often take on heightened focus. Fortunately, these concerns can be alleviated by following some reasonable guidelines.

In general, the best practices of adhering to standards and regulations for safe in-person care apply to TMH care, and it should never be implied that delivering

---

[☆] Disclaimer: Any opinions or assertions contained herein are the private views of the authors and are not to be construed as official or reflecting the views of the Department of the Army or the Department of Defense.

[*] Corresponding Author: Greg M. Kramer, National Center for Telehealth and Technology, 9933 West Hayes Street, Joint Base Lewis-McChord, Tacoma, WA 98431. Tel.: +1-253-968-3228, Fax: +1-253-968-4192, E-mail: gregory.kramer@us.army.mil

Telemental Health. DOI: http://dx.doi.org/10.1016/B978-0-12-416048-4.00006-3

care from a distance removes the established ethics, knowledge, or past training of a health-care provider. This means that practitioners who are comfortable following accepted standards of practice and ethics should not view TMH care as so different, exotic, or even frightening. However, as a newer mode of delivery, the ability to practice TMH has outpaced some regulatory reforms necessary to fully address the adoption and modification of current mental health standards to this mode of practice. However, there are some standards to follow and common recommendations to consider that can help ensure safe and effective care delivery.

This chapter is intended to cover some of the key risk-management issues in today's TMH environment, with specific emphasis placed on licensure, malpractice, credentialing and privileging (C&P), patient's privacy, data security, informed consent, and emergency management of patients. The focus is on clinic-based TMH, with some space at the end of the chapter devoted to future TMH applications beyond the traditional clinic setting. The aim is to point out the core legal and regulatory areas facing the TMH professional and to provide the requisite knowledge to make informed decisions on managing risk in common situations so that one feels as comfortable providing TMH care as one does providing care face-to-face. Given the evolving environment for TMH, it is important that those engaged in its practice remain aware of developing trends as well as current rules, guidelines, and regulations.

Legal and Regulatory Issues

Licensure

A unique TMH benefit is its ability to reach across geographic boundaries to facilitate care between a clinician at one location and a patient at another, sometimes very distant, location. This is especially helpful in addressing the unmet health-care needs of those living in rural, remote, and underserved populations as many individuals who need care cannot access that care without traveling great distances (Kazal & Conner, 2005). While helpful for addressing gaps in care for specific populations, TMH fundamentally allows for any patient with the appropriate equipment to connect to a health-care provider whether to fill a basic need, provide specialty care, or to facilitate continuity of care. A 1998 American Psychiatric Association report spoke of the promise of telehealth, "[O]riginally conceived to enhance access to health care for the geographically hard-to-reach and the underserved... telemedicine is much broader and will become the way we are all served—whether underserved or not—with greater efficiency, continuity, and timeliness." TMH therefore provides the opportunity to cross jurisdictional boundaries, most notably state lines, to connect providers and patients.

The current regulatory environment presents some barriers to fulfilling all of these opportunities, particularly for those who may provide or need to receive care across state lines. Traditionally, the United States has primarily given the States, rather than the federal government, control over establishing and enforcing licensure requirements for a wide range of health-care professionals, including mental health professionals (U.S. Department of Health and Human Services, Health Resources and Services Administration, 2010a). Prior to the advent of telehealth and the expansion of telecommunications technologies, questions over the jurisdiction of states to regulate health care rarely arose because diagnosis and treatment almost exclusively occurred face-to-face within one state (Ameringer, 2011). The emergence and increased use of telehealth have changed the care-delivery system, with increased commentary on the limitations of a state-based licensure system (Ameringer, 2011; Gupta & Soa, 2010; Miller et al., 2005). One reason for the perceived barrier is that obtaining multiple licenses is often a financial and administrative burden for many health-care professionals (Miller et al., 2005). While there has been activity over the years to modify the state-based licensure system to better address telehealth services, the debate on potential solutions continues. Understanding the developmental history of this system is helpful to understand the current environment.

Background and History of Telehealth Licensure Reform Attempts

The Tenth Amendment states, "The powers not delegated to the United States by the Constitution, nor prohibited by it to the States, are reserved to the States respectively, or to the people."[1] Historically, the authority for states to regulate the practice of health care comes from this Tenth Amendment "police power" granted to states (*Gibbons v. Odgen*, 1824; defining police powers of the states under the Tenth Amendment to include an "...immense mass of legislation, which embraces everything within the territory of a State, not surrendered to the general government: all which can be most advantageously exercised by the States themselves. Inspection laws, quarantine laws, health laws of every description, as well as laws for regulating the internal commerce of a State..."). Police powers have been defined as those that states should exercise in order to protect the health, safety, and welfare of citizens within their borders (U.S. Department of Health and Human Services, Health Resources and Services Administration, 2010b). Following this definition, most state statutes delegate authority for regulating and enforcing licensure to state medical, psychology, social work, or other health-care boards.

Although the power of states to regulate health care has been strongly supported over the years, the power of states to regulate health care is not absolute (Gupta & Soa, 2010; U.S. Department of Health and Human Services, Health Resources and Services Administration, 2010a). For example, the Commerce Clause of the United States is interpreted to place limits on states in creating interstate trade barriers (U.S. Department of Health and Human Services, Health Resources and Services Administration, 2010c) and the Supremacy Clause of the Constitution preempts state laws that are contrary to the laws of the federal government.[2] Consistent with this interpretation, certain federal government agencies (e.g., Department of

[1] U.S. Constitution, Amendment X.
[2] U.S. Constitution Art. VI, cl.2.

Defense, Veteran Affairs, and Indian Health Services) have preemption approaches based on statute and/or case law that allow some categories of health-care practitioners licensed in one state to practice within their federal duties in any state. This approach effectively allows the licensure policy or regulation of the federal agency to preempt individual state licensure requirements. However, in general, explicit statutory language must exist to demonstrate Congressional intent to preempt state law, and there is a strong presumption against federal preemption of state law absent that specific language (U.S. Department of Health and Human Services, Health Resources and Services Administration, 2010a). Also, though the practice of health care across state lines may constitute interstate commerce, the potential legal argument that might arise between the power of the states to regulate health care within their state and restraints in interstate commerce in not allowing a health professional to practice across state lines remains an open question subject to legal debate beyond that which this chapter can offer (Federation of State Medical Boards of the United States, 1996).

Given the apparent legal ambiguity and the call for licensing reform in telehealth, various national health regulation authorities have proposed alternative strategies to address the issue. The Federation of State Medical Boards (FSMB) was one of the earliest organizations to address the issue of telehealth and licensure in the United States. Recognizing that the use of telehealth technology would make it increasingly possible to deliver health care across broad geographical areas, the FSMB issued a Model Act in 1996 as a proposal to regulate the practice of medicine across state lines (Federation of State Medical Boards of the United States, 1996). That report proposed a special telemedicine (note this is not specific to TMH) license allowing practitioners to provide telemedicine across state lines with certain limitations. As proposed in the Model Act, the special license would extend to those who "regularly and frequently" practice telemedicine but would not cover a physician who physically enters another state to provide care. The report also stated that the practice of medicine occurs in the state where the patient is located and that physicians would remain under the jurisdiction of the medical board in the state where the patient resides. States did not rush to adopt the Model Act and more recent FSMB efforts, supported by licensure portability grants from the Office of the Advancement for Telehealth, have focused on developing a uniform application and a common credential verification service (Federation of State Medical Boards; U.S. Department of Health and Human Services, Health Resources and Services Administration, 2010a).

The Association of State and Provincial Psychology Boards (ASPPB) also has undertaken efforts to facilitate professional mobility of psychologists through licensure recognition programs. One of those programs is an Interjurisdictional Practice Certificate, the intent of which is to allow licensed psychologists to practice temporarily and provide short-term psychological services in another state in lieu of obtaining full licensure. Theoretically, this could cover a situation where a patient moves temporarily to another state, e.g., a college semester or a short-term work assignment. Only a few states currently accept this certificate for temporary practice, but it does provide a potential solution for promoting cross-state telemental heath practice. The ASPPB also developed a model act for psychologist licensure; the most recent version approved in 2010 included new language to address the "delivery of psychological services by electronic or other means (i.e., telepsychology)" (The National Council of State Boards of Nursing, 2000).

Another approach to address interstate licensure is the Nurse Licensure Compact (NLC) that was developed by The National Council of State Boards of Nursing (NCSBN) in 2000. The NLC is a mutual licensing recognition agreement among member states that allows a licensed nurse to practice in another state, if that state has agreed to the compact. Essentially, if a state agrees to the compact, then it agrees to recognize the nursing license granted by all other states that have signed the compact. This model had some initial momentum though it appears to have slowed as only a few states have agreed to the compact in the last several years.

More progressive licensure reform has occurred outside the United States. In 2005, the European Union enacted a system of mutual recognition of professional qualifications that allows appropriately trained and qualified medical providers to practice their profession in all European Union member states (European Commission). The agreement was meant to ensure the free circulation of services and goods within a single European market (American Telemedicine Association, 2011), though exactly how this system works is beyond the scope of this chapter. In addition, Australia recently moved to a national occupational licensing system to begin with certain professions (Information on Australia National License). Along with that system, Australia created national boards for 10 health professions to implement national registration and accreditation (Australia Health Practitioner Regulation Agency). How this national system is eventually implemented is worth watching.

However and as previously noted, there remains much controversy and conflicting opinions within the United States as to the best approach for licensing health-care providers. This is further complicated by the lack of consistency across licensing boards such that a proposed solution for physicians may not be similar to those for psychologists, social workers, or nurses. For example, the American Medical Association has opposed a national telemedicine license and supports the current state-based system that requires a full and unrestricted license in any state a physician practices, including the practice of telemedicine (American Medical Association). The FSMB has indicated support for preserving the state-based licensure system, while also providing some support for license portability or license endorsement for telemedicine (as described above), resulting in a rather complicated position (Telemedicine and License Portability). The American Bar Association (ABA), 2008, Health Law Section issued a report in 2008 that argued against multiple state licensure for telemedicine and recommended a system of mutual license recognition. Under that model, they recommended one application that would permit a physician to practice telemedicine in all other states subject to compliance with those states' licensure fees, discipline and regulations. Recently, the Federal Communications Commission (FCC) 2010 National Broadband Plan included recommendations to reduce regulatory barriers (Federal Communication Commission). One such recommendation was for states to revise their licensing requirements to enable e-care to include some form of an interstate licensing agreement. The FCC concluded, "If states fail to develop reasonable e-care licensing policies by the next 18 months (by September, 2011), Congress should consider intervening to ensure Medicare and Medicaid beneficiaries are not denied the benefits of e-care" (Federal Communication Commission). And lastly, one of the most prominent telehealth organizations, the American Telemedicine Association (ATA), has long urged the policy makers to change the current state-based licensure system. Over the years, the ATA has outlined various alternatives to the current system, without specifically recommending one. Most recently, the ATA launched a web site called www.fixlicensure.org that is dedicated to reform the state-based medical licensing system in favor of a national license portability system (American Telemedicine Association).

The licensure issue, especially within the United States, has recently become more pressing and complicated, with the activities of numerous states to legislate the provision of telehealth within their boundaries. At least 20 states currently have some form of legislation on the practice of telehealth and additional states have introduced or are considering telehealth legislation. Similar to concerns at the national level, there is lack of consensus among states as to the best approach. Many of these state telehealth laws address licensure requirements and define whether and to what extent someone may practice telehealth within their state on a temporary or limited basis. Some require obtaining a full license to provide services within that state, while others offer some form of a consultation exception that allows an out-of-state licensed provider to consult on patients in a different state who are under the care of a provider in that state (Gupta & Soa, 2010). Adding to the confusion is that some state laws cover a broad range of telehealth providers, while some cover a single type of provider (e.g., psychologist specific); some discuss very specific requirements (e.g., for informed consent); some amend how they define the practice of medicine; and some define what types of communications are covered. These laws are so wide ranging in terms of how they define telehealth services and address specific requirements to practice telehealth in the state as to lack a consistent theme. Fortunately for the active telehealth provider, reviews of these state laws do exist (American Psychological Association, 2010; Gobis).

Real Case Scenario and Licensure Risk Management

As discussed above, the attempts at reform and the positions of national organizations on the issue of cross-state licensure remain varied. For the TMH professional, cross-state licensure remains a challenge without a widely accepted solution, and while it is helpful to know about the licensure debate, it is more pressing for telemental health providers to understand how to safely provide care under the current system. It is believed that the vast majority of telehealth encounters, even across state lines, are conducted safely and within the scope of existing regulations. This does not mean, however, that case examples of unsafe practices do not exist. *Christian Ellis Hageseth v. The Superior Court* of San Mateo illustrates one such case. In this case, the defendant, Christian Hageseth, M.D., a psychiatrist licensed to practice medicine in Colorado (though interestingly but not of legal consequence in this case, his license in Colorado was restricted so that he could not prescribe at the time), wrote a Prozac (fluoxetine) prescription for a California resident that he had never examined but had only administered on an online questionnaire. The California resident committed suicide soon after obtaining the Prozac (fluoxetine) and Dr. Hageseth was charged with and convicted of the crime of practicing medicine in California without a license. He was sentenced to 9 months in county jail for practicing medicine without a license. While many facets of this case focus on online prescribing (covered elsewhere in this book) and jurisdiction (covered later in this chapter), this case indicates that states take licensure seriously, and it underscores the importance of understanding how various laws and regulations might apply to all forms of TMH care.

To help illustrate these complexities, two common professional scenarios are presented below, followed by key issues to consider.

Vignette A: Dr. Specialist

A well-known, and highly specialized, psychiatrist (Dr. Specialist), located and licensed in Chicago, IL, often gets inquiries about her availability to serve patients in Indiana and Iowa. This psychiatrist is both affiliated and employed with a hospital clinic and has a private practice out of a rented office space. Both the hospital and her private office have video-teleconferencing capabilities and she is considering offering telepsychiatry services as a means of increasing her efficiency and reaching out to those eager to access her services without a long and costly commute. What issues does Dr. Specialist need to consider before deciding what services, if any, she can offer to patients in Indiana and Iowa, and under what circumstances?

Vignette B: Dr. Rural

A psychologist (Dr. Rural) licensed in northern California wishes to extend his practice to include rural and underserved areas similar to the small town where he grew up. He is aware of opportunities to reach out to individuals in rural areas of Oregon that have a limited number of providers and who often have to travel great distances to find these providers. His idea is to market his services out of state by offering video-teleconferencing and interactive Internet-based services so that patients can reach him at their convenience from the comfort of their own home. What issues does he need to consider before making this business decision?

1. *Consider cost and burden to obtain appropriate licensure.* The first concern for both is whether they can legally practice in another state. If only licensed in one state (Illinois and California, respectively), both need to consider whether it is worth the expense and burden to do what is necessary to become fully licensed in the neighboring states where they wish to extend their practice. The cost of obtaining and maintaining additional licenses can vary based on profession, years of experience, and individual state

requirements. Since obtaining a full license in any state in which one wishes to practice is one of the safest risk-management strategies, it is worth investigating what is required to do that before automatically deciding against it. If either has determined that the cost and burden (e.g., having to keep up with continuing education requirements specific to neighboring states) are too prohibitive, other options may exist for certain situations.

2. *Examine relevant state laws, including telehealth and professional practice statutes.* If obtaining additional licenses is too prohibitive, a recommended next step for TMH providers is to investigate the laws that may exist in any state that they wish to practice and consider whether they can make an independent determination of what provisions, if any, apply to their practice. For example, in the case of Dr. Specialist, according to an American Psychological Association Telehealth 50-State Review, Indiana, does have statutory language that includes services provided through electronic communications as medical practice that requires a license, while Iowa does not yet have a telehealth statute (American Psychological Association, 2010). While specific language in a state statute may seem definitive on the licensure issue, it is important to highlight that the absence of a state telehealth statute or statutory provision does not usually signal a free pass. The absence of a specific state law or regulation on the issue does not shield one from liability or unethical practice; there are other sources of information that may bear on what is considered malpractice or unethical behavior beyond a specific telehealth or TMH statute or regulation.

An additional resource to examine is state health practice statutes. Some state statutes allow mental health professionals to practice within their state for a maximum number of days per year under certain conditions. They may provide some assurance for one who wishes to simply contact patients on a limited basis, when either the patient or provider is out-of-state due to work, education, or vacation. But in terms of licensure, the risk-management analysis will likely go further.

3. *Determine applicability of laws based on profession, type of service, and frequency of service.* According to the American Psychological Association Good Practice article, only three of the 22 states that have telehealth laws apply specifically to psychologists (although interpretation may generalize); "laws in the additional 19 states with telehealth laws do not appear to apply to psychologists at this time (American Psychological Association Practice Organization, 2010)." Considering our two vignettes, this could have different impact for our psychiatrist Dr. Specialist than for our psychologist Dr. Rural, though it is important to note that the full extent of that impact is not clear. Some statutes also speak to the technologies/type of services covered, while others do not define it with any specificity, and many statutes have licensure exceptions for consultative services including guest or temporary license availability for out-of-state practitioners. Considering these variations, Dr. Specialist might decide to limit her out-of-state activity to consulting with out-of-state clinicians on their treatment of certain patients as this type of service might not require additional licensure and might meet Dr. Specialist's need. Dr. Rural, on the other hand, may wish to do more than simply consult and there may be relevant provisions that could meet his needs. For example, in the case of Dr. Rural, the American Psychological Association Telehealth 50-State Review indicates that Oregon allows a licensed out-of-state psychologist to practice for a period of no more than 180 days in any 24-month period with certain conditions (American Psychological Association, 2010). This could meet the immediate needs of Dr. Rural who may want to try seeing patients in Oregon via videoconferencing on a part-time and limited basis to further assess if it is worth considering in the future full licensure in Oregon.

4. *Consult local counsel and/or opinion of local licensing board.* A local attorney who is familiar with the relevant issues can assist in helping to fully research the issues and offer

legal opinions based on their research and knowledge. An alternative or additional risk-management step is contacting the applicable state professional boards. State professional boards are a potential resource for clarifying what regulations may or may not apply to you when providing care in a particular state and some have issued written opinions addressing what services require a license (American Psychological Association Practice Organization, 2010). It is a good idea to check with a respective state professional board within any state that you wish to practice *before* providing services in that state to confirm whether the board has any written policies on what constitutes legal and ethical TMH practice within that state (American Psychological Association Practice Organization, 2010). Also, TMH "services" across state lines are potentially considered furnished in *both* the state where the provider is located and in the state where the patient is located, so knowledge of more than just the state law of where the patient is located is essential, as the patient can attempt to bring a licensing complaint in either or both states.

Malpractice

While licensure is one major concern of TMH practitioners, malpractice liability is an equal or even greater concern especially when practicing across state lines. To date, most cases of "telemalpractice" have occurred when a physician has issued a prescription over the telephone or Internet without first examining the individual (Natoli, 2009). However, as the range of technologies used to deliver care increases (e.g., video-teleconferencing (VTC), Internet, mobile phone), it is anticipated that the courts will further address malpractice issues that may arise over the emerging technological forms of TMH care delivery. This section will describe the main malpractice issues to consider and provide some recommendations for how to manage malpractice liability risk in TMH.

Similarly to licensing, states have the authority to regulate health insurance within their borders and vary in their insurance requirements and regulations (Gupta & Soa, 2010). One common thread is that many states require a health-care professional to have some form of malpractice insurance if providing care in their state (Kazal & Conner, 2005). For federal government employees, that requirement is usually met through the coverage under the Federal Tort Claims Act which protects government employees from personal liability by substituting the United States government as a defendant in any case brought against them for care provided in their federal employment.[3] In addition, many malpractice insurance companies have long established policies that were designed to cover traditional "face-to-face" encounters within the state where the professional practices and is licensed. Many of these policies, however, have neither considered the issue of telepractice nor have they considered the issue of providing care in another state. Since liability can arise in any situation, there are some overarching key issues to consider from a malpractice liability and a risk-management perspective.

The initial legal issues that can arise in the TMH context are jurisdiction and choice of law. Jurisdiction relates to a state's ability to exercise authority over persons within its territory, including the power to require persons to appear in court

---

[3] 28 U.S.C. (United States Code), 1346(b).

to allow adjudication of legal claims (Gupta & Soa, 2010). Once jurisdiction is established, the next issue is which law to apply to the case in question—the law of the state where the case is being heard or the law of the state where the alleged injury occurred. In the typical medical malpractice case, these issues are rather straightforward as the alleged "injury" occurs in the state where the treatment occurred; in other words, the state where both the patient and the provider are located. The cross-state TMH practice scenario raises complex jurisdictional and choice of law issues as it poses questions both for where the treatment occurred and where the alleged injury occurred (Chee, 2010). While fully describing the legal analysis that could occur to resolve this issue is beyond the scope of this chapter, there is some general guidance to highlight.

One issue that courts will likely consider in determining jurisdiction is whether the provider has established "minimum contacts" in the state. Under that doctrine, a court may apply jurisdiction over a defendant who has no physical presence in a state as long as the defendant has engaged in purposeful actions in the state (Gupta & Soa, 2010). Legal analysis requires consideration of several factors, but one scholar argues that it is reasonable to assume that a TMH provider who "remotely treats and diagnoses patients" in another state is establishing minimum contacts in that state for purposes of jurisdiction of that state to adjudicate claims against that provider (Chee, 2010). However, according to that scholar, provider-to-provider *consultations* on an out-of-state patient may not subject the provider to foreign jurisdiction (Chee, 2010). Another point of view suggests that it is debatable whether all the requirements of "minimum contacts" will allow jurisdiction in every cross-state telehealth malprac-tice claim, and that it is unclear whether adjudicating interstate telehealth claims in one state is the most reasonable policy course (U.S. Department of Health and Human Services, Health Resources and Services Administration, 2010a).

The *Hageseth v. The Superior Court* of San Mateo case presented earlier focused on the issue of jurisdiction, but within the context of a criminal complaint, noting that "minimum contacts," though well settled in civil matters, is not the appropriate means of determining jurisdiction in a criminal case (a malpractice claim is usually a civil complaint). However, it is noteworthy that the court, in determining that California had jurisdiction for criminal adjudication based on the "detrimental effect theory," held,"[a]ccordingly, in the circumstances of this case, jurisdiction is not precluded by petitioner's physical absence from the state and the fact he did not act through an agent located in California". This case suggests that at least with criminal matters, it might prove difficult to assert lack of jurisdiction simply because a defendant has not entered the state where he or she has committed some TMH action toward a state resi-dent. Accordingly there does appear to be some general precedent for courts to give primary consideration to the law of the state where the injury occurred (Chee, 2010).

Additional issues to consider for liability risk-management center around an understanding of the legal definition of what constitutes malpractice. The generally accepted elements of negligence are what courts consider in malpractice actions. Those elements are (a) duty owed, (b) breach of that duty, (c) injury as a result of breach of duty, and (d) proximate cause between the breach and the injury. Generally, it is safe to assume that TMH providers have the same duty of care to patients as when providing face-to-face care (Natoli, 2009), though as described later, some states have additional regulation on informed consent.

However, again, especially for cross-state practice, the use of technology does create additional considerations. For one, when is a professional relationship for which a duty of care is owed established in TMH? Does a provider-to-provider consultation establish a relationship with a patient in another state? What about an initial phone consultation, email, or even live Internet connection to establish professional contact or arrange an initial visit? Analysis of case law by the authors of one book suggests that provider-to-provider consultations about a patient would not establish a patient relationship for purposes of malpractice liability (Fleisher & Dechene, 2004). And while there is still little legal guidance on how to know if one is establishing a professional relationship, it seems reasonable to assume that a professional relationship can be established through any medium. In the absence of clear guidance, a TMH provider should consider that any mental health service that a patient may reasonably rely upon as professional advice could establish a professional relationship (Chee, 2010).

Another unanswered question in TMH is when is a duty of care breached? As discussed above, jurisdiction and choice of law are complex legal issues that remain largely unresolved in cross-state TMH care. So what is the appropriate standard of care that is allegedly being breached in a malpractice claim? Unfortunately, there is no clear consensus answer to the question as the appropriate standard of care varies from state to state, with some states following a local "community" standard while other states look to a national standard (Chee, 2010). Of note, the American Medical Association (1999) has stated that certain online interactions, medical questionnaires, and Internet prescribing without examining the patient fall "well below a minimum standard of medical care." What about alleged injury that results from technical malfunction or from insufficient training? Given there are some questions without currently clear responses, we offer some general malpractice liability risk-management recommendations for TMH providers.

1. *Ensure up-to-date knowledge of current malpractice coverage.* Read the coverage to determine if there is any mention of coverage for telecare or any mention of coverage for care provided in another state. If there are any questions, concerns, or omissions, contact your malpractice insurance carrier. Since many malpractice insurance policies are silent on some or all of these issues, attempt to get clarification in writing, from your carrier. Understand that many of these issues are unresolved and unaddressed by traditional insurance carriers and that they may not have or easily divulge sufficient answers. For example, Hyler and Gangure (2004) conducted an informal survey of professional liability insurance companies by phone to ask questions about their telepsychiatry policies. The general answer they received was that such requests are handled on a case-by-case basis and that there was no standard approach. Returning to our vignettes above, both Drs would be wise to contact their respective malpractice insurance carrier before initiating new TMH service, describe exactly the new TMH service(s) they wish to provide, and ask if their carrier will cover it. Remain assertive in attempting to get answers, try to get them in writing, document any verbal conversations, but recognize that you may have to consider other avenues to get the answers you want.

2. *Familiarize yourself with all applicable law and consider obtaining the advice of local legal counsel.* Do not make any assumptions about which state laws will apply and familiarize oneself with the laws of both where the provider and the patient are located. This should include any specific telehealth laws and general health-care malpractice liability laws for each state of practice. It bears repeating that advice from a local attorney can help ease concerns about TMH malpractice issues in each state, and as technologies evolve and TMH practice becomes more common, local counsel is often the best source for information about legal clarifications and development. In particular, Dr. Rural from the vignette could benefit from consulting the counsel to obtain a more complete legal analysis of where and when care might be established depending on the type of services he wishes to provide (e.g., videoconferencing vs live Internet). Even if he finds no specific law on telepsychology in the states, he wishes to extend his practice, what existing telemedicine laws say about general medicine or psychiatry could have bearing in establishing the standard of care for a psychologist.

3. *Become involved in or establish a local community of TMH providers for ongoing consultation.* Often one person in the community will have already encountered similar issues. Community groups are great sources of information sharing and also a good source of support for thinking about difficult issues. Industry organizations, such as the ATA and local practice organizations, can offer a wide range of relevant information from online sources, conferences, and committees.

4. *Consult existing national and state TMH guidelines.* The Telemental Health Special Interest Group of the American Telemedicine Association has published two resources for TMH practice: *Practice Guidelines for Videoconferencing-Based Telemental Health and Evidence-Based Practice for Telemental Health* (American Telemedicine Association, 2009; Grady et al., 2011). In addition, the American Academy of Child and Adolescent Psychiatry published *Practice Parameter for Telepsychiatry with Children and Adolescents* (Myers & Cain, 2008). Other professional mental health organizations such as the American Psychiatric Association, the American Psychological Association, and the National Association of Social Workers have also produced some information on TMH (American Psychological Association Ethics Committee; National Association of Social Workers; Resource Document). It is helpful to consult their web sites on an ongoing basis for further TMH specific information. Also, check with appropriate state professional organizations for information and resources, e.g., Ohio Psychological Associations recently created telepsychology guidelines.

5. *Obtain appropriate training and education.* Ensuring appropriate training and education is always a good risk-management strategy. This can include training on any equipment and technologies you plan to use as well as educational offerings on best TMH practices. Having established back-up and emergency plans for technical malfunctions and patient emergencies is vital and covered later in this chapter.

Credentialing and Privileging

C&P is another regulatory issue that specifically impacts TMH especially within hospital settings. Hospitals owe a certain duty of care to their patients and one way this is exercised is by ensuring that providers in a specific hospital meet certain education and training requirements (Fleisher & Dechene, 2004). The process of ensuring the qualifications of hospital care providers is called C&P. Credentialing generally refers to the procedure for evaluating and verifying the qualifications of health-care providers who wish to provide care in a facility (e.g., diploma and transcripts to prove completion of necessary education and license). Privileging generally refers to the process of evaluating those qualifications in order to determine the level of competency each provider has to provide certain services and to care for certain types of patients. That way, providers are only "privileged" to provide services for medical specialties (e.g., surgery and radiology) in which they possess the necessary credentials and competency. This process requires producing documentation and involves having a hospital body review the documents in order to make appropriate decisions. Typically, this occurs at each hospital in which privileges are sought and hospitals tend to have their own local administrative process for verifying credentialing and granting privileges. As such, there is great variability in the pace and efficiency in which clinicians are ultimately granted privileges to practice.

The key issue for TMH is whether a provider needs to be credentialed and privileged at the hospital where they are located, where the patient is located, or both. This can create a significant administrative and financial burden for both providers and hospitals. Accrediting organizations such as The Joint Commission have specific requirements for C&P health-care providers. The Centers for Medicare and Medicaid Services (CMS) also has standards for certifying hospitals, and until recently did not have any special regulation for C&P telehealth providers. Instead, CMS requirements were for telehealth providers to follow existing regulations that required local privileging at each patient site hospital. This was identified as a significant burden for providers and a barrier to the expansion of telehealth services within the United States. After much public comment on the issue, CMS released a new regulation on telemedicine C&P in 2011 (42 CFR).

The new rule streamlines the telehealth C&P process by essentially allowing the hospital receiving the telehealth services (the patient or "originating site") to "privilege by proxy" and rely upon the C&P decision of the distant site facility if certain conditions are met including (a) there is a written agreement in place to do this between the sites; (b) the distant site (provider) hospital is a Medicare-participating hospital; (c) the distant site provider is privileged at the distant site hospital, with the distant site hospital having a list of privileges; (d) the distant site provider holds a license issued or recognized by the State that is receiving the telemedicine services; and (e) the originating site hospital must have evidence of internal review of the distant site provider's performance, including any adverse events and complaints. The new rules are specific to telemedicine but include a broad definition of telemedicine that includes "overall delivery of health care" (42 CFR). In addition, the new rules extend "privileging by proxy" to other telemedicine non-hospital entities providing services to hospitals (e.g., teleradiology, teleICU, and teleneurology). The new regulation was seen as an improvement by organizations such as the American Telemedicine Association, who wrote that the "rule will reduce the burden and duplicative nature of the traditional privileging process for Medicare-participating hospitals and CAHs that are engaged in telemedicine agreements, while still assuring accountability to the process." Awareness of this new rule is important for the TMH practitioner who works in a hospital setting or wishes to provide TMH services to a hospital, as this may make the process easier.

Consider again the case of Dr. Specialist. If Dr. Specialist is interested in providing care as part of her practice to patients located in other hospitals, Dr. Specialist will likely have to gain privileges at those other hospitals. If Dr. Specialist is going to provide that care as part of her hospital practice (where she is presumably already privileged), the new CMS regulations might make it easier for her to gain privileges at new hospitals implementing the CMS regulations. However, if Dr. Specialist is seeking to provide care from her private office to patients located in other hospitals, the new CMS regulation may not help her streamline the process. Consideration of C&P issues could impact her decision on where to and from she can provide additional TMH services.

Security and Privacy Considerations

Patient's rights to privacy, confidentiality, and security are prominent concerns of TMH practitioners, as with any type of health-care delivery. While most practitioners have an understanding of these terms, Hyler and Gangure (2004) have provided the following specific definitions within the context of telepsychiatry: *Privacy* is an individual's claim to control the use and disclosure of personal information; *Security* involves the safeguards in an information system that protect it and its contents against unauthorized disclosure and limit access to authorized users in accordance with established policy; *Confidentiality* is the status accorded to information that indicates it is sensitive for certain reasons and must therefore be protected and access to it controlled.

The most well-known federal standard covering privacy and security in the United States is the United States Health Insurance Portability & Accountability Act HIPAA of 1996 (Public Law 104-191), which was intended to improve efficiency in health-care delivery by standardizing electronic data interchange and to protect confidentiality and security of health data through setting and enforcing standards (Centers for Medicare and Medicaid, U.S. Department of Health and Human Services). HIPAA contains both a privacy rule, which "... provides federal protections for personal health information held by covered entities and gives patients an array of rights with respect to that information," and a security rule, which "specifies a series of administrative, physical, and technical safeguards for covered entities to use to assure the confidentiality, integrity, and availability of electronic protected health information" (U.S. Department of Health and Human Services). HIPAA applies to "covered entities" that include health-care providers, health plans (e.g., insurance companies, HMOs, government health care programs), and health-care clearing houses that electronically process health information (U.S. Department of Health and Human Services).

It is important to note that compliance with HIPAA alone may not fully suffice to ensure maximum privacy and security, as there are also state laws on the topic. While HIPAA will likely preempt state laws that have less stringent privacy and security requirements, state laws that have more stringent privacy and security requirements might preempt HIPAA (Hyler & Gangure, 2004; Genomics Law

Report). It should be remembered that HIPAA compliance is a set of processes rather than a defined set of rules and as such requirements for new services are not always absolute.

Data Security for Electronic Protected Health Information

By its very nature of transmitting communication through the use of technology, the confidentiality of TMH patient information poses the inherent risk of being intercepted by third parties (Clark, Capuzzi, & Harrison, 2010; Luxton, Kayl, & Mishkind, in press). TMH professionals should take steps to ensure that all transmission of electronic patient information meets applicable security standards. The ATA has provided guidance on requirements to comply with HIPAA and overall good practice during TMH care delivery (American Telemedicine Association, 2009). The guidelines specify that synchronous audio/video sessions shall be secured to the greatest practical extent and that protected health information (PHI) shall be secured through use of a private, point-to-point circuit, Integrated Services Digital Network, or Advanced Encryption Standard (AES) encryption or Virtual Private Network (VPN) for Internet transmissions (American Telemedicine Association, 2009). In addition to specific compliance with State and foreign privacy requirements for TMH services provided in other countries, the guidelines specify the need for network and software security protocols, accessibility and authentication protocols, and for measures to safeguard data against intentional and unintentional corruption during both transmission and storage of data.

Current HIPAA standards require a minimum of 128-bit encryption of electronic PIH (this may change with advances in technology). HIPAA-covered entities have several options to meet the data encryption requirements and those options generally depend on what technology or infrastructure is to be used. The AES (National Institute of Standards and Technology) was developed for use by both the federal government and by private organizations. AES uses cryptographic keys of 128, 192, and 256 bits to encrypt and decrypt data in blocks of 128 bits. Popular video-conferencing software companies may describe encryption at 256-bit AES. However, encryption alone does not fully determine HIPAA compliance. TMH care delivered over the Internet can be secured by Transport Layer Security and its predecessor, Secure Sockets Layer by using asymmetric cryptography with 128 bit or 256 bit encryption protocols. VPNs are also an option for transmitting voice, video, or data over the Internet. VPN provides a secure connection to a private local area network at a remote location by using the Internet or any public network to transmit encrypted network data packets. Mobile VPNs can be used in situations where the endpoint of the VPN moves across different networks such as cellular networks or between multiple Wi-Fi access points.

Special Considerations for Mobile Devices in TMH Care

The emergence of mobile devices such as smartphones and tablet PCs has brought new possibilities for TMH care delivery (Luxton, McCann, Bush, Mishkind, &

Reger, 2011; Luxton, Mishkind, Crumpton, Ayers, & Mysliwiec, in press). As discussed by Luxton, Kayl, and Mishkind (in press), there are a number of particular issues that threaten the privacy and the security of patients' data with the use of these devices, notably wireless capabilities of these devices. Use of wireless technology, such as Wi-Fi and cellular networks, can make it easier for third parties to monitor and record unencrypted data than it is with hard-wired networks. Although there are current security standards such as Wi-Fi Protected Access (WPA and WPA2), there is no guarantee that these security features have been enabled by the end user or whether they are in place in public environments. Ultimately, electronic data must be encrypted before transmission in order to prevent threats to privacy in most wireless environments. Thus, smart phone applications should have HIPAA compliant encryption features built-in (Luxton, Kayl, & Mishkind, in press). It should be noted that HIPAA does not apply to end users who store or share data between other end users on a personal mobile device. If the user transmits or shares PHI with a health-care professional who is a HIPAA-covered entity, however, the professional must assure HIPAA compliance (Luxton, McCann et al., 2011).

The increased use of mobile devices is also contributing to increased regulatory attention. In particular, the Food and Drug Administration (FDA) recently issued a draft guidance document advising about regulating certain applications that meet the definition of a "medical device" as contained in section 201(h) of the Federal Food, Drug, and Cosmetic Act and either (a) is used as an accessory to an already regulated medical device or (b) transforms a mobile communication device into a regulated medical device (Food and Drug Administration, 2011). The draft guidelines also state, "When the intended use of a mobile app is for the diagnosis of disease or other conditions, or the cure, mitigation, treatment, or prevention of disease, or is intended to affect the structure of any function of the body of man, the mobile app is a device." Mobile applications that act only as electronic medical textbooks or reference materials or are used solely to log, track, and make recommendations on developing or maintaining records are not likely to be considered medical devices according to the draft guidance. While the FDA has issued examples of the types of devices that might fall under their regulation, it is unknown at the time of this writing how the final regulation will read.

Other Privacy Considerations

The location of the room for the encounter at both the originating site and patient's location should ensure comfort, privacy, and confidentiality. For example, one might consider a "... quiet room, located away from busy hallways and receptions areas with lots of noisy office equipment and congregating patients" (Kramer, Ayers, Mishkind, & Norem, 2011). In addition to room location, there are other considerations for protecting patient's privacy that professionals should consider prior to initiating care and before each TMH session. For example, a TMH professional might identify to the patient all people who are in the room on the provider end, and if the provider is alone, scan the camera around the room to show the patient that no one else is there. The provider might also explain to the patient the extent of audio privacy present in the environment. Ideally, the audio should be loud enough at each end so that both the patient and provider can be easily heard, but not so loud that the TMH session can be overheard by people outside passing by the room or in adjacent rooms. Visual privacy is also important and the TMH professional should consider the windows within the patient's room. The use of blinds can help to protect privacy as well as control for sunlight which could cause glare.

Lastly, to ensure health information remains confidential, a TMH professional might consider using space that is secure enough to prevent tampering or unauthorized use of equipment. On the patient's end, this may prove more difficult, depending on where the patient is located at the time of the encounter (particularly if the patient is at home). And while it may prove difficult for the provider to secure equipment on the patient's end, the provider can take steps to maximize privacy on the patient's end. For example, at the initial encounter, the provider can discuss with the patient the importance of privacy and inquire about the environment where the patient is during the encounter. The provider can ask patients prior to initiation encounter if they are alone, or expect to be interrupted, or if privacy is a concern (Luxton, O'Brien, McCann, & Mishkind, in press). For encounters in which the patient is at home, a provider can suggest to the patient that they choose a room that they expect to be free of interruption and is private (i.e., can close the door and has adequate sound proofing).

In sum, it is important for the TMH professional to use approved telehealth technologies, and to be knowledgeable of the privacy requirements for their use, as well as be cognizant of potential liability issues (e.g., HIPAA noncompliance and possible negligence for failure to operate the technology appropriately to avoid patient harm). Any TMH professional should possess a basic technical knowledge, obtain appropriate training if necessary, and know where to seek the help of technical experts to assure patient privacy and data security. Also, TMH professionals should feel comfortable that any electronic means chosen to communicate or exchange information with patients is sufficient enough to allow them to make accurate clinical decisions.

Clinical Practices to Manage Risk

Informed Consent

Informed consent is generally considered a necessary and ethical standard of care when initiating mental health treatment. Numerous professional mental health organizations have statements, guidelines, and ethical codes that describe the requirements for informed consent. As TMH is mental health, there is no reason to believe that requirements for informed consent are any less than they are for traditional face-to-face mental health encounters. Thus, in the absence of any explicit guidance, it is safe to assume that written, informed consent prior to an initial TMH encounter is a standard of care, even in cases where written informed consent for face-to-face mental health exists. In fact, several states have specific statutory requirements for what constitutes valid informed consent in telehealth (e.g., Arizona, California, Georgia, Kentucky, Oklahoma, Texas, Vermont, and Wisconsin per an American Psychological Association article) (American Psychological Association Practice Organization, 2010). Large federal government organizations such as Veteran Affairs and the military have created sample informed consent forms for telehealth, and many additional ones exist on the Internet (American Telemedicine Association). It is recommended to first investigate any specific statutory requirements for informed consent, but in the absence of specific guidance, some elements that a TMH consent form might contain include the following as per a TMH Guidebook (Kramer et al., 2011).

- The nature of TMH using VTC and what it entails;
- The risks and benefits of TMH using VTC and that there is an empirical literature base on its application, effectiveness, and potential risks;
- That there are two sites participating in their care, along with the roles and responsibilities of each site with respect to their care;
- The security measures taken to ensure compliance with HIPAA and protect patient's privacy when documentation and information are shared between the two sites;
- That they are not being recorded, and separate written approval and consent are needed in order to videotape a session;
- That there are policies and procedures in place in case of technical breakdown or clinical emergency; and
- Informing the patient that they have an option to refuse TMH care and if so, they retain the option of receiving face-to-face care.

Safety Plans and Emergency Management

Safety planning in order to resolve emergencies is a necessary component of TMH care delivery and our experience reviewing standard operating procedures (SOPs) from government agencies suggests that emergency protocols are always an area of special attention. The ATA Practice Guidelines for Videoconferencing-Based Telemental Health states that TMH care providers shall establish SOPs or protocols for emergency issues and provides specific recommendations for managing psychiatric emergencies to include administrative issues, legal issues, and general clinical issues. In this section, we describe and elaborate on these general guidelines (American Telemedicine Association, 2009).

Administrative Issues

As a first step, it is necessary to assess the resources available at the patient's site, including obtaining information on local regulations and emergency resources and identifying potential local collaborators to help with emergency management. This information should then help the development of emergency protocols for all TMH services with clear explanation of roles, responsibilities, and procedures in emergency situations. We add that it is vital that emergency protocols clearly delineate how two geographically distant sites will collaborate in technical, clinical, and medical emergencies. SOPs often take into account local, patient's site emergency plans, as emergencies are generally handled consistent with already existing emergency protocols at the patient's site. But emergency plans should also clearly assign responsibility for contacting emergency and other necessary personnel in the event of an emergency. Furthermore, both sites should have immediate access to emergency contact numbers that can respond to the originating (patient) site in the event of an emergency (e.g., local law enforcement, facility security, and emergency medical response teams) (Kramer et al., 2011). Collection of patient information needed by law enforcement, including the details of the situation, the patient's diagnosis and how it could influence interaction with law enforcement officers, and contact information for local mental health support and follow-up care, is also recommended (Gros, Veronee, Strachan, Ruggerio, & Acierno, 2011; Luxton, O'Brien et al., in press).

The ATA Practice Guidelines for Videoconferencing-Based Telemental Health specifically states that clinicians shall be aware of the potential impact of disclosures made during emergency management on patient confidentiality and relationships in small communities (American Telemedicine Association, 2009). The guidelines also state that clinicians shall consider involving family members in emergency treatment situations when possible and clinically appropriate, while also being sensitive to potential family tensions in small communities when family members may become involved (American Telemedicine Association, 2009). These issues should be discussed during the informed consent process with the patient.

Legal Issues for Emergency Management

TMH providers need to be familiar of civil commitment as well as duty to warn/protect requirements. Criteria and procedures for hospitalization vary by state, however, and as noted previously in this chapter, providers should therefore familiarize themselves with procedures in both their own jurisdiction as well as the patient's jurisdiction (Godleski, Nieves, Darkins, & Lehmann, 2008). In the event that a patient threatens to harm a specific other person, TMH providers should also know whether they have a legal duty to either warn or protect the third party. In the landmark 1974 *Tarasoff v. Regents of the University of California* case, the California Supreme Court ruled that mental health professionals have a duty to warn third-party individuals who are being threatened bodily harm by a patient. This ruling was amended in 1976 to specify "duty to protect," a duty which may be carried out in a number of ways including but not limited to notifying law enforcement, warning the intended victim, or having the patient hospitalized (*Tarasoff v. Regents of the University of California*). The *Tarasoff* rulings quickly spread to additional states and have seen additional interpretations and applications since the 1970s (Walcott, Cerundolo, & Beck, 2001). More than half of the states have enacted statutes for mandatory duty to warn. These states vary, however, in how they specify who can be warned (law enforcement and/or the intended victim) and according to how much discretion the clinician has in applying his or her own judgment to the case. Several states and the District of Columbia has given permission to warn but do not impose duty to warn. For example, Texas statutes neither require nor permit disclosure of patient threats to anyone other than law enforcement, including the intended victim. That is, psychologists in Texas may disclose to law enforcement but are not required to do so; should they disclose to the intended victim, they could be liable for breach of confidentiality (Herbert, 2002). Finally, some states have no duty to warn statutes; within that group of states, some have case law that imposes a duty, while others have no clear case law or statute on the topic.

General Clinical Issues

The ATA guidelines also state that "Clinicians *shall be* aware of safety issues with patients displaying strong affective or behavioral states upon conclusion of a session, and how patients may then interact with remote site staff" (American Telemedicine Association, 2009). The primary concern here involves risk of patient harm to self or others self-harm. There are several key steps in safety planning that can help to mitigate risk. Review of patients existing clinical record for history of adverse interactions, as well as assessment of suicide risk prior to initiating and during treatment is also advised (Luxton, O'Brien et al., in press).

Potential problems with the telehealth technology and network infrastructure also have implications for patient's safety in emergency situations if the quality of the sessions is inadequate or connection is lost (Luxton, O'Brien et al., in press). Not only should the TMH provider have a secondary method for immediately contacting the patient and staff at the originating site in case of equipment failure but should also discuss with the patient up front in an initial encounter what both parties will do in the event of technical malfunction. Discussing all emergency procedures (for technical, clinical, and medical emergencies) with the patient as part of informed consent or additionally in the initial encounter is good TMH clinical practice.

Risk Issues in Home-Based TMH

The provision of TMH care to clinically unsupervised settings, such as to a patient's home, is an emerging area of care delivery. In particular, home-based TMH can provide improved access to mental health care for those unable or unwilling to seek traditional care due to barriers associated with mobility, geography, or concerns about stigma (Luxton, O'Brien et al., in press). A recent review by Luxton, Sirotin, and Mishkind (2010) of in-home care safety data provides initial evidence that TMH services delivered to clinically unsupervised settings can be safely managed by following the regulatory and risk-management guidelines already discussed in this chapter. To date, however, there has been limited empirical investigation on these types of settings, and there are few guidelines that address specifically appropriate and safe care within these environments. As such, there are unique risk issues associated with home-based TMH that require particular attention.

In-person care and TMH services that are delivered to clinically supervised settings (i.e., hospitals or outpatient clinics) have appropriate on-site treatment staff available to resolve safety issues that may occur. TMH care delivered directly to a patient's home, however, likely does not have clinical staff immediately available to respond to adverse events that might occur during or at the end of treatment sessions. Of particular concern is the risk of patient's harm to self or others. In some situations, a patient with a history of adverse reactions to treatment may not be suitable for home-based TMH care because potential reactions cannot be addressed without additional on-site staff (Luxton, O'Brien et al., in press).

The identification and use of a local collaborator, such as a family member or close friend of a patient, should also be considered as part of home-based TMH safety planning (Shore, Hilty, & Yellowlees, 2007; Luxton, O'Brien et al., in press). Local collaborators can provide TMH providers an additional mechanism to contact their patients should they be unable to communicate with them if a connection is lost or during an emergency situation, and may also be able to provide technical assistance in the event that a connection is lost, and when appropriate, provide support to a patient during certain emergency situations. It might also make sense to consider the use of a second care provider to help with care coordination in the event of psychiatric crises during home-based TMH care (Gros et al., 2011; Luxton, O'Brien et al., in press). As an example, the successful management of a suicidal patient during home-based TMH treatment was recently reported by Gros et al. (2011). The patient, who was being treated for posttraumatic stress disorder, reported suicidal ideation during a session and stated that he could not guarantee his own safety. A secondary clinician coordinated with emergency dispatchers while the primary TMH clinician maintained contact with the patient and his family. Also, as noted by Luxton, O'Brien et al. (in press), it is important for TMH clinicians to consider the risks of involving local collaborators when managing crisis situations. In some scenarios, it may be best to rely only on local 911 responders if there is potential risk to the safety of local collaborators.

Home-based TMH has the potential disadvantage of relying on the network limitations of the patient's location as well as the patient's equipment (e.g., personal computer and camera). Luxton, O'Brien et al. (in press) therefore recommend assessment of technology and infrastructure prior to initiating home-based TMH treatment. Technology issues include the adequacy of bandwidth (the rate of data transfer) for synchronous communication as well as adequacy and reliability of telehealth equipment (e.g., computers, monitors, video cameras, and audio equipment). The loss of connection during a crisis situation is a primary concern of patient's safety. Connection loss can be caused by inadequate transmission bandwidth or other equipment failure. It is therefore especially important to consider the basic minimal technical requirements for conducting home-based TMH and to have a plan to test and troubleshoot the technology prior to initiating in-home TMH treatment.

Conclusion

There are many known and assumed benefits of providing access to mental health care via telecommunications technologies, and this chapter was intended to provide an overview of the primary legal, regulatory, and risk-management issues associated with the safe and effective delivery of TMH services. With this chapter, we have attempted to alleviate common concerns and remove hesitancy that some may have about the delivery of mental health care from a distance. The information and guidelines presented in this chapter should give any new or seasoned TMH provider the foundation necessary to effectively mitigate any real or perceived risk associated with TMH care.

As a provider of TMH services, it is important to be aware of and actively manage these regulatory issues; however, the overarching principles for providing good clinical care using established practice standards for the broader mental health field remain the core of safe and effective practice. TMH is a dynamic field and it is a very exciting time to be not just a part of but also a driver of its growth. This dynamism requires clinicians to remain current and up-to-date on TMH issues. With knowledge and a little bit of background work to remain knowledgeable, new TMH clinicians can manage risk just as successfully as it is being managed by many clinicians who are currently engaged in TMH practice.

References

American Bar Association. Health law section. Report to the House of Delegates. (2008). <http://www.americanbar.org/content/dam/aba/migrated/health/04_government_sub/media/116B_Tele_Final.authcheckdam.pdf/> Accessed 18.03.12.

American Medical Association. Advocacy resources. Physician licensure: An update of trends. <http://www.ama-assn.org/ama/pub/about-ama/our-people/member-groups-sections/young-physicians-section/advocacy-resources/physician-licensure-an-update-trends.page/> Accessed 18.03.12.

American Medical Association. Report of the Board of Trustees, 35-A-99, internet prescribing. (1999). <http://www.amaassn.org/meetings/public/annual99/reports/>.

American Medical Association. Policy statement H-480.969: The promotion of quality telemedicine. <http://www.ama-assn.org/resources/doc/council-on-med-ed/cme-rep6-a10.pdf/> Accessed 18.03.12.

American Psychiatric Association. Telepsychiatry via videoconferencing. (1998). <http://archive.psych.org/edu/other_res/lib_archives/archives/199821.pdf/> Accessed 07.12.11.

American Psychological Association. Practice Directorate, Legal & Regulatory Affairs. Telehealth 50-state review. (2010). <http://www.apapracticecentral.org/advocacy/state/telehealth-slides.pdf/> Accessed 18.03.12.

American Psychological Association Ethics Committee. APA statement on services by telephone, teleconferencing, and internet. <http://www.apa.org/ethics/education/telephone-statement.aspx/> Accessed 18.03.12.

American Psychological Association Practice Organization. Telehealth: Legal basics for psychologists. Good Practice. 2010. Available to members of the APA Practice Organization at <http://www.apapracticecentral.org/update/2010/08-31/telehealth-resources.aspx> Accessed 18.03.12.

American Telemedicine Association. Practice guidelines for videoconferencing-based telemental health. (2009).<http://www.americantelemed.org/files/public/standards/

PracticeGuidelinesforVideoconferencing-Based%20TelementalHealth.pdf/ Accessed 18.03.12.

American Telemedicine Association. Medical licensure and practice requirements. (2011). <http://www.americantelemed.org/files/public/policy/ATAPolicy_StateMedicalLicensure. pdf/> Accessed 18.03.12.

American Telemedicine Association (ATA). ATA holds congressionalbriefing on national licensure. (2012). <www.americantelemed.org/> Accessed 18.03.12.

American Telemedicine Association. Comments on proposed changes affecting hospital and critical access hospital conditions of participation: Credentialing and privileging of telemedicine physicians and practitioners. <http://www.americantelemed.org/files/ public/policy/CMS%203227P.pdf/> Accessed 18.03.12.

American Telemedicine Association. Fixlicensure.org. Remove medical licensure barriers: Increasing consumer choice, improving safety and cutting costs, for patients across America. <http://www.fixlicensure.org/> Accessed 18.03.12.

American Telemedicine Association, Telemedicine forms. <http://www.americantelemed.org/ i4a/pages/index.cfm?pageID=3471/> Accessed 18.03.12.

Ameringer, C. F. (2011). State-based licensure of telemedicine: The need for uniformity but not a national scheme. *Journal of Health Care Law and Policy, 14,* 55–85.

Association of State and Provincial Psychology Boards. <http://www.asppb.net/> Accessed 18.03.12.

Australia Health Practitioner Regulation Agency. <http://www.ahpra.gov.au/> Accessed 18.03.12.

Centers for Medicare and Medicaid. U.S. Department of Health and Human Services. Health insurance portability and accountability act of 1996 (HIPAA). <http://www.cms.hhs.gov/ HIPAAGenInfo/> Accessed 18.03.12.

42 CFR (Code of Federal Regulations) Part 482 and 485. Changes Affecting Hospital and Critical Access Hospital Conditions of Participation: Telemedicine Credentialing and Privileging; published May 5, 2011; effective July 5, 2011.

Chee, J. (2010). Tele-medical malpractice: Negligence in the practice of telemedicine and related issues. Center for Telehealth and e-Health Law <http://www.ctel.org/research/ TeleMedical%20Malpractice%20Negligence%20in%20the%20Practice%20of% 20Telemedicine%20and%20Related%20Issues.pdf/> Accessed 18.03.12.

Clark, P. A., Capuzzi, K., & Harrison, J. (2010). Telemedicine: Medical, legal, and ethical perspectives. *Medical Science Monitor, 16,* 261–272.

European Commission. EU singlemarket, directive 2005/36/EC on the recognition of professional qualifications. <http://ec.europa.eu/internal_market/qualifications/policy_developments/ legislation_en.htm/> Accessed 18.03.12.

Federal Communication Commission. National Broadband Plan, Chapter10, Health Care. <http://www.broadband.gov/plan/10-healthcare/> Accessed 18.03.12.

Federation of State Medical Boards. <http://www.fsmb.org/ua-history.html/> Accessed 18.03.12.

Federation of State Medical Boards of the United States. Model act to regulate the practice of medicine across state lines. Report of the ad hoc committee on telemedicine. (1996).<http://www.fsmb.org/pdf/1996_grpol_Telemedicine.pdf/> Accessed 18.03.12.

Fleisher, L. D., & Dechene, J. C. (2004). *Telemedicine and e-health law.* New York, NY: Law Journal Press. <http://www.lawjournalpress.com/player/default.aspx#bppkid=70/> Accessed 18.03.12.

Food and Drug Administration. Draft guidance for industry and food and drug administration staff: Mobile medical applications. (2011). <http://www.fda.gov/downloads/

MedicalDevices/DeviceRegulationandGuidance/GuidanceDocuments/UCM263366.pdf/>
Accessed 18.03.12.

Genomics Law Report. *Don't forget about state law: Michigan decision reminds health care providers of HIPAA preemption issue*. Isidore Steiner, DPM, PC v. Marc Bonanni, No. 294016 (Mich. Ct. App. Apr. 7, 2011). <http://www.genomicslawreport.com/index.php/2011/06/28/dont-forget-about-state-law-michigan-decision-reminds-health-care-providers-of-hipaa-preemption-issue/> Accessed 18.03.12.

Gibbons v. Odgen, 22 U.S. 1. (1824).

Gobis, L. An overview of state laws and approaches to minimize licensure barriers. *Telemedicine Today Magazine*. Vol. 5, #6 and Vol. 6, #1. <http://www2.telemedtoday.com/statelawguide/index.shtml/> Accessed 09.12.11.

Godleski, L., Nieves, J. E., Darkins, A., & Lehmann, L. (2008). VA telemental health: Suicide assessment. *Behavioral Sciences and the Law*, 26, 271−286.

Grady, B., Myers, K. M., Nelson, E. L., Belz, N., Bennett, L., & Carnahan, L., et al. (2011). Evidence-based practice for telemental health. *Telemedicine Journal and e-Health*, *17*, 131−148.

Gros, D. F., Veronee, K., Strachan, M., Ruggerio, K. J., & Acierno, R. (2011). Managing suicidality in home-based telehealth. *Journal of Telemedicine and Telecare*, *17*, 332−335.

Gupta, A., & Soa, D. (2010). The unconstitutionality of current legal barriers to telemedicine in the United States: Analysis and future directions of its relationship to national and international health care reform. *Health Matrix: Journal of Law-Medicine*Social Science Research Network <http://ssrn.com/abstract=1549765/> Accessed 18.03.12

Hageseth v. Superior Court, 150 Cal. App. 4th 1399 (2007).

Herbert, P. B. (2002). The duty to warn: A reconsideration and critique. *Journal of the American Academy of Psychiatry and the Law*, 30, 417−424.

Hyler, S. E., & Gangure, D. P. (2004). Legal and ethical challenges in telepsychiatry. *Journal of Psychiatric Practice*, 10, 272−276.

Information on Australia National License. <http://nola.gov.au/> Accessed 18.03.12.

Kazal, L. A, & Conner, A. M. (2005). *Planning and implementing a statewide telehealth program in New Hampshire: A white paper*. Endowment for Health. <http://www.telehealthworld.com/images/knowleadgecenter/kc_whitepapers_dms.pdf/> Accessed 18.03.12.

Kramer, G. K., Ayers, T, Mishkind, M, & Norem, A. (2011). *DoD telemental health guidebook*. National Center for Telehealth and Technology. <http://t2health.org/sites/default/files/cth/guidebook/tmh-guidebook_06-11.pdf/> Accessed 18.03.12.

Luxton, D. D., Kayl, R. A., & Mishkind, M. C. (in press). mHealth data security: The need for HIPAA-compliant standardization. *Telemedicine and e-Health*.

Luxton, D. D., McCann, R. A., Bush, N. E., Mishkind, M. C., & Reger, G. M. (2011). mHealth for mental health: Integrating smartphone technology in behavioral healthcare. *Professional Psychology: Research and Practice*, 42, 505−512.

Luxton, D. D., Mishkind, M. C., Crumpton, R. M., Ayers, T. D., & Mysliwiec, V. (in press). Usability and feasibility of smartphone video capabilities for telehealth care in the U.S. military. *Telemedicine and e-Health*.

Luxton, D. D., O'Brien, K., McCann, R. A. and Mishkind, M. C. (in press). Home-based telemental healthcare safety planning: What you need to know, *Telemedicine and e-Health*.

Luxton, D. D., Sirotin, A. P., & Mishkind, M. C. (2010). Safety of telemental health care delivered to clinically unsupervised settings: A systematic review. *Telemedicine and e-Health*, *16*, 705−711.

Miller, T. W., Burton, D. C., Hill, K., Luftman, G., Veltkemp, L. J., & Swope, M. (2005). Telepsychiatry: Critical dimensions for forensic services. *Journal of the American Academy of Psychiatry and the Law*, *33*, 539–546.

Myers, K., & Cain, S. (2008). Practice parameter for telepsychiatry with children and adolescents. *Journal of American Academy of Child and Adolescent Psychiatry*, *47*, 1468–1483.

National Association of Social Workers *and Association of Social Work Boards Standards for Technology and Social Work Practice*. <http://www.socialworkers.org/practice/standards/NASWTechnologyStandards.pdf/> Accessed 18.03.12.

Natoli, C. M. (2009). *Summary of findings: Malpractice and telemedicine*. Center for Telehealth & e-Health Law. <http://www.ctel.org/research/Summary%20of%20Findings%20Malpractice%20and%20Telemedicine.pdf/> Accessed 18.03.12.

Ohio Psychological Association. Telepsychology guidelines. <http://www.ohpsych.org/resources/1/files/Comm%20Tech%20Committee/OPATelepsychologyGuidelines41710.pdf/> Accessed 18.03.12.

Resource Document, Telepsychiatry Via Videoconferencing, American Psychiatric Association. <http://www.psych.org/lib_archives/archives/199821.pdf/> Accessed 18.03.12.

Shore, J. H., Hilty, D. M., & Yellowlees, P. (2007). Emergency management guidelines for telepsychiatry. *General Hospital Psychiatry*, *29*, 199–206.

Tarasoff v. Regents of the University of California, 529 P.2d 553 (Cal. 1974).

Tarasoff v. Regents of the University of California, 17 Cal. 3d 425, 551 P.2d 334, 131 Cal. Rptr. 14 (Cal. 1976).

Telemedicine and license portability policy documents 140.001–140.007. Federation of State Medical Boards Public Policy Compendium. <http://www.fsmb.org/pdf/GRPOL_Public_Policy_compendium.pdf/> Accessed 18.03.12.

The National Council of State Boards of Nursing. Nurse licensure compact. (2000). <https://www.ncsbn.org/nlc.htm/> Accessed 18.03.2012.

U.S. Department of Health and Human Services, Health Resources and Services Administration. Health licensing board, report to congress. (2010a).<http://www.hrsa.gov/ruralhealth/about/telehealth/licenserpt10.pdf/> Accessed 18.03.12.

U.S. Department of Health and Human Services, Health Resources and Services Administration. Health licensing board, report to congress, citing Goldfarb v. Virginia State Bar, 421 U.S. 773, 792 (1975). (2010b).<http://www.hrsa.gov/ruralhealth/about/telehealth/licenserpt10.pdf/> Accessed 18.03.12.

U.S. Department of Health and Human Services, Health Resources and Services Administration. Health licensing board, report to congress, citing Maine v. Taylor, 477 U.S. 131, 137 (1986). (2010c). <http://www.hrsa.gov/ruralhealth/about/telehealth/licenserpt10.pdf/> Accessed 01.03.12.

U.S. Department of Health and Human Services. Understanding health informationpolicy. <http://www.hhs.gov/ocr/privacy/hipaa/understanding/index.html/> Accessed 18.03.12.

Walcott, D. M., Cerundolo, P., & Beck, J. C. (2001). Current analysis of the Tarasoff Duty: An evolution towards the limitation of the duty to protect. *Behavioral Sciences and the Law*, *19*, 325–343.

Section Three

Establishing a Telemental Health Practice

7 Business Aspects of Telemental Health in Private Practice

*Dehra Glueck**

Department of Psychiatry, Washington University School of Medicine, St. Louis, MO

Introduction

As technology improves and costs decrease, many traditional mental health practices are considering the use of technological approaches to increase their patients' access to care and to change their professional and personal lifestyle balance. There is a growing evidence base supporting the validity of diagnoses (Elford, White, & Bowering, 2000; Shore, Savin, & Orton, 2007; Singh, Arya, & Peters, 2007) and efficacy of treatment (Cuevas, Arredondo, & Cabrera, 2006; Modai, Jabarin, & Kurs, 2006; Nelson, Barnard, & Cain, 2003; O'Reilly, Bishop, & Maddox, 2007; Ruskin, Silver-Aylaian, & Kling, 2004) provided through telemental health care. Mental health providers are now looking for specific answers to questions of licensure, risks, malpractice coverage, and other legal and regulatory issues regarding telemental health practice. The goal of this chapter is to provide a directed review of the literature and to share professional experiences relevant to meeting the unique challenges to establishing a successful telemental health private practice. First, this chapter walks readers through the decision-making process regarding whether to start an independent telemental health practice or to join an established group telemental health practice. This is followed by a discussion of the different models of telemental health care that range from consultation to direct ongoing treatment. Specific practical considerations such as licensure, liability coverage, staffing, billing, and sharing of records are addressed. Additional sections address decisions regarding the choice of technology and obtaining adequate support. Practical suggestions for growing a telemental health business and joining a community of telemental health providers are discussed. As providers move into telemental health, there are many ways that they can adapt current models of care to enrich their new practice style. Throughout this chapter, clinicians are

* Corresponding author: Dehra Glueck, Department of Psychiatry, Washington University School of Medicine, 660 South Euclid, Campus Box 8043, St. Louis, MO 63110. Tel.: +1-314-747-2156, Fax: +1-314-747-3443, E-mail: glueckd@pschiatry.wustl.edu

Telemental Health. DOI: http://dx.doi.org/10.1016/B978-0-12-416048-4.00007-5

encouraged to ask thoughtful questions of themselves and companies with whom they are considering working. A careful understanding of their own technological and business comfort can help clinicians make decisions that will result in a rewarding telemental health practice.

Throughout this chapter, the term "provider site" is used to refer to the telemental health practitioner's services. The term "patient site" refers to the place where the patient receives care. Videoteleconferencing (VTC) refers to the use of secure videoconferencing technology to facilitate a provider meeting with patients in real time, i.e., using synchronous technology in which there is a mutual exchange of information rather than the review of recorded-patient encounters at a later time, referred to as asynchronous evaluations. Face-to-face (FTF) refers to traditional care settings in which both the patient and the provider meet in the same-room.

Choosing a Telemedicine Group or Technology-Only Support

When telemedicine became technologically feasible for clinical practice, costs were so prohibitive that it was generally practiced only within large academic settings. However, in the past several years, many new companies have developed, which offer mental health clinicians everything from a "virtual" private practice group to just a secure Internet connection they use on a desktop computer. These companies represent an ever-changing landscape of options, and the choice of which company to use rests largely on understanding what the individual teleclinician will need to feel comfortable in practice. On one end of this spectrum are companies that simply provide a secure Web site that can be accessed by downloading their software onto the user's desktop and using it with a basic desktop camera and commercial Internet found in most communities. In this model, the clinicians are responsible for identifying a patient base for their telemental health practice, making sure that patients can access their service, and all aspects of business and legal functioning. At the other end of this spectrum, there are full-service commercial models that hire clinicians to work for their company. These companies provide the patient contracts, hardware, software, and technical support along with the business support of a traditional private practice.

When deciding whether to join a group or to start an independent telemental health practice, there are some basic questions to ask:

- How much financial risk can I comfortably undertake? Will this be adequate to cover my expected start-up expenses?
- Will I have access to an adequate patient base to support my costs? Do I have a targeted patient group and allies in developing this practice?
- How comfortable am I with day-to-day operation of the technology and specifically videoconferencing technology? Do I have rapid and responsive access to technological assistance?
- How comfortable am I with the business aspects of a practice, such as policies and procedures, legal and regulatory considerations, and collecting payment?

In general, the more aspects of telemental health that clinicians feel comfortable managing, the less support they will need. For example, a clinician who has a high level of comfort with technology and has been commuting to a distant site for a number of years with an established patient base and wants to add telemental health to this practice might consider contracting with a technology-only company for the software and connectivity as the existing infrastructure would supply the patient base and administrative activities. In this arrangement, clinicians use the scheduling, patient protocols, and payment structure of the original FTF model and the only change is that patients are treated through videoconferencing equipment rather than FTF. Alternatively, clinicians who are newly out of training and do not have experience operating their own business may elect to join a telemedicine group practice that provides more comprehensive support. In this model, the telemedicine group, or company, provides access to a specific patient base and payment for contracted time. In comparing technology-only models to group-practice models, it is important to understand the advantages and disadvantages from both a provider and a patient perspective.

Technology-Only Models

Technology-only models are based on the idea that the clinician only requires a secure means of contacting patients. Any telemedicine or telemental health session involves a set of videoconferencing equipment at each site. In addition to the obvious need for a camera, an equally important aspect is the Internet connection itself. The Internet connection starts from a camera at the patient site, goes through a satellite or cable network provider, and ends at the camera in the provider's office with many intervening steps that make secure or wireless connections possible. Generally speaking, each of these aspects, from camera to Internet line, has to have a clear person who is responsible for care and maintenance, especially in the event of a technical disruption. Providers need to know who to call when the video does not work. When looking at technology-only options, it is important to have the potential vendor demonstrate the entire process from the camera at one end all the way through to the camera at the other end in order to understand what the vendor controls and maintains and what the provider can expect to maintain.

Additional questions arise as to the company's ability to guarantee that the provider will be using a secure connection when conducting a telemedicine session. The definition of what constitutes a secure connection is evolving as regulations that were originally developed for older technologies, such as fax machines, are adapted to newer technologies, such as videoconferencing. Again, this is a process of understanding exactly how the information is transmitted and ensuring that there is no unseen third party access to telemedicine sessions. Details regarding security protocols are covered in this book. Suffice it to say that the potential telemedicine provider should inquire whether the vendor provides a connection that is compliant with the Health Insurance Portability and Accountability Act (HIPAA). The vendor should then discuss how the methods of encryption and security compare against the national standard for patient care. Additional discussion of bandwidth and technology as it relates to assessment and treatment of patients appears later in this chapter.

Technology-only companies vary significantly in terms of what services and equipment they provide. In the past, the majority of telemedicine setups involved had a dedicated room for telemedicine, with a free-standing camera, TV monitor, and separate technical equipment, such as routers and code−decode (CODECs) that were used to maintain a secure Internet connection for televideo. In this setting, some technology companies simply sell cameras and the clinician then needs to have their own technical support team help them make the camera work on their network and establish a secure and stable connection to the Internet. In this setting, clinicians may also be responsible for maintaining the equipment purchased as well as for purchasing the additional support equipment needed, such as TV monitors routers. This scenario is still common in academic or large-volume telemedicine settings, not only because of the high-quality video it can provide but also because of significant cost and technical support needs associated with it. It is important for clinicians who are considering telemental health to carefully consider the support needs that a large free-standing system will require. For instance, in this setting it is often helpful to have access to an on-site rapid response team or significant personal comfort with technical equipment. If a provider does not have access to on-site support, some hardware companies now contract with independent service providers who will maintain and service the camera and Internet connections of the equipment they sell. With the many equipment options available to clinicians, the most important step is to ask detailed questions about what is included with any equipment purchase and how support needs are handled. Additional discussion of the impact of bandwidth on patient encounters is discussed later in this chapter.

For providers who feel less comfortable managing the Internet connections or hardware, there are several new companies that maintain Web sites with downloadable software to establish a "virtual meeting room" that utilizes a clinician's and patient's desktop computers and cameras. In this model, providers generally contract for a flat monthly fee and the vendor provides a Web site with secure connections between the provider's desktop or laptop system and the computer at the patient site. This usually requires a minimal financial investment in a desktop camera system and the connection can be made through commercially available Internet speeds. In this setting, it is important to make sure that both the provider and the patient have adequate bandwidth to allow for synchronous video that is free from frequent breaks or disruptions. No matter what equipment is purchased, the bandwidth available through the Internet service provider will be a primary determinant of whether or not the video is continuous without frequent breaks. While there is significantly less financial investment in the camera and the basic equipment, there are still significant demands on the Internet connection to allow good video quality. It is important that the vendor demonstrates its technology with a bandwidth that is similar to what the provider and patient will have at their practice site so that the provider can assess whether the connection speed is adequate to establish rapport, make accurate diagnoses, and conduct treatment. It is equally important to ensure that both the provider site and the patient site feel comfortable with the desktop technology and software interface and have adequate technical supports from the vendor to make it feasible. Both sites will need to be able to do basic troubleshooting to make the connection work. Additional information on the interface of technology and clinical care can be found in Chapter 3.

There has been significant debate in telemedicine communities about the relative security of "free" VTC options, such as Skype or "Google Talk." At the time of this writing, there have been significant concerns voiced about the security of these options for patient care. Their encryption appears adequate. The majority of concerns relate to the structure of the connection, whereby it would be possible for the vendor's employees to monitor a session. Practitioners are encouraged to discuss the issues of patient privacy with any technology company they are considering. Additionally, it is important to openly discuss and document the possible security limitations with patients as part of informed consent for telemental health.

Group-Practice Models

There are several new businesses emerging that connect telemental health providers to patients, while providing comprehensive technical and administrative support. These businesses can use the Internet for recruitment of both providers and patients as well as for the provision of services through videoconferencing Web sites. Providers can contract with one or more of these companies for a number of hours or for a specific patient panel. The company connects the provider with patients through secure Internet connections over desktop computers or may install hardware in the provider's office that integrates with the company's existing infrastructure. This arrangement may especially appeal to providers who want to increase their patient panel but do not want to manage the technology and do not have a system for referral of patients to their telemental health practice. The downside is that profits are shared with the contracted business, although there is also minimal overhead expense. Although this business sector is evolving, some general description of the process is possible. In general, there are two types of practices these companies tend to support: (i) institution-based telemental health practice and (ii) direct-to-consumer practice.

Institution-Based Practice Model

In this model, the company develops contracts with distant health institutions in need of mental health expertise and links them to the telemental health providers they have hired. For example, a company may develop a contract with a rural community mental health center to provide 4 h of psychiatric consultations per week at a specified hourly or block rate. The company will then use its own or another Internet-based videoconferencing service to connect one of its contracted providers with the community mental health center. The company then pays the telemental health providers for their dedicated time. As another example, a company may develop a contract with a rural emergency room to provide 5 h of weekend psychiatric consultation by one of their contracted telemental health providers. Although the company is not itself a health-care institution, it functions as a virtual institution and the consultation seeks to provide an "institution-to-institution telemental health consultation." This type of institution-based practice requires careful coordination of electronic medical records (EMR) as well as an understanding of the legal, regulatory, and clinical protocols necessary for good patient care at a distance. It has the advantage of having skilled clinicians at the patient site to assist the telemental health provider in evaluation and patient care.

Direct-to-Consumer Model

In this model, the company contracts with providers and individual patients to allow patients to directly access care from a given provider through the Internet. This model can differ considerably from the institution-based model. A key difference is that patients are treated without other clinicians being present or involved in their care, such as in the aforementioned example of the emergency room or mental health center consultation. This difference is particularly relevant when there are safety concerns or complex regulatory issues. For instance, companies vary in the degree to which they manage issues of cross-state licensure and emergency management. Some companies only allow patients to access providers licensed in the patient's location. Others leave it to the providers or the patients to manage this issue. A clinical challenge, and potentially an ethical issue, is that patients are receiving care in clinically unsupervised settings. Therefore, emergency management relies predominantly on the cooperation of the patient. This practice is controversial and has led to the development of practice guidelines by the American Telemedicine Association (Grady, Myers, & Nelson, 2009). However, these companies continue to grow. One explanation for their success is their popularity with patients. Internet-delivered telemental health has brought a new definition to the term "patient-centered care," in terms of access, flexibility of appointments, patient decision making, and even privacy in that patients may elect to separate these sessions from other health care and their health insurance coverage. It is unclear how many insurers cover this modality of care.

When considering whether to become a part of a telemedicine group, it is important to also take a consumer point of view and evaluate the companies not only in terms of their financial and professional benefits but also in terms of their provision of telemental health care. Although there are no hard and fast rules, some generalizations can be made. It is important that a company has adequate input and collaboration from actual health-care providers when developing its business model. Generally speaking, companies started by experienced mental health clinicians understand clinical practice. However, some companies are not led by health-care providers. This may be acceptable, as long as the company adequately addresses the key clinical concerns in providing care through videoconferencing to distant sites. Thus, it is important to evaluate companies in terms of how well they (i) adhere to licensure laws, (ii) have a clear emergency management protocol, (iii) protect patients' privacy, and (iv) have a process for documentation and billing comparable to that found in traditional care. Although these companies provide comprehensive administrative and technical support, it is the individual providers' responsibility to ensure that their care adheres to the ethical and legal guidelines established by their profession and by their state licensing board.

Deciding on the Model of Care—Direct Care Versus Consultation

When considering a telemental health practice, the next decision is which model of care to be provided, and this can vary along a spectrum from ongoing direct care of patients (Cuevas et al., 2006; Grady et al., 2009; Modai et al., 2006; Nelson et al., 2003; Ruskin et al., 2004) to consultation with primary-care providers (Myers, Vander Stoep et al., 2010; O'Reilly et al., 2007). In direct-care models, the mental health provider is responsible for establishing the diagnosis and rendering ongoing treatment including services such as medication management and psychotherapy. In consultation models, the provider evaluates the patient and makes treatment recommendations, but the primary responsibility for ongoing care remains with the referring physician. Part of this decision rests on the telemental health provider's comfort with using the technology for ongoing care as well as on preferences of referring physicians, patients, and reimbursement mechanisms. There is also relevant research from which to draw.

Direct Care—Evaluation of Patients

The first step in beginning the treatment is to establish a reliable diagnosis, and many telemental health providers have questions about their ability to do this through VTC. Studies in this area began by comparing the diagnoses obtained from an FTF evaluation of a patient to the diagnosis obtained from a telemental health evaluation of that same patient. In general, the methodology has been to compare assessments of the same patient through both VTC and FTF while randomizing the psychiatrist performing the evaluation and the order in which the assessment is provided (i.e., half of the patients having VTC first and the other half receiving FTF first). Studies have differed on whether they used naturalistic assessments, i.e., the psychiatrists own practice style and management similar to what is typically done in private practice or whether they used structured instruments that are more commonly used in research settings. Both methods have consistently shown good reliability (Shore, Savin, & Orton 2007) and agreement (Singh et al., 2007). Studies with adults comparing naturalistic assessments (Singh et al., 2007) versus structured diagnostic interviews (Shore, Savin, & Orton 2007) have shown substantial agreement on Axis I diagnoses. Similar findings have been found with children.

Elford et al. (2000) completed a randomized controlled trial comparing naturalistic diagnostic interviews made in person or by VTC for 23 patients aged 4–16 years. They found 96% agreement across the five psychiatrists completing the evaluations. One way to adapt this research to clinical practice is to conduct a naturalistic diagnostic evaluation augmented by more structured rating scales to reinforce the telemental health provider's differential diagnostic thinking or to establish baseline data for monitoring treatment.

Direct Care—Ongoing Treatment of Patients

Once a diagnosis has been established, treatment interventions can begin. As the evidence base for making reliable diagnoses through telemental health expanded, the literature began looking at the effectiveness of treatment. As one example, Ruskin et al. (2004) examined the treatment of 131 depressed male veterans using a combination of techniques commonly employed in private practice: medication management, psychoeducation, and brief supportive counseling. Patients showed significant improvement in both FTF and VTC settings and had no difference in adherence, medication compliance, or patient satisfaction. Similar results have been found in children including a study by Nelson et al. (2003) that randomized 28 depressed children to receive cognitive-behavioral therapy (CBT) through either FTF or VTC. Results indicated comparable remission rates across both conditions and, interestingly, the group treated through VTC had a greater rate of decline in depressive symptoms. Attendance at sessions and satisfaction with care were comparable in the two groups. In addition to these studies in which patients received all their care through one or the other modality, Modai et al. (2006) completed a study looking at the experiences of patients who changed from FTF to VTC. They found that the adherence ratios were twice as high in the VTC setting and that patients endorsed high satisfaction for care delivered via VTC. Overall, the expanding literature continues to support the effectiveness of treatment provided through direct telemental health care including its ability to serve the significant need for medication treatment in rural and other underserved communities. For further information on treatment, please see Section Five including Chapters 15 and 16 and Section Six, Chapter 19.

Consultative Care

There has also been growing interest in consultative models that strengthen the care provided by local physicians in providing mental health care and in expanding their prescribing capabilities through consultation with psychiatrists (Hilty, Yellowlees, & Nesbitt, 2006), especially in settings where there are inadequate resources for the psychiatrist to practice independently (Shore & Manson, 2005). Thus, telepsychiatry is one of the most requested telemental health services (Hilty, Yellowlees, & Cobb, 2006). In this model, the local physician maintains primary responsibility for the patient while the telepsychiatrist conducts evaluations and makes recommendations for treatment but does not directly manage the patient's care or prescribe medication. Proponents of this model cite continuing education of primary-care physicians (PCPs) and their increased skills and knowledge in caring for a broader range of patient diagnoses as the key benefits of this model (Hilty, Yellowlees, & Cobb, 2006; Hilty, Yellowlees, & Nesbitt, 2006). A study examining the referral patterns of PCPs participating in a consultation model showed a gradual transition over time from their requesting assistance in making diagnoses to increased requests for assistance with developing or modifying treatment plans (Hilty, Yellowlees, & Nesbitt, 2006). This study also found that PCPs increased their compliance with national dosing standards. In another study of consultation models, O'Reilly et al. (2007) examined change from dysfunctional to functional scores on the Brief Symptom Inventory for a broad range of diagnoses. They found equivalent results across the two settings (VTC and FTF), supporting usefulness of the consultative model.

Deciding on a Model: Strength and Needs Assessments

Overall, the database supporting telemental health as an effective service delivery model is encouraging, but still limited. Thus, the decision regarding which model of care to provide is based less on the existing guidelines and more on the provider's comfort with each model and the respective community's needs and resources. Since the success of a telemental health program rests on good relationships with the patient's community, it is recommended that telemental health providers reach out to the local community over a series of meetings to concretely establish their unique needs and abilities to provide ongoing mental health care (Shore & Manson, 2005).

Important questions to consider include the following:

- Are there local clinicians who can provide psychotherapy that the telemental health provider may recommend? Do they have experience with the evidence-based techniques, such as CBT?
- Are there local providers who are comfortable prescribing psychotropic medications if indicated? Do they have experience with the medications the telemental health provider commonly prescribes, including access to and familiarity with requirements for laboratory monitoring?
- Are there local options for case management and financial assistance?
- Are their liaisons with schools or employers?
- Are there formal structures for crisis management and emergent evaluations and/or hospitalizations?
- Who are the stakeholders who will help to make the telemental health service successful?

In addition to the community's needs and resources, it has been the author's experience that the ability to make an informed decision regarding the type of telemental health practice to implement is based on a realistic assessment of the provider's risk tolerance and the availability of good partners at the patient's site. Some providers find that they are uncomfortable with the distance between the sites and elect to have a local clinician retain primary responsibility for the patient.

Part of this decision depends on the ability to have concrete plans for emergencies and ability to provide high acuity care. Related to this, it can be helpful to make a list of prominent "fears" regarding telemental health services and then to develop protocols to address these "fears." For instance, a common "fear" is how to handle patients who are suicidal or have emergencies during a telemental health session. These are concrete scenarios that can have very practical solutions by arranging access by phone to local emergency room physicians during and after hours and/or having a staff member in the room with the patient during the encounter. It is also important to ensure that either the institution or the patient, depending on the service delivery model, has adequate access to the telemental health provider between scheduled sessions. For example, if a patient's condition worsens or side-effects to medication develop, a contracted institution will need to triage the patient to a local clinician who may want to discuss the care with the telemental health provider. Or, in a direct-to-consumer model, the patient/consumer will need access to the provider. This can often be handled by having pager access to the provider and establishing protocols for emergent evaluations of patients with local resources, such as emergency departments (Shore, Hilty, & Yellowlees, 2007).

Financial Feasibility

Regardless of whether a clinician contracts with a group practice or practices independently, it is important to understand the factors that affect the financial feasibility of telmental health endeavors. Cost can be understood from both the patient and the provider perspective as well as understanding how volumes and no-show appointments affect sustainability. The landscape of insurance reimbursement is rapidly evolving and the historical dependence on grants is changing.

Understanding Costs: Patient and Provider Perspective

Reviews of the literature on the costs associated with telemedicine have noted problems associated with a lack of consistency in the methodology used to determine cost. Part of this inconsistency relates to whether the study considers costs from the provider's perspective (Myers, Sulzbacher, & Melzer, 2004) or the patient's perspective. In practice, these can be quite different especially if providers pay for their travel to patient sites in FTF models. Interestingly, studies that looked at providers' travel costs have found that costs from VTC are generally equivalent to FTF care in the distant community if the provider has to travel more than 22 miles (Ruskin et al., 2004) and can be less than FTF care if travel to the distant sites involves airfare or lodging (O'Reilly et al., 2007). The ability to eliminate travel costs can be a substantial financial benefit. In addition, when providers are no longer using hours to travel to a patient site, those same hours can be used for additional patient-care hours, thus potentially increasing revenue as well as increasing the hours available for scheduling.

Patients experience similar revenue loss when they are required to take time away from work to travel to remote sites. Additional expenses such as paying for childcare, cost of gasoline, or transportation also have a significant impact. Studies examining costs from the perspective of the patient (Modai et al., 2006) have found that accounting for patient costs such as travel, lost wages, and paying for childcare resulted in decreasing the disparity between FTF and VTC care from 32% to 10%. Telemental health providers at the University of Kansas Medical Center were able to decrease their costs per consult from US$168.61 to US$30.99 when they accounted for the patient's cost of travel, other expenses, and time away from work (Spaulding, Belz, DeLurgio, & Williams, 2010). These cost savings to patients can be an incentive for them to use the VTC services and can be part of marketing to the local community.

Impact of Patient Volume on Costs

One important proactive strategy for ensuring the financial feasibility of telemental health is to ensure an adequate volume of patients. Each telemental health encounter will have costs for the provider's time as well as the technology. Thus, maximizing the number of patients seen within that time helps to ensure there is adequate income to offset both types of costs. Studies have noted that increased volume disperses technology costs over a greater number of paid visits (Hyler & Gangure, 2003) as well as improves cost minimization per day (Ruskin et al., 2004). For example, telemental health can be used to service multiple sites within a single day, with no loss of time for travel. Thus, a 4-h block of time could potentially serve four different sites that only had a single patient at each site. Rather than losing billable time traveling between sites or sitting at a site without referrals, telemental health allows for maximum efficiency. Rabinowitz et al. evaluated the costs of a telepsychiatry consult service for rural nursing home residents and found that savings were closely tied to whether visits were clustered together. One substantial benefit of telemental health is this ability to provide care to patients at multiple sites within the same day. Thus, a private practitioner can evaluate and treat patients across multiple settings with the visits being dictated by need instead of the convenience of the provider's on-site presence.

Many new telemental health providers are concerned that they will not have adequate volume to establish their practices. It is clear that some marketing and cooperation with local providers are important in maintaining adequate referrals and community visibility. In communities where there is a high need for mental health services, utilization may be more dictated by availability of hours. A study by Myers, Vander Stoep et al. (2010) found high saturation of additional visits when blocked time was made available suggesting that availability might play a key role. Telemental health providers who are practicing outside of a group or block funding are encouraged to use financial modeling to determine the number of baseline visits required to offset fixed technology and staffing costs. With this model in place, they can use targeted strategies to increase their patient volume and number of referrals.

Impact of No-Show Appointments on Costs

Telemental health practices are impacted by no-shows in much the same way a traditional FTF practice would be; however, telemental health practices also have the additional financial consideration of technology and connectivity costs. These costs will vary significantly depending on what kind of practice and technology is used. Impacts on this cost include the amount being charged for patient visits and the cost of Internet connections. For providers who are contracted on the basis of an hourly rate independent of billing, no-shows may have little or no financial impact, other than whether the patient site will be able to continue to pay for telemental health services. Other providers that maintain high-speed connections may have significant charges for their basic Internet connection that they will need to offset. No-show appointments are rarely seen as a completely fixed event. Instead, there are multiple patient and provider variables that impact them. Studies by Krupinski (2004) found that the majority of missed VTC sessions were completed eventually, suggesting that some of this income may ultimately be captured, although costs are still impacted by missed visits. Factors noted to impact the rate of failed appointments include patient travel, convenience of appointment time, ease of contacting the provider to reschedule, and reminder calls. Transferring responsibility for scheduling to the patient site has been shown to decrease the no-show rate (Hilty, Cobb, & Neufeld, 2008), in one case from 21% to 13% (O'Reilly et al., 2007). Interestingly, some studies report lower no-show rates in the telemental health setting when patients do not have to travel for services (Ruskin et al., 2004). Many private practices implement strategies such as appointment reminder calls the day prior to the appointment, leaving a message after a missed visit or contacting the referring physician if an appointment is missed. These strategies can be adopted in telemental health settings as well.

Reimbursement: Insurance

The reimbursement landscape has been changing rapidly over the last several years. Reimbursement is influenced by federal programs such as Medicare as well as local and state laws. Navigating this landscape can seem overwhelming. National organizations, such as the American Telemedicine Association (www.americantelemed. org), have set aside portions of their Web site (Telemedicine Reimbursement Central) and created downloadable documents to aid telemedicine providers in understanding the reimbursement landscape. These documents are regularly reviewed and updated by knowledgeable telemedicine providers and provide an important first starting point.

When looking at national programs such as Medicare and private payers, there are often some differences between codes for FTF mental health and telemental health. Sometimes this is as simple as adding a modifier, e.g., a "gt modifier," to the usual Current Procedural Terminology (CPT) code, and in other cases, there are certain CPT codes that are not allowed. Providers are encouraged to contact Medicare directly with any questions (http://www.medicare.gov/navigation/help-and-support/

contact-medicare.aspx) or the Center for Telehealth and e-Law (http://ctel.org/expertise/reimbursement/medicare-reimbursement/). More information on CPT codes often used by telepsychiatrists and Center for Medicaid and Medicare Services (CMS)-compliant templates used to document services provided under each code can be found in Chapter 16.

As for private payers, Medicare rules are often the starting point for private payers' policies regarding reimbursement, but there can be significant variations by state. Thus, it is important that telemental health providers first review the Center for Medicare Services guidelines directly (www.cms.gov/Manuals/) prior to billing. Then, providers can determine guidelines that are state-specific. For instance, California has developed a reimbursement handbook (www.nrtrc.org/wp-content/uploads/Telemedicine-Reimbursement-Handbook1.pdf) (Telemedicine Reimbursement Handbook, 2006). Many times these state guidelines can be easily found through Internet searches of the individual state. If these state-specific guidelines are not in place, reviewing documents by other states can aid in advocacy efforts within the provider's home state. As a final step, telemental health providers are encouraged to make a list of all insurance carriers with which they intend to work and contact them with a letter describing their intent to bill for telemental health services, including the list of CPT codes they will use. This allows for verification of the insurance company's acceptance of specific telemental health codes and confirmation of the amount that they will reimburse for each visit.

Many providers report comparable reimbursement rates for CPT codes billed FTF and VTC. Some investigators found that their telemental health practice had a less favorable case mix than did their on-site clinic, largely reflecting the larger Medicaid population represented in rural areas which telemental health typically serves (Myers, Sulzbacher, & Melzer, 2004). When Hilty, Cobb, and Neufeld (2008) examined the rate of reimbursement, they did not find problems specifically with reimbursement but found that 60% of claims had been paid, 30% were pending at the time of service completion, 3% were denied, and 8% were uninsured. Informal surveys indicate that this is roughly comparable to claims statistics for FTF care. Understanding the case mix at the intended patient site and the reimbursement rates of individual insurance companies will help telemental health providers to decide with which companies they will work. This information can become part of informed financial modeling that allows telemental health providers to understand their relative costs.

Reimbursement: Private Payment

Some mental health providers have elected not to bill insurance carriers in their private practice and this is an option in telemental health practice as well. Additional considerations arise for transmission of payment at a distance. Although there are not published standards for accepting direct payment, telemental health providers at national meetings indicate they use a variety of techniques including accepting credit cards, mailed payments, and establishing a PayPal account through secure Web sites. There is also an option for cash to be accepted if there are staff at the distant site to manage the payment. Additional accounting support can be obtained to help manage patient bills as would traditionally be done in a FTF practice.

Reimbursement: Contracted Time

Telemental health providers who do not want to bill insurance carriers can pursue contracts with organizations such as community mental health providers or federally qualified health centers that allow for block funding, often at an hourly rate. This contracted work requires finding mental health agencies that can afford to pay the telemental health provider's time and having adequate staffing to manage insurance billings. Many new providers are unsure of the rates they should charge for services. One approach to calculating an hourly rate is to obtain the average insurance reimbursement for a FTF visit in that community and extrapolate. For example, if psychiatrists at the remote site would generally charge US$80 for a FTF medication management visit and typically conduct two to three visits in an hour, they would make from US$160 to US$240 per hour. Then, accounting for no-shows, the rate could be averaged around US$200 per hour. Some providers note that this may be an overestimation as there will be some administrative costs at the patient site and so they charge around US$150 per hour. One advantage to telemental health providers from block funding is having a stable income stream regardless of the no-show rate. Calculations that take into account an expected percentage of no-shows and the administrative costs at the patient site will help to keep the hourly rate financially feasible for a patient site that is billing for these encounters.

Sometimes the full hourly rate for a provider's time is cost prohibitive to the community mental health provider. In this setting, some telemental health providers have pursued a hybrid option in which the telemental health provider charges a lower hourly rate to the patient site for availability and then bills the insurance carrier themselves for visits that are completed. In keeping with the previous example's cost assumptions, in the hybrid model, the provider conducting two medication visits per hour would bill US$75 per hour for availability and then submit two insurance claims for the two completed visits. This would result in an hourly rate of US$75 + US$80 + US$80 = US$235. An advantage of this hybrid model is that providers do not operate at a total loss when visits are not kept, and outside agencies are able to purchase services at a decreased rate. Regardless of the funding model, the feasibility rests on the providers understanding how much financial risk they can assume and how many patients or contracted hours are required to offset their fixed costs.

Practical Considerations—Malpractice, Licensure, and Consent

There are a number of practical considerations when considering telemental health practice including obtaining malpractice that covers telemental health, licensure, and informed consent. Of primary importance is obtaining adequate liability coverage. There is growing awareness of telemental health practice by major liability insurers, and many national plans, including those sponsored by professional organizations, will provide coverage to telemental health providers. Providers should contact several liability insurers to obtain comparative pricing. It is also helpful to compare reimbursement rates for FTF with VTC practice. Informal surveys at national meetings indicate that rates are not substantially different for telemental health coverage. Generally, liability insurers require notice that providers will be using telemental health in their practice and may ask for additional information regarding risk management. Providers are encouraged to write out their risk management polices and send these to their carrier to aid in obtaining informed practice coverage.

There is an evolving literature that specifically addresses risk management issues in telemental health, including a review by Cash (2011) and also in Chapter 6. These authors review licensure requirements and recommend contacting state licensing boards to ensure that the provider has adequate licensure for practice in that state and is conforming to the state's practice guidelines. Related to this, it is important to contact both the licensure board where the provider practices as well as the licensure board where the patient obtains care in order to determine whether the practice crosses state lines. These reviews indicate that state licensing boards and legislatures view the location of the patient as the place where the practice of medicine occurs, and thus, where issues of malpractice and licensure will be determined. Generally, the most conservative approach is to obtain full medical licensure in both the patient's and the provider's states. From a risk management perspective, licensing board statements are particularly important in case patients file complaints, as they are likely to file in the state where they reside.

Informed Consent and Standard of Care

Issues of informed consent are an important aspect of providing high-quality telemental health care. Informed consent involves a competent patient being informed of the risks, benefits, and alternatives of a given treatment and expressing agreement with planned treatment. It is important to have both ongoing conversations as well as legal documentation of informed consent when treating patients through telemental health. Potential risks of telemental health may vary with practice setting but can include limitations of technology, including disruptions in care or decreased resolution of the visual image or auditory signal. Attorneys note that the standard of care in telemental health is the same as the standard of care for patients receiving care FTF (Cash, 2011). Thus, telemental health providers are encouraged to identify ways of obtaining information if technological limitations are present, such as using rating scales or collateral from other providers. These kinds of adaptations can be included in the comprehensive risk management policies that are provided to liability insurance carriers. Telemental health providers often offer patients the option to be evaluated FTF or referred to a local provider if telemental health is not meeting their needs for mental health care. There is some debate over the adequacy of general consent forms to cover telemental health care. It is recommended that providers obtain legal review of the consent forms to determine their suitability in a given state. Alternatively, some states provide sample telemental health consent forms, such as those found in the California reimbursement handbooks (www.nrtrc.org/ wp-content/uploads/Telemedicine-Reimbursement-Handbook1.pdf). Telemental health providers are encouraged to seek legal consultation regarding development of consent policies.

Staffing

When providing care at a distance, there are a certain fixed tasks that must be accomplished, just as in FTF care. These include scheduling visits, handling patient calls, making referrals to the community, obtaining signed consent forms, assisting with technology and completion of physician-ordered tasks such as laboratory assessments when indicated. Telemental health practices differ substantially in how they handle these tasks. Again this varies along a spectrum. At one end of this spectrum, all tasks are completed by the telemental health provider. At the other end of the spectrum, the patient site hires dedicated staff to assist the practice. Providers who have time and adequate staffing at their own site may consider handling these tasks themselves. Patients then mail consent forms and other relevant documents to them directly. If providers do not have this kind of support or are contracting with a remote community health organization, they can consider using staff at the patient site to complete these tasks. One common model involves having a dedicated staff person, often called a telemedicine coordinator, who is hired by the patient site that communicates with the telemental health provider regularly and completes all of the above tasks. In this model, the coordinator is the primary point of contact for patients and completes all scheduling tasks and community referrals. In this model, if the telemental health provider is a psychiatrist, the coordinator can also handle requests for medication refills, laboratory monitoring, and patients' prescriptions. There are some insurance companies that will allow the patient site to bill a "facility fee" for each encounter and this can be used to offset salary costs for the coordinator. Additional considerations for staffing, including education level, have been previously discussed by Glueck (2011) and the reader is encouraged to discuss this specifically with patient sites when developing contracts.

Sharing Records

Discussions among telemental health providers reveal considerable variability in the ability to send and receive medical records. Telemental health providers must follow all HIPAA requirements for release of patient information and patient privacy. On a practical level, meeting this obligation depends on the record keeping practices at both sites. When one site uses a paper chart, evaluations are generally faxed back and forth as needed. Some providers also use encrypted e-mail documents to transmit information, and there are options to purchase software that automatically encrypts e-mails. When web-based electronic records are used, providers can be given access to and trained to use the EMR at the patient's site. Many telemental health providers report that the transmission of records is most complete, timely, convenient, and reliable when using web-based EMRs. Personal health records, in which patients have access to their EMR, may also be informative.

Technology—Selection, Use, and Technical Support

Private practice telemental health providers have access to an abundance of new technologies. Some of these technology decisions are taken on when deciding which kind of practice to join. Specific technical requirements will be discussed in detail in other chapters. When considering technology for private practice settings, several options exist to obtain competitive pricing, including options to go to national telemedicine meetings and meet vendors of multiple types of equipment. Costs must be balanced with concerns regarding quality of service. Overall, these considerations should guide decisions regarding which equipment to purchase when comparing costs across vendors. Direct observation of the equipment at these national meetings can also help providers to ascertain quality across a broad array of options. When telemental health providers are unable to afford the equipment, some providers have also been successful in obtaining grant funding to purchase the initial equipment, thus minimizing or eliminating up-front costs altogether. Further information can be obtained from the United States Department of Agriculture, Rural Development (http://www.rurdev.usda.gov/Utilities_LP.html). Also, refer Appendices II and III.

The primary determinants of costs in this setting can again be divided into costs related to camera equipment and Internet connectivity. Providers who purchase larger room systems that involve high-definition endpoints and cameras will have significantly greater up-front costs than providers who use desktop systems and cameras. Additionally, providers who use dedicated high bandwidth through a T1 line offered through commercial communications companies will have higher costs than providers who use commercial Internet services that share bandwidth. Each of these decisions regarding endpoints, cameras, and connectivity significantly impact both cost and quality of the transmission.

When considering equipment, it is important to consider the needs of both the provider site and the patient site. Many providers will make modifications to their existing office to accommodate telemental health practice. This can include choosing desktop systems that allow them to use their existing computer equipment. This often reduces costs but can have trade-offs, e.g., if the bandwidth is not reliable, the resolution of the computer screen is not sufficient for clinical work, or the system does allow remote control of the camera at the patient site. Purchasing cameras with pan—tilt—zoom functionality will allow the telemental health provider to follow the patient's movements throughout the room and zoom in when additional clarity is needed regarding abnormal movements, dysmorphology, affect, or other aspects of the mental status. When setting up the patient site, it can be beneficial to use larger monitors such as high-definition, flat-screen monitors so that the clinical encounter more closely approximates the size and perspective of FTF care. When using monitors for display of video transmission, they should be placed at a comfortable height so that seated patients are looking directly at the provider. In practice, considerations that decrease the noise and ensure adequate lighting of facial features are helpful in increasing providers' and patients' comfort. Setups for both providers and patients should emphasize functionality and comfort.

It is also important to make sure that both sites have adequate technical support for the equipment and interface they purchased. In general, when telemental health sites purchase equipment-only options, there will be increased need for on-site technical support if the systems have significant complexity, such as that found in a free-standing room system that requires a camera, TV monitor, and router. Providers in this setting are encouraged to have dedicated support provided by their own technical team, if they are in an academic or hospital setting, or consider contracting with vendors for equipment support. Providers who are using desktop systems with web-based software will require support for the Web site as well as the camera. It is important to get detailed information about the availability of support when contracting with web-based companies and have information on how to contact camera manufacturers or purchase a back-up camera in case of malfunction. Regardless of whether they are using a desktop or free-standing room system, all videoconferencing systems rely on a stable Internet connection, and providers will need access to support to handle Internet connection problems. Clinicians are encouraged to inquire about response times and contact numbers for support before contracting with an Internet service. Some clinicians have found it helpful to make a list of all the equipment they use for telemedicine and have a contact number for support of each item.

Technology: Bandwidth

Bandwidth is a primary determinant of the costs for Internet connectivity required to provide telemental health. When providers contract with a cable or satellite Internet company, they will typically be given a range of bandwidths to purchase. Often, the higher the bandwidth, the higher will be the cost. Options range from low-cost and generally lower bandwidth options to higher cost options with higher fixed bandwidth. Advantages associated with lower bandwidth (128 kBs) often include lower monthly costs, especially for relatively infrequent use of VTC. Potential disadvantages relate to greater pixilation and/or decreased synchrony of the audio/video signals. At lower connections speed, providers may feel less comfortable detecting nonverbal cues and have decreased reliability of observations of patient behavior. In addition, lower bandwidth options rarely have guaranteed response times by the Internet service providers if there are technical disruptions, and this can result in delays and further lost revenue before services are resumed after a disruption. Some Internet providers do not guarantee a minimum connection speed. This means that the quality of the connection can vary significantly depending on the use of the community where the lines are based, such as decreased audio and video quality at times of peak use for neighboring offices or community users. Getting this information from Internet providers up-front can aid in making decisions about bandwidth. Generally, it is the provider's bandwidth that will affect the quality of other commercial products such as secure telemental health sessions, as each of these products rely on the Internet connection to determine some aspects of the transmission quality. No matter how good the camera or software is, all telemedicine equipment relies on having a stable and fast Internet connection to be able to provide a continuous videoconference. There can be additional disruptions if the videoconferencing software does not have features that prioritize a stable connection. This problem with dropped calls can be significant in some "free" VTC options. Providers considering the use of low-bandwidth technologies may find that it impacts their comfort level with diagnoses or may find the need to augment traditional diagnostic observation with rating scales that focus on patient report.

Potential advantages associated with higher cost and higher fixed bandwidth are improved audio and video continuity with enhanced ability to detect nonverbal cues or more subtle symptoms (Grady et al., 2009; Zarate, Weinstock, & Cukkor, 1997), such as distinguishing the blunted affect of depression from neuroleptic-induced akinesia. Additional advantages offered by some high-speed dedicated lines, such as T1 lines, are mandatory response times of less than 24 h if there is technical disruption. A significant disadvantage of using T1s is the cost, which can range from US$300 to US$800 per month depending on the location. There are programs available through the Federal Communications Commission (2012), including the Rural Healthcare Program, that match line charges so that rural areas have rates that are competitive with urban rates in that state. Information about this program can be obtained through their Web site: http://transition.fcc.gov/wcb/tapd/ruralhealth/. Options now exist for skilled technical support to use a single high-speed connection, such as a T1 line, for all the data needs of a private practice (e.g., Internet, fax, telephone, and video) and simply dedicate priority for video. This can allow uninterrupted transmission of video while still allowing a single line to serve the data needs of the entire practice. Telemental health providers are encouraged to seek skilled technical support to help assess and design the technological setup for their practice.

Technical Support

It is important for providers to develop a skill set which includes familiarity with the videoconferencing equipment that they will use and an ability to do basic troubleshooting. Most equipment comes with manuals that outline basic use and options for working through technical disruptions. It is also important to obtain adequate technical support. Many Internet service providers now provide dedicated technical support. Telemental health providers are encouraged to contact local communications companies to inquire about design and support services that are available to them. When considering potential support for Internet technologies (IT), it is important to assess their availability and their experience with technology specific to VTC. Technical disruptions can result in compromised care and lost revenue if patient visits are not completed. Thus, it is important to negotiate a guaranteed response time by which the IT team will work to remedy the situation. Many providers also recommend having a suitable backup in place such as the ability to conduct the visits by phone if VTC is not available and the patient cannot be rescheduled.

Building a Referral Base and Growing a Practice

Once the initial setup is completed, there are a number of ways to build relationships with referral sources in the patient community. Some providers schedule regular visits to the patient site so that they can meet patients and other providers directly. In addition to the option to schedule FTF visit during the time on-site, a remote visit can also involve setting up open house hours where local community leaders, such as judges or hospital executives, can meet with the telemental health provider informally. When direct travel is not feasible, other techniques can be employed, such as getting local newspapers online and talking informally with staff and patients about local events over time. Patients are often excited to discuss local events and can enjoy comparing settings and weather across the telemedicine encounter. Other successful strategies to increase relationships with referral sources include making sure that the provider's records are reliably sent to the referring clinician and calling when there are relevant events in patient care. Some providers recommend routine meetings with community stakeholders to assess whether services are meeting the community's needs and monthly e-mails showing utilization rates (Shore & Manson, 2005). One option to do this is to provide staffing via VTC which has a dual advantage of more informal contact with the telemental health provider as well as allowing stakeholders to directly experience VTC for themselves. In the author's experience, good communication with referral sources and other stakeholders along with adequate transmission of records can also go a long way to building a referral base. Additional information about building relationship with distant clinicians can be found in Chapter 3. Providers also now use social networking sites or blogs to increase the name recognition of their service and to provide education to local clinicians. Conducting lectures or other presentations on mental health topics can also increase visibility within a community.

Lifestyle Benefits

The potential lifestyle benefits of a telemental health practice are limited only by the individual provider's creativity. Once basic considerations such as security, privacy, and safety for patient care are adequately addressed, multiple options exist for the provider's practice. Some providers have decided to practice from home, thus eliminating commutes and time spent away from loved ones. This has allowed providers who have young children to spend lunches and no-shows times with their children who are at home with another caregiver during the provider's work hours. Other providers have used telemental health to come up with creative practice locations, such as living on a boat and using a small office onshore to set up the VTC equipment. Some providers use telemental health to allow the seamless transition from two different practice sites, such as a winter practice in a warmer climate or transitioning from rural to urban settings during the week. Understanding these different options and lifestyle priorities for a given clinician can help them make decisions on which style of practice to pursue.

Conclusion

Telemental health is becoming an acceptable approach to meeting the nation's needs for mental health care, particularly in traditionally underserved areas. Although factors affecting the adoption of telemental health practice are profound and dynamic, perhaps the greatest impetus for private practitioners to consider telemental health practice is that people want it. Communities want telemental health to meet their citizens' needs, individuals want it as a personal choice, providers want it as a lifestyle enhancer and a way to reach new populations, while policy makers and insurers are increasingly considering it as a viable option. This field will continue to grow. The best way to make that growth sustainable is to understand the individual factors that will affect a given provider. Understanding what providers need in terms of financial security and technical support can help them to choose the option that best suits their practice needs. As this field evolves, many of the technical considerations outlined in this chapter will change dramatically as will reimbursement strategies. What will remain constant is the desire to provide high level of care to patients and providers who have enough flexibility to adapt to this new environment.

References

American Telemedicine Association. (2012). <www.americantelemed.org/> Accessed 31.03.2012.

California Telemedicine and eHealth Center. Telemedicine reimbursement handbook. (2006). <www.nrtrc.org/wp-content/uploads/Telemedicine-Reimbursement-Handbook1.pdf/> Accessed 31.03.2012.

Cash, C. (2011). Telepsychiatry and risk management. *Innovations in Clinical Neuroscience, 8*, 26–30.

Center for Medicare Services. Center for Medicare and Medicaid Services online manual. (2012). <www.cms.gov/Manuals/> Accessed 31.03.12.

Center for Medicare Services. Center for Medicare and Medicaid Services contact information. (2012). <http://www.medicare.gov/navigation/help-and-support/contact-medicare.aspx/> Accessed 28.05.2012.

Cuevas, C., Arredondo, T., & Cabrera, M. (2006). Randomized clinical trial of telepsychiatry through videoconference versus face-to-face conventional psychiatric treatment. *Telemedicine Journal and e-Health, 12,* 341−350.

Elford, R., White, H., & Bowering, R. (2000). A randomized, controlled trial of child psychiatric assessments conducted using videoconferencing. *Journal of Telemedicine and Telecare, 6,* 73−82.

Federal Communication Commission. Universal service rural health care program. (2012). <transition.fcc.gov/wcb/tapd/ruralhealth/> Accessed 31.03.2012.

Glueck, D. A. (2011). Telepsychiatry in private practice. *Child and Adolescent Psychiatric Clinics of North America, 20,* 1−11.

Grady, B., Myers, K., Nelson, E. L., & Telemental Health Standards and Guidelines Working Group (2009). *Practice guidelines for videoconferencing-based telemental health.* American Telemedicine Association. <http://www.americantelemed.org/i4a/forms/form. cfm?id=24&pageid=3717&showTitle=1>.

Hilty, D., Cobb, H., & Neufeld, J. (2008). Telepsychiatry reduces geographic physician disparity in rural settings, but is it financially feasible because of reimbursement? *Child and Adolescent Psychiatric Clinics of North America, 31,* 85−94.

Hilty, D., Yellowlees, P., & Cobb, H. (2006). Models of telepsychciatric consultation−liaison service to rural primary care. *Psychosomatics, 47,* 152−157.

Hilty, D., Yellowlees, P., & Nesbitt, T. (2006). Evolution of telepsychiatry to rural sites: Changes over time in types of referral and in primary care providers' knowledge, skills and satisfaction. *General Hospital Psychiatry, 28,* 367−373.

Hyler, S., & Gangure, D. (2003). A review of the costs of telepsychiatry. *Psychiatric Services, 54,* 976−980.

Krupinski, E. A. (2004). Telemedicine consultations: Failed cases and floundering subspecialties. *Journal of Telemedicine and Telecare, 10,* 67−69.

Modai, I., Jabarin, M., & Kurs, R. (2006). Cost effectiveness, safety and satisfaction with video telepsychiatry versus face-to-face care in ambulatory settings. *Telemedicine Journal and e-Health, 12,* 515−520.

Myers, K., Sulzbacher, S., & Melzer, S. (2004). Telepsychiatry in child and adolescent psychiatry: Are patients comparable to those in usual outpatient care? *Telemedicine Journal and e-Heath, 10,* 278−284.

Myers, K., Vander Stoep, A., McCarty, C. A., Klein, J. B, Palmer, N. B., & Geyer, J. R., et al. (2010). Child and adolescent telepsychiatry: Variations in utilization, referral patterns and practice trends. *Journal of Telemedicine and Telecare, 16,* 128−133.

Nelson, E. L., Barnard, M., & Cain, S. (2003). Treating childhood depression over videoconferencing. *Telemedicine Journal and e-Health, 9,* 49−55.

O'Reilly, R., Bishop, J., & Maddox, K. (2007). Is telepsychiatry equivalent to face-to-face psychiatry? Results from a randomized controlled equivalence trial. *Psychiatric Services, 58,* 836−843.

Rabinowitz, T., Murphy, K., Amour, J., Ricci, M., Caputo, M., & Newhouse, P. (2010). Benefits of a telepsychiatry consultation service for rural nursing home residents. *Telemedicine Journal and e-Health, 16,* 34−40.

Ruskin, P., Silver-Aylaian, M., & Kling, M. (2004). Treatment outcomes in depression: Comparison of remote treatment through telepsychiatry to in-person treatment. *American Journal of Psychiatry, 161,* 1471−1476.

Shore, J., Hilty, D., & Yellowlees, P. (2007). Emergency management guidelines for telepsychiatry. *General Hospital Psychiatry, 29*, 199–206.

Shore, J., & Manson, S. (2005). A developmental model for rural telepsychiatry. *Psychiatric Services, 56*, 976–980.

Shore, J., Savin, D., & Orton, H. (2007). Diagnostic reliability of telepsychiatry in American Indian Veterans. *American Journal of Psychiatry, 164*, 115–118.

Singh, S., Arya, D., & Peters, T. (2007). Accuracy of telepsychiatric assessment of new routine outpatient referrals. *BioMed Central Psychiatry, 7*, 55–68.

Spaulding, R., Belz, N., DeLurgio, S., & Williams, A. R. (2010). Costs savings of telemedicine utilization for child psychiatry in a rural Kansas community. *Telemedicine Journal and e-Health, 16*, 867–871.

Zarate, C., Weinstock, L., & Cukkor, P. (1997). Applicability of telemedicine for assessing patients with schizophrenia: Acceptance and reliability. *Journal of Clinical Psychiatry, 58*, 22–25.

8 Technology Options for the Provision of Mental Health Care Through Videoteleconferencing[1]

Garret Spargo[a], Ashley Karr[b] and Carolyn L. Turvey[c],*

[a]Alaska Native Tribal Health Consortium, 4000 Ambassador Drive, Anchorage, AK, [b]Iowa City VA Medical Center, 601 U.S. 6 West, Iowa City, IA, [c]Department of Psychiatry, University of Iowa Carver College of Medicine, Psychiatry Research-MEB, Iowa City, IA

Introduction

Videoteleconferencing (VTC) has long been recognized as a staple technology in the telehealth community. In the past, VTC was limited to specific networks, locations, and/or computers. Today, health care providers are increasingly comfortable with VTC and are moving toward anytime, anywhere VTC availability. Demands are being placed on organizations to offer VTC to their providers, patients, and partners with reliable, easy-to-use video capabilities. Manufacturers have responded by creating a variety of VTC software applications that support real-time audiovisual communications and that operate on personal computers (PCs). These new technologies are requiring organizations to assess needs, product capabilities, and risks posed by new venues for communication in health care.

As the concepts and operations involving VTC are the same across all health care applications, this chapter utilizes the broad and inclusive term telehealth to designate uses of VTC in medical, mental health, and educations applications. This chapter explains the concepts and terms behind VTC solutions with emphasis on desktop, or computer-based, solutions. It includes discussions on various types of desktop VTC products, bandwidth, cloud computing, audio technology, privacy concerns, and the costs and benefits of certain videoconferencing options. It also discusses the need for backup technologies and protocols in the event of VTC failure. In short, after reading this chapter, health care providers of modest

---

[1] The views expressed in this chapter are those of the authors and do not necessarily reflect the position or policy of the Department of Veterans Affairs or the US government.

* Corresponding Author: Carolyn L. Turvey, Department of Psychiatry, University of Iowa Carver College of Medicine, Psychiatry Research-MEB, Iowa City, IA 52242. Tel.: 1319353-5312, Fax: 1 319 353-3003, E-mail: Carolyn-Turvey@uiowa.edu

Telemental Health. DOI: http://dx.doi.org/10.1016/B978-0-12-416048-4.00008-7

technological knowledge and skills should be able to make an informed choice about which types of VTC equipment and programs will best serve them and their patients, how to use this equipment as efficiently and effectively as possible, how to protect the privacy of their patients, and how to ensure continuity of care if the technology fails.

Hardware and software VTC technology encompasses a wide range of devices and standards. Standardization has helped connect networks and systems more easily than in the past, but one particular, best configuration for a VTC program does not exist (Polycom, 2012; The Computer Technology Documentation Project, 2012). VTC equipment often needs to work within a larger organizational network. It is important to take the time to consider the best options available and make an informed decision based on how the equipment will be used, the technical, personnel, and space resources of all sites making use of the technology, and resource availability for technical support and upgrades in the future. Health care providers should consult information technology (IT) and privacy and security specialists in the earliest planning stages of a telehealth program.

Standards-Based Versus Consumer-Grade Software

Computer-based VTC software applications fall into one of two broad categories: standards-based or consumer-grade (Polycom, 2001). Standards-based applications communicate with existing VTC end points and other VTC systems that use standards defined by the International Telecommunications Union (ITU), their standardization sector (ITU-T), and other standards-issuing bodies (National Institute of Standards and Technology, 2001). These standards are open (nonproprietary) and can be used to facilitate communication between products from different manufacturers.

Consumer-grade software applications only communicate through consumer-grade networks—the most common being the Internet. Connections are only available between PCs that are running the manufacturer's software. These applications may follow some standards but do not support the range of ITU-T standards that would allow a full audio–videoconference with another manufacturer's VTC product. The protocols used to communicate between these software clients are mostly closed (proprietary). Servers and computers that facilitate communication between consumer-grade clients are controlled by the manufacturer.

Standards-based applications are generally more secure, more expensive, and more complicated to set up than consumer-grade. Standards-based applications support higher definition video and higher quality audio, allow for multipoint conferencing, encrypt communications, may require additional infrastructure for connecting outside of firewalls, and may necessitate using a virtual private network (VPN) or proxy device. Conversely, consumer-grade applications are generally less expensive, putatively less secure, and offer lower quality audio and video streams. They do not communicate with other VTC applications and equipment, do not require additional infrastructure for connecting outside of firewalls, and are most suited for communication outside of protected networks. Although consumer-grade applications have lower quality than standards-based applications, their quality has improved enormously in recent years and their level is often acceptable to patients, particularly in light of the current widespread use of programs such as Skype or Google Talk.

Hardware-Based Codecs

Many VTC users may not be aware of all the system's working parts but are familiar with the term *end point*. The end point is a unique location on a network that can engage in a VTC with another end point and is made up of a codec, camera, and monitor. A codec is a hardware that codes and decodes audiovisual data sent during a VTC session, acting as the brains of a VTC end point. It takes video data from the camera and transmits a video signal to the monitor, takes in audio and video information from peripheral devices (i.e., the microphone) and communicates with core infrastructure or other end points (Telehealth Technology Assessment Center, 2010). Codecs come in many shapes and sizes, from small, all-in-one units to large, computer-like boxes. Benefits of hardware-based codecs over software-based applications include greater control of security and potential for customization. Setbacks include relatively complex security and firewall issues and difficulty connecting with out-of-network users and end points if desired.

Software-Based Applications

Although many industries now use the improved software-based applications to fill their VTC needs, using consumer-grade VTC software within health care has been a point of concern. Health care professionals must be sure that applications are secure, private, and reliable enough for use in the delivery of care. The software should provide an appropriate level of security and a usable platform. The decision to implement a particular solution will depend on organizational policies and procedures, risk management, and existing technical infrastructure. If an organization chooses to use a software-based application, it should centrally manage the software installation, use, and maintenance. Before installing, it is important to know which personnel and devices need VTC access and to ensure that users outside of their network have VTC access. Policies and procedures related to account creation, software features to enable or limit, regular software updates, and security protections are needed. Despite these concerns, there are many benefits to software-based applications, such as easy integration into an organizational system, ability to communicate with users outside of the network, and low overall cost.

Mobile

Mobile products, such as tablets and cell phones, use a software system that communicates with a videoconferencing infrastructure located elsewhere such as a PC, a remote server, or the Internet. The remote software, not the mobile device, manages calls with standard hardware-based conferencing platforms.

This software may be a variation of standard VTC software-based packages from the vendors, but it specifically facilitates the functions of the mobile device. Concerns regarding using mobile products for VTC health care delivery are similar to concerns with software-based applications. Benefits include greater mobility of the VTC program, access to hard-to-reach patients, such as the homeless or those living in rural areas, ease of setup on the patient end, and low cost (Luxton, McCann, Bush, Mishkind, & Reger, 2011).

Dedicated, Direct Connections to VTC Equipment and End Points

There are a number of ways that VTC users can connect to other users and end points. A VPN allows a user outside of a network to secure and login to an open channel between the user and the network. The user is then able to access servers, programs, and files within the network.

A T1 line is a digital telecommunications line capable of sending large quantities of data relatively quickly. An important measure for digital telecommunications lines is bandwidth, which refers to how many bits can be transferred each second. A bit is the basic unit of data used in computers and can be loosely compared to the way a letter is the basic unit of data in a book. A letter makes up words, then sentences, paragraphs, chapters, and eventually an entire book. A T1 line includes 24 channels with each channel providing bandwidth of 64 kilobits per second (kbps). A full T1 can transmit data at 1.5 megabits per second (Mbps), even with multiple simultaneous users. The line can be split between transmitting voice (telephone) and data (Internet). Dedicated, direct connections to VTC equipment can occur either by working within a VPN or through a proxy edge product. A VTC proxy device that functions on the "edge" of a network allows users to access the network from the public Internet without having to use a VPN connection into the network. Whether using a VPN or proxy device, the VTC session can be done over a very fast and powerful connection (Myers, Cain, & Work Group on Quality Issues of the American Academy of Child and Adolescent Psychiatry, 2008).

Bandwidth

In computer networks, bandwidth refers to the rate that information is transmitted during online communication. It is most often measured in bits per second (bps), and the higher the bandwidth, the more seamlessly information can pass through a network. VTC can require immense amounts of bandwidth, and the amount of bandwidth required for a VTC program depends upon a number of factors. These factors create such variation in bandwidth requirements that a true standard cannot be set. Taking examples from existing VTC programs, the minimum bandwidth for a simple program was found at 128 kbps (Nelson, Barnard, & Cain, 2003) and a maximum bandwidth for a more complex system was found at 5 Mbps. The American Telemedicine Association's Practice Guidelines for Videoconferencing-Based Telemental Health recommends bandwidth of at least 384 kbps (Yellowlees, Shore, Roberts, & The American Telemedicine Association, 2010).

Bandwidth requirements vary by manufacturer of the specific videoconferencing technology, video resolution sent and received, the number of end points in a single call, the number of simultaneous calls within the larger system, and what other systems will be requiring bandwidth during the VTC. Communicating with outside organizations and patients at home will also require sufficient bandwidth to ensure connectivity and audio—video quality. To optimize existing bandwidth, some organizations may implement quality of service (QoS) tools to help control traffic and prioritize the delivery of particular content. For example, VTC content may be sent in real time, while e-mail and asynchronous communication may be sent as bandwidth is available. While QoS tools can be useful, they will add more costs to a VTC program. Organizations should consider factors such as budget, VTC product manufacturer recommendations, minimum bandwidth requirements, and computer requirements to ensure sufficient quality and operability during sessions.

A technique to estimate needed bandwidth is as follows: First model various common transmissions that will occur between two end points, and then estimate the volume of those transmissions and the data size for the type of transmission. This information can be used to recommend bandwidth needed between two end points. Second, consider the types of transmissions that occur on the organization's network beyond VTC for telemedicine, such as the general office systems and electronic medical record usage, transmission of clinical images and patient vitals, live video transmissions for administrative meetings, and voice-over Internet protocol (VOIP) traffic and calculate the bandwidth requirements of those transmissions. Third, add together the results of step one and step two to show how much bandwidth the system will require. Fourth, calculate the difference between existing bandwidth and the answer to step three. This difference represents the bandwidth needed currently not available within the organization's system. This process may not be extremely precise, but it allows for a reasonable estimate of bandwidth needs (Myers et al., 2008; Yellowlees et al., 2010).

Impact of Cloud Computing

Significant discussion has occurred regarding the use of cloud computing in personal, business, and health care applications. Many manufacturers and service providers use the term, though there does not seem to be a consensus as to exactly what constitutes "the cloud." Generally speaking, the cloud refers to using the Internet and public networks to provide access to services and resources, such as e-mail or intranet hosting, videoconferencing facilitation, and enterprise-wide backup systems. Some service providers emphasize the redundancy of cloud resources, providing multiple servers in disparate locations to reduce the likelihood of a single catastrophe or network failure from curtailing access to resources. Other service providers highlight ease of maintenance for their customers by providing and hosting all-inclusive, fully supported solutions that do not require any local staff or technical expertise. Cloud computing will facilitate telehealth in two broad ways. First, networks that are run on redundant systems "in the cloud" will be less prone to network failures due to local problems. Second, small providers will be able to offer telehealth services due to cost savings on technology resources.

Audio

Poor audio quality can be a frustrating problem with a larger negative impact than a poor video signal. This means that high-quality audio is one of the most important components of a successful VTC session. To get high-quality audio, a number of considerations must be taken into account when recording, storing, converting, and playing auditory information. These considerations allow a balance to be struck between the sound quality and the amount of audio information to be transmitted.

Microphones

Manufacturers have responded to the interest in computer-based VTC capabilities by creating a variety of software-based desktop VTC software applications that support real-time audio–video communication and operate on PCs. Microphones that may be used in VTC software applications come in a variety of styles, each with its own costs and benefits. The two main areas of difference in these microphones exist between the output type Universal Serial Bus (USB) (USB and direct) and their transducer properties (dynamic or condenser). Condenser microphones, though highly sensitive to sound, are expensive and break easily. Dynamic microphones are of adequate quality for the purposes of telehealth and they are more durable. The output type refers to the mechanism used to connect the microphone to the computer. USB outputs either can be dedicated, audio-only connections or may be a part of a combined audio–video device that sends both video and audio data to the computer.

It is important to note that these microphone outputs will typically appear as different inputs on the VTC software's configuration pages. Microphones that are connected to either the computer's direct line-in or microphone inputs on a computer will often be available as the default microphone or appear as the computer's sound card, while USB microphones will typically appear in the software settings as a specific microphone model number or manufacturer name. Most of the modern software will automatically detect a USB microphone and use it by default, if it is available.

Using external microphones may be problematic in a limited number of settings. Some computers may struggle with simultaneously processing the audio from a USB microphone and a live video source, though most modern computers are capable of handling this (Telehealth Technology Assessment Center, 2010). Problems are often manifested as a slightly delayed audio source in speakers or headphones, which can be quite disorienting to the person speaking. Note again that most modern computers are capable of handling audio from a USB microphone and do not pose any problems. Microphones with a 3.5 mm connection may be too quiet or may be prone to degradation of audio quality if the connector is overly worn or damaged.

Both primary transducer types used in microphones can be found in USB and direct varieties of microphones. Dynamic microphones provide the benefit of being sturdier and more capable of withstanding abuse, while condenser microphones are capable of providing a much more accurate capture of sounds. Dynamic microphones lose some of their sensitivity to sound in comparison to condenser microphones, while condenser microphones are more prone to damage by loud noises, moisture, and physical shock. An additional concern for condenser microphones is their need for a power source, which is not a requirement of a dynamic microphone. This power is called "phantom power" and may be delivered by a battery, external source, or USB cable. Both varieties of microphones are capable of producing an audio signal that is sufficient for use in telemedicine, and each is likely to be rugged enough to handle daily use in a controlled setting. When deciding upon which type of microphone to purchase for a VTC system, the following are a few practical considerations:

- Dynamic microphones cost less than condenser microphones. While a very expensive condenser microphone can produce finer quality sound, this difference will not greatly affect the perceived quality of sound in a VTC session. A moderately priced dynamic microphone can produce a sound quality that is acceptable during VTC sessions.
- Dynamic microphones handle abuse better than condenser microphones. If the microphone will be used daily, it is best to purchase a dynamic microphone, as it will last longer.
- Condenser microphones are more sensitive than dynamic microphones and distort and create feedback more aggressively than dynamic microphones.

Microphone placement can be very important to the overall quality of the audio in a VTC session (Wootton et al., 2003). When using a microphone that is positioned closely to the individual speaking, it may be necessary to provide a pop filter to reduce the percussive and sibilant sounds of particular vocal noises. Note that this is not often required but may be an issue if "p" or "sh" sounds result in excessively distorted or loud audio for the recipient. Moving further away from the microphone can reduce some of those sound issues but may result in reduced audio quality as many microphones will produce better sounds as the audio source gets closer to the microphone.

Other common problems with microphone placement can be the result of personal habits that may inadvertently be picked up by the microphone, such as the tapping of fingers or feet against the surface supporting the microphone, or the failure to realize that microphones may be more capable of picking up quiet audio than the human ear, rendering whispers or side conversations clear to the far end of the consulting room. Appropriate configuration of audio settings may counteract all of these problems, either by reducing microphone sensitivity or by allowing use of the mute function when needed.

Echo Cancelation

Echo is the reflected, delayed copy of an original sound. *Acoustic echo* occurs when a microphone picks up sound from a loudspeaker in the same-room, such as when a telephone's microphone picks up sound generated from the same telephone's ear-piece (Telehealth Technology Assessment Center, 2010). When direct sound from the loudspeaker enters the microphone, it is called *direct acoustic path echo*. The sound will be returned to its origin if it is not canceled, and the acoustic echo can be extremely distracting due to the slight round-trip transmission delay. This problem exists in many situations where there is a speaker and a microphone and can cause difficulty when telecommunication technology is used in patient care.

Removing echo from audio information to improve sound quality is termed *echo cancelation* and is available with most microphones. Echo cancelation occurs when an *echo suppressor* or *echo canceler* recognizes the original sound as separate from the echo or delayed copy in the transmitted or received signal. It then removes the echo by "subtracting" it from the transmitted or received signal. There are a number of ways to ensure that a microphone has echo cancelation. One is to check the product before purchase, and as always, the more expensive the microphone, the more likely it will have an echo cancelation feature clearly advertised. If the microphone is built-in or connected to a computer, VTC system, or sound system, there may be an option within the computer or system to enable echo cancelation. Additional auditory issues include "garbled" audio that is unintelligible, "delayed" audio where the audio does not come through for several seconds and then is played back at a faster or out-of-sync rate, audio feedback, quiet audio, and no audio. Garbled and delayed audio are both typically the result of connectivity problems and rarely occur unless there are also significant video problems at the same time. These problems should be treated as network connectivity issues.

Audio feedback can range from hearing an echo of your own voice to a swelling, high-pitched noise that results from the microphone picking up and playing back the audio from the speakers. Both of these issues stem from having either the speakers up too loud or too near the microphone. Note that some microphones are more prone to picking up feedback signals than others, and that this problem may be especially pronounced in laptops with built-in microphones and speakers. The problem of feedback can be resolved in a number of ways: turning down speaker volume at all end points, reducing the microphone sensitivity in a computer's *settings and options* menu, using headphones, and or purchasing a higher end professional-grade webcam or microphone.

Video

Video Standards

Consumer-grade VTC systems typically use closed-source or proprietary codecs for handling video compression and encoding of the video signal to facilitate transmission. The compression process is similar to that of making a zip file, where information is stored in fewer bits of data that can be expanded upon after transmission (Harte, 2007). Currently, the most widely used VTC video standard for standards-based VTC systems is H.264. It is used for video encoding in many consumer products and includes a number of optional components. *Scalable video coding* is one such optional component and is implemented by only a handful of vendors. This means that an additional piece of hardware or software, known as a gateway device, may be needed to convert or translate the video to a format that can be used with other products.

H.264

Video standards are an evolving concept in VTC. As new methods of optimizing, sending, and receiving video signals are developed, these methods become refined and standardized for use across various systems. One of the more frequently used standards is *H.264*, which is a standard format for compression of high-definition (HD) video data (Polycom, 2012). As stated earlier, a video signal is typically compressed, resulting in a video that requires fewer bits of data for viewing and sending. Older standards exist within the VTC world, such as the H.261 and H.263 standards. These old standards are less effective at reducing file size and are used less often by modern systems. New developments are being implemented by VTC systems as they are made available and as they can be accommodated by videoconferencing equipment. Newer standards introduced to VTC present some difficulties, however, as there may be a need to use an intermediary translator device. This device will allow two computer end points to communicate when a device using a newer standard is incompatible with a device using an older standard.

Screen-in-Screen

Also known as *picture-in-picture*, screen-in-screen refers to the VTC function that allows a user to view multiple VTC participants simultaneously (Yellowlees et al., 2010). For example, the health care providers see the patient in a large window (remote end view) and a video of themselves in a smaller window (local view) in the bottom corner of the screen. Some software allows for a split screen where one can view oneself and the person at the remote site. Sometimes, sharing content will remove the local view, putting the content on the main screen and the remote end in a small window. These windows can be turned off and not every VTC program offers these features. The content sharing standard, H.239, allows users to stream an additional video channel over an H.323 multimedia call. One feature included in this standard is often referred to as *screen sharing*, where a user can send a video image of his or her computer desktop and applications to another user. The content can appear on a secondary monitor or in a picture-in-picture layout. This feature may come in handy if a provider wants to review some written material with a patient at a remote site. The provider can call up the text file then share it with the patient at the remote site.

Camera Options and Clinical Implications

Computer-based VTC software requires a webcam to capture and send images. Some computers have built-in cameras, while others need external cameras that connect via a USB cable. Camera quality will play an important role in the VTC session's image quality. Consequently, a strong network connection will lose much of its benefit if the video quality is too low (National Center for Telehealth and Technology, 2011).

Some webcams provide HD video streams; however, there are limitations to how much video data can be sent through a USB connection. While camera sensors may be able to capture an image that qualifies as HD, extensive compression must be applied and/or frame rate must be reduced to one that falls within the limitations of the USB standard. Additionally, the stream of HD video places an enormous strain on a computer's central processing unit (CPU), which may be a limiting factor regarding image quality. To overcome this issue, some cameras contain internal hardware support and image processing that reduce the strain on the CPU and the limits of the USB transfer speed.

When using VTC for telehealth applications, it is recommended to purchase cameras that have remote control, so the clinician can pan, tilt, and zoom the camera on the patient end to allow for close-ups and for scanning of the consultation room.

Screen Size

Clinicians and personnel involved in creating a telehealth program will have to decide upon optimal screen size for their VTC sessions (Major, 2005). There is no one best screen size for videoteleconferences; instead, there are a number of considerations to make while deciding on the best screen size. The following is a list of questions based on these considerations:

- What is the patient population and what is its needs?
- What type of organization is creating the telehealth program?
- What are the security requirements for the organization?
- What other preexisting technology and equipment are available and are they compatible with all new devices?
- What cameras will be used on both patient and clinician and what are their resolutions? If a low-resolution camera is used, a high-resolution screen will be irrelevant.
- What is the budget for purchasing, maintaining, and updating new equipment?
- Where will the clinician be located during the VTC?
- Where will the patient be located during the VTC?
- What type of screen and camera will the patient have?
- Will the VTC equipment need to be mobile and portable, or will they be fixed in one particular area?
- Will overall setup give adequate representation of patients to get the necessary clinical data?

Based on the responses to these questions, decision makers can identify which screen sizes and corresponding pixel resolution will best suit their needs. Screen size is specified by units of length, such as centimeters, millimeters, or inches. Number of rows and columns of pixels describe resolution. In general, a higher resolution gives clearer images, but this also requires greater bandwidth because more information is being sent. The following table briefly describes the most common respective pixel ratios. Selection of screen size should be guided by the resolution in pixels of the VTC software:

Screen Name	Resolution in Pixels	Notes Regarding Screen Size
VGA (Video Graphics Array)	640×480	Base resolution available on the first PCs from the 1980s
SVGA (Super Video Graphics Array)	800×600	
XGA (eXtended Graphics Array)	1024×768	
SXGA (Super eXtended Graphics Array)	1280×1024	
SXGA + (Super eXtended Graphics Array Plus)	1400×1050	
WSXGA + (Wide Super eXtended Graphics Array Plus)	1680×1050	
Full HD (High Definition)	1920×1080	Resolution of Full HD movies. Note that "HD Ready" does not mean "Full HD" or "HD 10080." Most common size of computer monitors currently
WUXGA (Wide Ultra eXtended Graphics Array)	1920×1200	Many 24″ monitors come in with this resolution and are convenient for document editing because of the taller vertical axis
WQXGA (Wide Quad eXtended Graphics Array)	2560×1600	Only a few 30″ monitors that support this resolution are available

In purchasing a large HD monitor, a decision about where the monitor will be placed must also be considered. Monitors, particularly large flat screens, can be permanently fixed to a wall in the room designated for telehealth consultation. However, often flexibility about where the consultation takes place is desired. For example, consultation to busy primary care clinics with a premium on space (in short, 95% of primary care clinics) may not have the luxury of cordoning off a room for VTC alone and this may lead to scheduling conflicts. In this case, screens affixed to mobile carts may be best. Carts for VTC equipment can be designed to hold both the computer or codec and the monitor and be wheeled to wherever consultation is needed. The screens size is not limited to PC-sized monitors. Larger screens can also be mounted on carts, yet may reduce mobility (National Center for Telehealth and Technology, 2011).

As a final note, whether purchasing an HD expensive system or a commercial software package, it is important to test the system before making any final decisions and purchases. End points at both the clinician's and patient's location should be tested. If clinicians and personnel involved in creating a telehealth program develop good relationships with manufacturers, they will often be sent and allowed to test equipment before purchase. Other telehealth sites may also loan their equipment for testing during slow or off-hours. When purchasing equipment, it is advised to keep all receipts, tracking numbers, warranties, and packing materials, and take note of any policies and procedures for returning equipment for refunds or replacements. Lastly, equipment, maintenance, updates, and support vary by manufacturers and should be well researched prior to any purchase. Many companies give free technical support and software updates, but some do not. Purchasing telehealth equipment from a company with excellent customer service records can save huge amounts of time and money over the life cycle of VTC equipment.

Video Issues and Troubleshooting

VTC is a bandwidth and processor-intensive method of communicating. As such, certain problems may arise if there are insufficient resources to support the conference. Symptoms of these insufficient resources include "blocky" video where portions of images appear to freeze or slow down, "out of sync" videos where the audio and video do not match up, or "dropped" video where the audio continues but the video is no longer available. Some of the products support voice-only calls, which allow users to disable video if there is insufficient bandwidth for video content. During some patient/provider VTC sessions, disabling the video and conducting an audio-only session may provide a short-term solution. In other situations, some troubleshooting may need to be carried out. First, all end-point users should close down any extra background applications that may be using system resources, especially if they also require large amounts of bandwidth. If that does not resolve the issue, all end-point users should reboot the VTC application and reinitiate the call. If that does not fix the problem, there may be other network issues, in which case users should treat this as a connectivity problem and resolve it accordingly.

Sometimes, there will not be video at the start of a videoconference. First, users should be sure that their camera is plugged in. Second, users should go to the computer's *settings and options* menu to ensure that the web camera is selected as the application's video input. Third, users should contact their IT team or the vendor supplying the virtual "meeting room" or other designated connection. If the problem continues, the health care provider should consider ending the call and following up either via telephone or in person. The lack of video may be a concern in some settings, as it removes the ability of VTC users to visually verify their identities.

Packet Loss

Performance issues with digital telecommunication technology, such as VTC, are often caused by something called *packet loss*. Packet loss simply means that one or more packets of data sent through a network do not reach their intended end point, and it is one of the main causes of error in digital telecommunications. Due to the fact that packet loss increases as traffic over a network increases, network performance is often measured in probability of packet loss and delay.

It is important to remember that packet loss does not necessarily mean that a network connection is bad or unreliable. If delay and minor packet loss of certain data are acceptable to users, then packet loss and delay can actually help the network to run more effectively and efficiently. The amount of acceptable packet loss depends on the type of data sent. For example, a single dropped packet when transmitting a text file means losing part of that text file. This could cause serious issues on the user end and would not be acceptable. Conversely, with technology such as VOIP, losing one or two packets of data over a short period of time will not affect performance; however, once packet loss reaches 5–10%, VOIP performance will be affected. Higher rates of packet loss are often caused by network problems, translating to extremely noticeable performance issues for all data types, as well as all other network applications. Ultimately, the clinician will have to decide whether packet loss sufficiently interferes with rendering care or collecting appropriate data.

There are various ways to manage packet loss, including a number of network transport protocols and QoS tools that provide packet delivery reliability. For example, transmission control protocol is designed to handle data bottlenecks with a *slow-start connection strategy*. This strategy creates perceived packet loss on the user end, which encourages users to stop flooding the network with data until the bottleneck is cleared. The data packets that users perceived as lost will be transmitted at a later time when the network is not flooded. When using HD systems through a T1 line, packet loss may be minimized by downgrading the bandwidth being used for that connection. When using a software package on a computer-based system, the vendor can be contacted to reroute the connection.

Technology and Privacy

HIPAA Compliance and Videoteleconferences

One of the most commonly asked questions about using VTC in telehealth applications is whether it is compliant with the Health Insurance Portability and Accountability Act (HIPAA) (US Department of Health and Human Services, 1996). In many ways, this is not the correct question to ask. The IT division of each health care organization, such as a hospital or medical office, has developed its specific methods to meet HIPAA regulations. Only the specialists for the organization can truly evaluate whether or not a VTC program meets its standards for remaining HIPPA compliant. That said, one can discuss some of the key features that must be evaluated when determining if a new communication technology meets one's organizational standards.

Any clinical telehealth program used within the US health care system must comply with relevant aspects of HIPAA and The Health Information Technology for Economic and Clinical Health Act (HI-TECH ACT) enacted as part of the American Recovery and Reinvestment Act of 2009 (US Department of Health and Human Services, 2009). Title II of HIPAA, known as the administrative simplification (AS) provisions, addresses the security and privacy of health data and requires the establishment of national standards for electronic health care transactions. The AS provisions encourage electronic data interchange throughout the US health care system to increase its efficiency and effectiveness. The use of consumer-grade VTC software within the US health care system has been a point of discussion and concern in recent years. The goal when implementing these products is to provide a safe, secure, usable platform. The decision to implement a particular solution will depend on organizational policies and procedures, risk mitigation plans, technical infrastructure, and VTC experience.

What Behaviors Are Important to Maintain Privacy

Health care organizations using VTC technology must properly educate their users about good computer habits to ensure the safety of their information, as much of the potential risk comes from the users themselves. In addition, user education can increase compliance with policies and procedures by informing users of the rationale behind them. Providers who will be interacting with patients via VTC should also learn how to teach patients about the new technology. Educational materials should be provided, and employees should be taught how to present these materials to the patient. Some patients will approach this technology with trepidation, while others may assume that their level of technical knowledge exempts them from learning about the intricacies of these applications, yet both groups can benefit from educational materials. Whether working with technically savvy patients or those who actively avoid using technology, a baseline of education is critical.

Patients should be encouraged to keep a clear delineation between health- and medical-related information by keeping health care data separate from all other information. When using a consumer-grade VTC application, such as Skype, or Google Talk, it is recommended that patients create a separate account focused on health care when possible. Another point of concern includes using clearly identifiable information as a part of a display or username. Should a patient communicate with a physician or hospital employee that is working from home, the patient's name and contact information will be placed within the contact list of the employee. This means that a personal, home-based computer of an employee would contain information about patients. Additionally, it should be reaffirmed frequently that organizations will not ask for personal account information in an e-mail or text format, and users should report suspicious links or e-mails to the organization.

Encryption plays an important role in ensuring that communication is private between two parties (National Institute of Standards and Technology, 2001). While the exact mechanics and standards of encryption may vary, encryption essentially renders communication between two points secure by "scrambling" data in a manner that can only be "unscrambled" by systems that have the appropriate token or key. If information is not encrypted, a third party may be able to intercept and view messages, audio, and video.

Different portions of a VTC call may be encrypted in different ways. End-to-end encryption refers to the encryption of call data from one end point to another. There are other encryption configurations where data might be encrypted only at the bridge between the sending network and the receiving network, or other infrastructure element, meaning that data may be unencrypted for part of the call. Additionally, some systems may only encrypt the data in the call itself, leaving the call initiation data unencrypted. Ideally, a system will support end-to-end encryption, though it may be acceptable within some organizations to utilize systems that do not provide such an option.

Not all VTC applications support encryption, but those that do are generally more secure than those that do not. VTC applications that support encryption sometimes require users to enable encryption manually. If there is a manual setting for enabling encryption, providers must ensure that it is turned on for all communication, including video, audio, and instant messages. A reasonable effort needs to be made to ensure that patients understand the risks of communicating over an unencrypted channel and to provide them alternative options for communicating with an organization in the event that the system is not using encryption. Organizations may provide resources for patients to choose and implement encryption on their own systems; however, this may go beyond the skills and abilities of many users and may not be a practical choice.

Beyond the use of encryption for VTC communications, an organization may also require either full disk or partial disk encryption. Disk encryption involves using a tool to encrypt the contents of a hard drive, subsequently securing log files or recordings that may have been left on the drive. Full disk encryption is regarded as being more secure than partial disk encryption and is generally recommended.

Two additional behaviors that can cause security concerns are phishing and spam. Phishing is the attempt to gather sensitive information by posing as a trusted source. This can come across as links to sites claiming to be run by a company and will often ask for credentials or other information to be submitted into a form or sent in an e-mail. Organizations should inform users to never share their account information via e-mail or phone. Spam is the sending of unsolicited messages to a user. These may appear as requests to add contacts, to view a file or web site, or to start a VTC session. Much of these can be avoided by informing users not to accept "friend requests" from unknown sources and by having them verify the identity of any incoming requests before accepting them.

Security Standards

Advanced Encryption Standard (National Institute of Standards and Technology, 2001) and Transport Layer Security (TLS) are standards that provide encryption when engaging in conference calls (Luxton, Kayl, & Mishkind, 2012; Luxton, Sirotin, & Mishkind, 2010). They render signaling, data transfer, video, and audio information secure against those who might try to intercept a VTC session. It is important to note the separation between signaling, data, video, and audio, as some software may only encrypt video, audio, and data, while leaving call signaling unencrypted. Another important term regarding online VTC security is *Hyptertext Transfer Protocol Secure* (HTTPS), which refers to the TLS protocol used with HTTP that provides encrypted communication and secure identification of a network web server.

Backup Technologies and Protocols Should VTC Equipment Fail

Telehealth systems delivering patient care should include a backup procedure in the event that the VTC technology fails. As network or computer problems may render VTC useless, health care providers should have a plan to connect with the patient via telephone to attempt to resolve the problem or propose a follow-up plan. It can be useful to establish who will call whom, and to determine if there are standard VTC problems that will necessitate a switch to a phone conversation. This may refer to a clear, easily identifiable problem, such as a dropped call; or may be much more subjective, such as a patient or a provider deciding that the technical problems are sufficiently severe to discontinue the session and to follow up with a phone call or an in-person visit (National Center for Telehealth and Technology, 2011).

Conclusion

Health care is a rapidly changing field due in part to the pace of technological advancements at large. Health care providers and organizations must strive to keep current with new trends in technology while continuing to provide high-quality care. This chapter discussed many of the considerations that health care providers must face when creating a telehealth program for their organization. The authors hope that after reading this chapter, health care providers of modest technological knowledge and skills should be able to make an informed choice about which types of VTC equipment and programs will best serve them and their patients, how to use this equipment as efficiently and effectively as possible, how to protect the privacy of their patients, and what steps to take to ensure continuity of care if the technology fails.

References

Harte, L. (2007). Introduction to IP video: Digitization, compression and transmission. Althos Press, Morrisville, NC.

Luxton, D. D., Kayl, R. A., & Mishkind, M. C. (2012). mHealth data security: The need for HIPAA-compliant standardization. *Telemedicine Journal and E-health, 18*, 284–288.

Luxton, D. D., McCann, R. A., Bush, N. E., Mishkind, M. C., & Reger, G. M. (2011). mHealth for mental health: Integrating smartphone technology in behavioral healthcare. *Professional Psychology: Research and Practice, 42*, 505–512.

Luxton, D. D., Sirotin, A. P., & Mishkind, M. C. (2010). Safety of telemental health care delivered to clinically unsupervised settings: A systematic review. *Telemedicine Journal and E-health, 16*, 705–711.

Major, J. (2005). Telemedicine room design. *Journal of Telemedicine and Telecare, 11*, 10–14.

Myers, K., Cain, S., & Work Group on Quality Issues of the American Academy of Child and Adolescent Psychiatry (2008). Practice parameter for telepsychiatry with children and adolescents. *Journal of the American Academy of Child and Adolescent Psychiatry, 47*, 1468–1483.

National Center for Telehealth and Technology. (2011). *DoD Telehealth guidebook.* <http://t2health.org/sites/default/files/cth/guidebook/tmh-guidebook_06-11.pdf> Accessed 24.05.12.

National Institute of Standards and Technology. (2001). *Federal information processing standards Publication 197.* <http://csrc.nist.gov/publications/fips/fips197/fips-197.pdf> Accessed 24.05.12.

Nelson, E. L., Barnard, M., & Cain, S. (2003). Treating childhood depression over videoconferencing. *Telemedicine Journal and E-health, 9*, 49–55.

Polycom. (2001). *Video communications: Building blocks for a simpler deployment.* <http://www.polycom.com/global/documents/whitepapers/video_communication_building_blocks_for_simpler_deployment.pdf> Accessed 24.05.12.

Polycom. (2012). *Video white papers: H.264 high profile: The next big thing in visual communications.* <http://www.polycom.com/products/resources/white_papers/index.html> Accessed 24.05.12.

Telehealth Technology Assessment Center. (2010). <www.telehealthtac.org> Accessed 24.05.12.

The Computer Technology Documentation Project. (2010). <http://www.comptechdoc.org/> Accessed 24.05.12.

US Department of Health and Human Services. (1996). *The Health Insurance Portability and Accountability Act of 1996 (HIPPA).* <http://www.gpo.gov/fdsys/pkg/PLAW-111publ148/pdf/PLAW-111publ148.pdf> Accessed 24.05.12.

US Department of Health and Human Services. (2009). *Health Information Privacy.* <http://www.hhs.gov/ocr/privacy/hipaa/understanding/coveredentities> Accessed 24.05.12.

Wootton, R., Yellowlees, P., McLaren, P., London, S., Trust, M. N., & Health, Q. (2003). Telepsychiatryand E-mental health. Royal Society of Medicine Press, London, UK.

Yellowlees, P., Shore, J., Roberts, L., & The American Telemedicine Association (2010). Practice guidelines for videoconferencing-based telemental health. *Telemedicine Journal and E-health, 16*, 1074–1089.

Improving Access for Special Populations Through Telemental Health

9 Telemental Health in Primary Care

Avron Kriechman and Caroline Bonham

Center for Rural and Community Behavioral Health,
University of New Mexico, Albuquerque, NM

The Rationale for Collaborative and Integrative Care

Telemental health (TMH) as discussed in this chapter is defined as the provision of behavioral health services through real-time videoteleconferencing (VTC) and telephone conferencing. To consider the utility of TMH in primary care, one must first consider evolving models of care in which patients receive behavioral health services from specialists who work in collaboration with primary care providers. This may also include models of care in which patients' mental and behavioral health services are integrated within primary care as part of their customary health care (Strosahl, 1998). Strosahl has noted that only 30% of primary care visits are for an identified medical condition. Other visits involve problems related to mental health, substance abuse, or lifestyle issues. Yet, primary care has traditionally not had access to models of care sufficient to meet these needs. Thus, Blount and Miller (2009) have summarized the rationale for developing collaborative and integrative models as follows: (a) most people with mental health needs rely exclusively on a primary care provider for care; (b) the majority of those who have been treated in primary care do not then receive care from behavioral health specialists and/or care in specialty settings; (c) the course of complex and/or chronic medical disorders is complicated by comorbid mental illness, substance abuse, and/or unhealthy behaviors requiring mental health/behavioral health intervention; and (d) if unaddressed, patients' problematic behaviors, lifestyles, and psychosocial problems inflate medical costs and impede optimal outcomes. Finally, primary care patients with mental/behavioral health concerns are often reluctant to discuss these problems with their primary care providers due to stigma and/or lack of motivation related to the underlying disorder (Thielke, Vannoy, & Unutzer, 2007). Mental health and physical health problems are intricately entwined. Collaboration between primary care and mental/behavioral health systems of care is the most viable way of closing the treatment gap and making sure people receive the mental/behavioral health treatment they need.

Telemental Health. DOI: http://dx.doi.org/10.1016/B978-0-12-416048-4.00009-9
© 2013 Elsevier Inc. All rights reserved.

A Continuum of Collaboration

Doherty, McDaniel, and Baird (1996) describe a Levels of Collaboration Model with a five-point continuum of collaboration between primary care and behavioral health providers from: (a) minimum collaboration in separate facilities and/or systems; to (b) off-site linkages; to (c) on-site collaboration; to (d) teamwork; to (e) close collaboration in a fully integrated system as members of the same multidisciplinary, colocated team. They "... suggest that the Levels of Collaboration Model can be used by organizations to evaluate their current structures and procedures in light of their goals for collaboration and to set realistic next steps for change."

Four Key Concepts in Collaborative Care

The Levels of Collaboration Model dovetails with four overarching concepts related to the implementation of mental and behavioral health services within primary care. The Milbank report (Collins, Hewson, Munger, & Wade, 2010) summarizes these concepts as follows:

a. *The patient-centered medical home* including: (i) patient tracking and registry functions; (ii) the use of nonphysician staff for care management; (iii) the adoption of evidence-based treatment guidelines; (iv) patient self-management support, (v) screenings, and (vi) referral tracking.

b. *A team of health care professionals* to share responsibility for a patient's care.

c. *Stepped care* on a continuum from: (i) basic educational efforts; to (ii) psychoeducational interventions; to (iii) behavioral health interventions provided by highly trained behavioral health care professionals within primary care; to (iv) specialty mental health services.

d. *The four-quadrant clinical integration* model in which Quadrant I patients have low mental health and physical health care needs and are served in primary care; Quadrant II patients have high behavioral health and low physical health care needs and are served in specialty behavioral health systems; Quadrant III patients have high physical health care needs and low behavioral ones and are served in primary care and/or medical specialty systems; and Quadrant IV patients have high needs in both categories, requiring a strong collaboration between specialty behavioral health settings and primary and medical specialty care settings. These patients are more likely to have co-occurring disorders in all categories as well as the lack of a stable medical home.

These models of collaborative care and integrated care are the ideal toward which many health care systems now strive. They are also a major focus for health services research in which investigators assess the effectiveness of these models in improving mental and behavioral health care and outcomes. However, many factors remain to be resolved. One core issue is how to provide the mental health and behavioral health specialists who will collaborate with or integrate into primary care. TMH provides one such approach by telecommuting a broad array of specialists across vast expanses of land and diverse communities to help build new models of care. However, this work is in its infancy.

The remainder of this chapter presents some of the current approaches, successes, and challenges in using TMH to provide specialty mental/behavioral health care. While these efforts are not yet fully collaborative nor integrative, they show the way.

Tailoring TMH to Models of Care

To optimally facilitate collaborative and integrative models of care, TMH must be tailored to the needs of the health care system with which it partners. Four models for the partnering of TMH with primary care have been described.

Direct care models: This model is often considered the traditional referral or replacement model in which the telepsychiatrist is the principal provider of mental health and/or behavioral health services after an initial TMH consultation (Hilty, Yellowlees, Cobb et al., 2006). Often, patients go to a telepsychiatry clinic, separate from their primary care clinic, at which a high-definition, secured network is available that approximates in-person care. Patients and providers have endorsed high satisfaction with this model and early research supports good outcomes in equivalency trials (Fortney, Pyne et al., 2007; Morland et al., 2010; O'Reilly et al., 2007). Primary care physicians (PCPs) may prefer this approach as the telepsychiatrist assumes primary responsible for mental and behavioral health care. This model is most consistent with Doherty's aforementioned "minimum collaboration in separate facilities" and/or "off-site linkages systems" and thus does not really advance collaborative or integrative models. If the telepsychiatry site could be colocated within the primary care space, this model would approach Doherty's third level of "on-site collaboration."

Consultation care model: This model is probably the most commonly used model in telepsychiatry practice. The PCP remains the principal provider of mental and behavioral health services following a telepsychiatric consultation (Hilty, Yellowlees, Cobb et al., 2006). The consultation may be consultee centered, i.e., the telepsychiatrist consults to a referring PCP, the "consultee," either with or without the patient present (Caplan & Caplan, 2000). This approach is geared to reinforcing PCPs' skills by incorporating some training and education regarding assessment, treatment planning, interventions, disposition planning, and resource navigation. In a variation of this model, the referring PCP accompanies the patient and makes final decisions regarding implementation of the consultant's (telepsychiatrist's) recommendations. The technology that is most appropriate to these two consultative approaches has not been addressed but may be especially appropriate for PCPs who have some expertise in mental/behavioral health or seek to expand their skills and can use their office desktop computers for ready consultation with the telepsychiatrist. Szeftel et al. (2011) describe such a model in which the telepsychiatrist at the hub site and the PCP at the spoke site provide consultation to a patient. This approach best fits Doherty's level of "on-site collaboration" or perhaps "teamwork" if the PCP or telepsychiatrist incorporate other health care staff in managing the patient's care, e.g., a care manager to track follow-up visits and health indicators.

Transition to these consultative models occurs only after a considerable investment by the telepsychiatrist in relationship building which confirms ongoing commitment to the support of involved clinicians, training of staff, and linkages to resources. It also involves consciousness raising with stakeholders regarding the scarcity of psychiatric resources, a population-based health perspective, community strategies to enhance local mental health services (Foy & Perrin, 2010), and the importance of providing culturally appropriate care, especially for rural, remote, and, underserved populations (Shore, Savin, Novins, & Manson, 2006).

Collaborative care model: In outpatient care, this model fits Doherty's level of "close collaboration in a fully integrated system as members of the same multidisciplinary, colocated team." It also utilizes the aforementioned core principles described in the Milbank report (Collins et al., 2010). Approaches may vary in how the collaboration is implemented. These issues have been minimally addressed in the telepsychiatry literature (Fortney, Pyne et al., 2007). The core issue is that after initial consultation, the telepsychiatrist follows patients jointly with the PCP, using frequent communication and/or a care manager who liaises between these clinicians and who tracks patients' visits, health indicators, and "steps up" care as clinically needed (Unützer, Schoenbaum, Druss, & Katon, 2006). The optimal technology remains to be addressed. Determining factors may include cost, number of PCPs involved in the collaboration, the frequency of use, and whether the collaboration can be done from a clinician's or care manager's office or requires dedicated space. Thus, choices vary from high-definition, secure, point-to-point end point systems using T1 lines to inexpensive, publically available commercial systems that operate on desktop computers.

A fully implemented model of collaborative care involves a major paradigm shift for PCPs, as well as other health care providers and systems. Making this paradigm shift concurrently with introducing telepsychiatry (Shore & Manson, 2005), or more generally TMH, for the provision of mental/behavioral health care will likely take considerable time and adjustment for participants, ideally led by committed TMH staff (Kessler, Stafford, & Messier, 2009; National Council for Community Behavioral Health Care, 2009).

Kriechman, Salvador, and Adelsheim (2010) have described a variant of this collaborative care model. Our model coordinates and supports the efforts of a patient's network of care. The network may include family members, peer supports, behavioral care providers, specialty care providers, educators, case managers, paraprofessionals, and other community supports in addition to referring PCPs. In this model, the collaboration is between specialty mental/behavioral health care and the patient's "medical home." It is consistent with Doherty's level of "close collaboration in a fully integrated system as members of the same multidisciplinary, colocated team." Our model transcends Doherty's levels as it also actively includes patients' families and community supports thereby basing care on patients' culture, language, and healing belief systems and practices (Bitar, Springer, Gee, Graff, & Schydlower, 2009; Foy & Perrin, 2010). Further, our model does not require the patient's support system to assemble in the same facility, nor even by videoconferencing, to integrate care. Working parents, providers, paraprofessionals, and community members may join by telephone, which is a more convenient modality for gathering the patient's network together, and is more likely to involve individuals who might otherwise not be able to join. Further, it precludes the technical difficulties that can be encountered when attempting to link multiple sites through videoconferencing.

When implementing one of these models of care and utilizing TMH as the mechanism to provide specialty mental/behavioral health care, appropriate steps need to be taken to ensure that TMH will be a "good fit," such as obtaining an assessment of the services needed, the population to be served, PCPs' comfort with TMH, and the technical and support resources available (Shore & Manson, 2005). Additionally, providers should be familiar with the evolving best practice guidelines for TMH (Telemental Health Standards and Guidelines Working Group, 2009).

TMH Consultation and Collaboration for Children, Adolescents, and Their Families

Case reports and program descriptions have generally supported the feasibility and acceptability to stakeholders of using TMH for the evaluation and treatment of children and adolescents. Mostly consultative models have been described.

Primary Care Sites

Several states have funded consultee-centered consultation services by telephone to aid PCPs in their management of children's mental/behavioral health problems. Sarvet, Gold, and Straus (2011) developed the first such program, the Massachusetts Child Psychiatry Access Project (MCPAP). MCPAP offers PCPs a range of services from answering a simple medication question to behavioral health training and continuing education, to accepting a referral for an acute psychopharmacologic or diagnostic concern. The program also provides outreach to school-based health centers.

In the State of Washington, the Partnership Access Line (PAL) program augments telephone consultation with a psychiatric assessment in-person or through VTC if clinical complexity precludes satisfactory telephone consultation to the referring PCP (Hilt, McDonell, Rockhill, Golombek, & Thompson, 2009). Selected sites across the state have telehealth clinics with high-definition/high-bandwidth VTC access that connects securely to Seattle Children's Hospital. Over 4 years, the PAL program has provided over 2000 such telephone consultations. The PAL program has been highly rated by participating providers and has expanded services into Wyoming.

This approach to supporting PCPs is being explored by multiple other states. Currently, 26 states are undertaking related efforts. The National Network of Child Psychiatry Access Programs at the Center for Mental Health Services in Primary

Care at Johns Hopkins Bloomberg School of Public Health is now coordinating information and interaction of these programs (www.nncpap.org) in order to train the next generation of child psychiatry consultants.

Another consultation program provides services to very rural and remote communities of First Nations people. The TeleLink Mental Health Program at The Hospital for Sick Children and the University of Toronto provides clinical consultation, education, evaluation, and research to primary care settings through VTC (Pignatiello et al., 2011). PCPs then continue care. This highly successful program connects to these remote sites at a maximum bandwidth of 384 kbits/s through integrated services digital network lines or Internet protocols (IP) without major technical difficulties. This group notes that key components of successful implementation include clear communication, the cooperation of both the children and parents, involvement of the schools and local health providers, and stability of the local agencies (Boydell, Volpe, Kertes, & Greeberg, 2007).

A somewhat different consultation model has been used by the TMH program at the University of California at Davis (Yellowlees, Hilty, Marks, Neufeld, & Bourgeois, 2008). This well-established and extensive program includes predominantly rural communities within a 33-county area. Both telepsychiatric and telepsychological consultation services are offered for children and adolescents. The consulting telemental specialist first meets with the patient and then the PCP joins for 5–10 min at the end of the consultation in order to discuss options for ongoing services. This program has found that 3 months after such consultation, parents reported improved behaviors on a standardized rating scale (Yellowlees, Hilty et al., 2008).

Seattle Children's Hospital in Seattle, Washington, offers a mixed model in which individual telepsychiatrists decide how to structure their services, i.e., either consultative or direct services even to the point that the patient "ages out" of the program (Myers, Vander Stoep, McCarty et al., 2010). Services are provided through high-bandwidth (512 kbits/s to 1 MB/s), high-definition, secured networks (IP/T1 lines) at several community clinics with VTC capability. The referring PCP remains involved through telephone feedback and written reports. Thus, the program is aimed at filling a service gap rather than building PCPs' skills or knowledge. This program reports that both parents (Myers, Valentine, & Melzer, 2008) and providers (Myers, Valentine, & Melzer, 2007) experience a high level of satisfaction with their care and that telepsychiatry is feasible for a large number of mental/behavioral health problems (Myers et al., 2007). Further, this program found that youth referred to telepsychiatry were comparable in terms of demographics, diagnosis, payer status, and reimbursement (Myers, Sulzbacher, & Melzer, 2004), to youth evaluated in a traditional face-to-face outpatient psychiatry clinic—suggesting that telepsychiatry treats a representative sample of children and youth in need of mental health care.

Telepsychology programs with children and adolescents do not appear to be as common as telepsychiatry programs. Van Allen, Davis, and Lassen (2011) have described several clinical efforts at the Kansas University Medical Center's (KUMC) Center for Telemedicine and Telehealth, including the "Healthy Hawks Clinic" for childhood obesity. This multidisciplinary clinic at KUMC brings together a pediatric dietitian, a physician or nurse practitioner, and a pediatric psychologist who use a disease management model (Collins et al., 2010) to evaluate and treat patients at distant sites through VTC. As most of these distant sites do not have access to high-bandwidth VTC equipment, the sessions are conducted at lower bandwidths with overall good connectivity and successful clinical practice. This innovative program appears to be the best TMH-mediated collaborative model that approximates Doherty's higher levels of "on-site collaboration" and "teamwork."

School-Based Health Centers

School-based health centers offer a naturalistic setting to provide health care services with unique opportunities for collaboration between educators, primary care clinicians, and mental/behavioral health care specialists. Thus, they expand the telehealth model across disciplines. Two models are presented here.

The University of Texas Medical Branch Telehealth for School-Based Mental Health Program (*The Brown University Child and Adolescent BehaviorLetter*, 2009) provides telemental consultation to underserved minority children and adolescents in Galveston County School-Based Teen Clinics. Approximately, one-third of their patients are Hispanics and another one-third are African-Americans. This program attests to the ability to use TMH to reach racial and ethnic minority youth.

As part of spectrum of TMH services provided to rural, remote, and underserved communities throughout the state of New Mexico, the University of New Mexico (UNM) Center for Rural and Community Behavioral Health (CRCBH) Telepsychiatry Program provides strengths-based, community-oriented, school-based mental/behavioral health services (Kriechman et al., 2010). This service involves school staff to improve their understating and management of children's difficulties. High-bandwidth VTC is used, with telephone connections as a backup as there is often a lack of technological supports at the school site when problems arise. Further, this program emphasizes the involvement of multiple members of the child's family and support system. The telephone allows all of these stakeholders in the child's network to participate without giving up work, traveling long distances, or compromising other important duties. The UNM CRCBH also teams psychiatrists, psychologists, social workers, and counselors to provide a continuing education training series via telephone and VTC targeted to schools, primary care, and behavioral health clinicians, as well as anthropologists and epidemiologists. Each session provides ample time for interdisciplinary case discussions and treatment planning.

TMH Consultation and Collaboration for Adults

Epidemiological data reveal increased rates of poverty and mental health conditions in rural areas compared to metropolitan regions (Simmons & Havens, 2007) and suggest that there are more barriers to mental health care in these communities (Hauenstein et al., 2007). TMH is a service delivery model with the potential to extend access to mental health care in rural communities and particularly to reach chronically mentally ill adults who are particularly underserved (Grubaugh, Cain, Elhai, Patrick, & Frueh, 2008). The following section reviews several TMH models used to facilitate consultation and collaboration between PCPs and mental health care providers.

Direct Care Models

Direct care models are a common approach described in the literature. Different levels of technology have been used. Direct services have elicited positive attitudes toward TMH among individuals who reside in rural areas and are seeking mental health care, in part due to the benefit of reduced travel time to distant mental health clinics (Grubaugh et al., 2008). Existing research suggests that clinical processes and outcomes are similar for patients who receive their mental health care in their primary care clinics via VTC compared to patients who receive in-person psychiatric treatment. Most reports of direct service TMH models fit Doherty's level of "minimum collaboration in separate facilities and/or systems." However, one study conducted at the Veterans' Administration (VA) has successfully implemented service delivery consistent with Doherty's description of "on-site collaboration." This randomized clinical trial conducted within the primary care system of VA showed comparable outcomes in medication adherence, patient satisfaction, and health care costs for veterans treated through TMH and those in usual treatment (Ruskin et al., 2004).

Consultation Care Model

Consultation models through TMH between primary care providers and mental health specialists have been developed in order to both expand workforce capacity in underserved areas and offer continuing education to primary care providers for common mental/behavioral health problems.

At the UNM, Project ECHO has utilized VTC to provide over 10,000 consultations on chronic disease management to PCPs in rural areas including mental illness and substance abuse management (Arora et al., 2011). Specialists offer regularly scheduled didactic presentations over high-bandwidth VTC with multiple PCPs participating across the state. In our experience, case-based learning is the most effective, skill-oriented, interactive training geared to increase the capacity of PCPs to address the mental health needs of their patients. At the beginning of each weekly 90-min teleconferencing training, we poll the attendees to learn their needs and whether they have particular patients they want to discuss related to the topic at hand. We then adapt the formal presentation to the needs of the attendees. PCPs have opportunities to ask specific guidance around de-identified cases and to share their own knowledge and resources with other participants. We emphasize the utilization of attendees as collaborators and coconsultants gradually creating multidisciplinary consultation teams in local communities.

Hilty, Yellowlees, and Nesbitt (2006) describe their experience with another TMH consultation approach. In this model, the telepsychiatrists conducted clinical assessments and then communicated with the referring PCPs in several ways: by a written consultation note within 10 min of the assessment, being available for telephone consultations, inviting PCPs to participate in joint TMH consultations, and/ or by offering continuing education lectures via VTC. They found that it may take time for providers to become accustomed to the new technology and consultation processes, but that over time, participating providers improved their knowledge about the use of psychotropic medications and reported increasing satisfaction over time with these consultations.

Neufeld, Yellowlees, Hilty, Cobb, and Bourgeois (2007) developed a TMH consultation aimed at increasing the availability of both psychiatry and psychology expertise in rural primary care clinics. This multipronged initiative involved access to telepsychiatric consultation, telepsychological assessment and short-term treatment, and continuing education on topics relevant to primary care. It also employed secure electronic messaging to enhance communication between off-site mental health specialists and PCPs through "rapid consultation" without the requirement for simultaneous (synchronous) availability of both the primary care provider and the specialist consultant. The clinic used a secure Internet-based messaging system providing password-protected authentication, encrypted access via any Internet browser, notification of waiting messages via fax or regular e-mail, and secure storage of messages. The authors report no difficulties maintaining the security of communications using this system. Patients' psychiatric symptoms improved over the course of this project. Interestingly, however, participating PCPs did not use the electronic messaging to consult with psychologists. One possible explanation could be that this group of PCPs had limited experience in working with psychologists and were unfamiliar with the expertise available. It is possible that offering interdisciplinary consults from a distance may necessitate further training of providers and/or a move toward more integrative models in which psychological services are embedded in the primary care clinic. Telehealth is amenable to such approaches.

In general, PCPs who receive teleconsultation for mental health topics express high levels of satisfaction. PCPs in rural areas may especially benefit from TMH. Hilty, Nesbitt, Kuenneth, Cruz, and Hales (2007) found that, compared to providers in suburban primary care sites, those in rural areas attended more teleconsultation sessions, indicated higher levels of satisfaction, and they made more changes in treatment based upon the recommendations of telepsychiatrists.

Collaborative Care Models

Collaborative care models developed for the treatment of depression and anxiety in primary care settings are associated with improved quality of care and health outcomes (Gilbody, Bower, Fletcher, Richards, & Sutton, 2006). These models embed mental health expertise in the primary care setting in innovative ways. For example, they train care managers to screen for depression and anxiety, to track cases to ensure that they receive timely follow-up, to assess treatment adherence, and to facilitate referral to a higher level of care if needed. Care managers liaise between the PCP and the collaborating psychiatrist in order to provide evidence-based medication management. On a weekly basis, the care managers meet with the psychiatrist to discuss patients' progress including reporting changes on symptom-based rating scales or other standardized measures used to monitor progress. These collaborative care models use systematic assessments and treatment protocols to ensure that treatment is progressing and, if not, to make needed changes in a timely manner. After the care manager reviews a patient's progress with the psychiatrist, the psychiatrist makes treatment recommendations which the care manager then conveys to the PCPs for implementation at their discretion. This includes intensifying, or stepping up, treatment for those patients who are not improving. In this model, the psychiatrists are not necessarily on-site with the care managers and their patient reviews may be conducted by telephone and other media, an obvious appeal for TMH. Investigation of the use of TMH in collaborative care models is just beginning.

Researchers at the University of Arkansas for Medical Sciences and the Veterans Administration have conducted a multisite, randomized clinical trial of collaborative care for the treatment of depression using TMH versus treatment as usual (Fortney, Pyne et al., 2007). On-site PCPs used TMH and electronic health records to collaborate with an off-site interdisciplinary team which included psychiatrists, pharmacists, and a nurse care manager. The nurse care manager contacted enrolled patients to: (a) assess their symptoms of depression; (b) provide psychoeducation; (c) make efforts to engage them in treatment; (d) assess medication adherence; and (e) systematically monitor medication side effects. Off-site pharmacists and psychiatrists reviewed this information and then used TMH to offer pharmacotherapy recommendations to the on-site PCPs. Patients receiving this collaborative care approach were more likely to adhere to their medication regimen, achieve remission of their depression, and experience improved quality of life (Fortney, Pyne et al., 2007). Cost-effectiveness analyses demonstrated that, compared to treatment as usual, patients in the intervention group had higher costs and utilization of mental health services; however, there was no difference in the total utilization or costs associated with all primary care encounters (Fortney, Maciejewski, Tripathi, Deen, & Pyne, 2011; Yeung, Hails, Chang, Trinh, & Fava, 2011). These findings suggest that depression treatment tends to be underutilized in primary care settings and that the addition of collaborative care via TMH is a cost-acceptable method for improving health outcomes. Yeung et al. have adapted this model to expand access to depression treatment for Chinese-Americans in primary care settings and report success in implementation (Ackerman, Pyne, & Fortney, 2009).

One of the critical components of collaborative care models is the role of the care manager. As described by Ackerman et al. (2009), the role of a care manager is generally quite complex and the responsibility of providing these services at a distance can be particularly challenging (Pyne et al., 2010). Care managers need extensive communication and interpersonal skills in order to pick up nuances in telephone consultations; the ability to balance competing demands involved in triaging requests for psychiatric consultation while simultaneously providing interim support; and the flexibility to follow scripted protocols aimed at obtaining consistent health outcome data while displaying empathy and active listening in order to build trust with patients. Some of the challenges involved in performing these duties remotely include professional isolation and a sense of burden associated with the responsibility of being the primary source of contact and support to a potentially vulnerable group of patients. In TMH applications of the collaborative care model, it may be preferable to colocate the care manager at the primary care site. This would provide collegial support, help foster the relationship with the PCPs, and possibly provide patients the opportunity for contact with an on-site staff. The challenge then is for the distant team, including the telepsychiatrist, to provide supervision for this complex role over VTC.

It is our experience that trainings that include role–play interactions achieve the best results when the care manager plays the role of the patient and the trainer (often the telepsychiatrist) plays the role of the care manager. The telepsychiatrist models the listening, communication, and liaison skills required in coconducting and collaborating in patient interviews. They can then switch roles to allow the care manager to demonstrate interviewing skills. After these role–play trainings, the care manager is asked to be present at the TMH interviews of the patients. With experience, care managers are encouraged to become increasingly involved in the interview process. For some patients who are "stepped up" in care, the telepsychiatrist will need to provide a direct assessment. An additional benefit of colocating the care manager at the PCP site is that the care manager becomes the "eyes" of the TMH consultant if the video link is lost and assessment must be completed by telephone. Hopefully, further exploration and examination of the use of TMH in collaborative care models will be forthcoming.

Asynchronous Telepsychiatry

The use of asynchronous (also known as "store and forward") TMH may also play a role in primary care. This technology records a clinical interview which can then be forwarded to a consulting mental health specialist who reviews the video at a later time. Many primary care sites are staffed by multiple providers who share a single full-time position. Providers are often overscheduled so that it becomes difficult to find a common time for a multidisciplinary collaborative team meeting. Asynchronous TMH avoids these scheduling difficulties.

Currently, the use of this technology has been limited because it is only reimbursable in the states of Hawaii and Alaska through federal demonstration projects. In a pilot study, nonpsychiatric clinicians recorded interviews of patients using a structured diagnostic assessment. The recordings of the interviews were then forwarded to telepsychiatrists who provided written feedback including diagnostic impressions and treatment suggestions (Yellowlees, Odor et al., 2010).

There may be some limitations to this approach. Specifically, there are some concerns that asynchronous telepsychiatry may not provide adequate diagnostic reliability (Singh, Arya, & Peters, 2007). Further, we have found that community clinicians are disinclined to employ structured diagnostic interviews because they are viewed as being overly rigid, insensitive to cultural and local understandings and languages, and inflexible to the demands of the patient—provider relationship. We have also found that local clinicians may view structured interviews as meeting the research needs of the consultant rather than the clinical needs of the community. This approach may be more acceptable if the interviewing clinician is a community member who is on-site with the patient so as to mix therapeutic contact with the inflexible structured interview. Further work is needed to address the feasibility of using asynchronous approaches to incorporate TMH services into primary care.

Cultural Considerations

Extending mental health services to primary care is an important method of reaching traditionally underserved populations since non-Caucasian individuals are less likely to seek care in specialty mental health settings (Gallo, Marino, Ford, & Anthony, 1995). When using any of these models to provide care to different cultural groups, it can be helpful to consider how TMH may help or hinder efforts to provide culturally appropriate care. As noted by Carpenter-Song, Schwallie, and Longhofer (2007), cultural competence involves being attentive to needs at the individual level, as well as the larger system level to ensure that programs are thoughtfully developed to meet the needs of the clients served. Therefore, telepsychiatrists working in primary care settings should reflect on their own clinical interactions as well as any implications of the model selected for the groups being served. Shore et al. (2006) have described some of the adaptations they have incorporated into their telepsychiatry work with Native American communities in order to establish rapport. For example, on an individual level, they have found it helpful to frame the camera image so as to include the entire torso rather than only the face. They suggest that this technique minimizes intense direct eye contact and provides more information about additional nonverbal cues. As an example of a clinic-level intervention, Yeung et al. (2011) were attuned to beliefs and practices of Chinese-Americans regarding mental health problems. Therefore, to make their clinical work culturally sensitive and meaningful, they altered their interview protocol to incorporate patients' beliefs and attitudes regarding the causes and treatment of mental health problems (Ackerman et al., 2009).

In the UNM CRCBH consultative programs, when presenters use telehealth to offer didactics and case consultations, they routinely ask all participants to share how local culture influences clinical presentations and treatment strategies. This deliberate attention to culture results in rich discussion and new insights for all participants—including the presenters and consultants.

Conclusion

Over the last decade, many organizations have used TMH to provide direct service and consultative models of care in an attempt to improve access to expert mental health services in primary care settings. In contrast, efforts to offer collaborative care models of chronic disease management via TMH represent a new direction in care. Currently, most of the research on the use of TMH with the collaborative care model has focused on the screening and treatment of depression. However, as evidence accumulates regarding the effectiveness of collaborative care in treating other psychiatric conditions (Myers, Vander Stoep, Thompson, Zhou, & Unitzer, 2010; Rollman et al., 2005), it will become important to determine how to incorporate TMH into these models so as to optimally redistribute the mental health workforce and to reach all populations in need of expert mental health care.

Finally, the financial implications of developing collaborative models of care through TMH must be considered. The preliminary work by Pyne et al. (2010) suggests that the financial burden of offering TMH care will come out of mental health budgets, whereas potential cost savings will be realized in primary care budgets (Fortney, Maciejewski et al., 2011). Additionally, the interdisciplinary structure of collaborative models does not fit easily into fee-for-service reimbursement mechanisms. Further, many rural and underserved patients who could benefit from TMH care are uninsured or covered by Medicaid programs possibly making TMH-mediated collaborative care models unsustainable. New approaches to financing will be needed.

Barriers remain. But, as national health care reform moves forward, consultative models of mental/behavioral health care will be expanded and collaborative care models will become more desirable, perhaps even mandated, for currently underserved populations. The role for TMH in a new collaborative, and eventually integrated, primary care paradigm needs to be defined—and grown.

References

Ackerman, B., Pyne, J. M., & Fortney, J. C. (2009). Challenges associated with being an off-site depression care manager. *Journal of Psychosocial Nursing and Mental Health Services*, *47*, 43–49.

Arora, S., Kalishman, S., Dion, D., Som, D., Thornton, K., Bankhurst, A., et al. (2011). Partnering urban academic medical centers and rural primary care clinicians to provide complex chronic disease care. *Health Affairs*, *30*, 1176–1184.

Bitar, G. W., Springer, P., Gee, R., Graff, C., & Schydlower, M. (2009). Barriers and facilitators of adolescent behavioral health in primary care: Perceptions of primary care providers. *Families, Systems and Health: The Journal of Collaborative Family Healthcare*, *27*, 346–361.

Blount, A., & Miller, B. (2009). Addressing the workforce crisis in integrated primary care. *Journal of Clinical Psychology in Medical Settings*, *16*, 113–119. doi:10.1007/s10880-008-9142-7.

Boydell, K. M., Volpe, T., Kertes, A., & Greeberg, N. (2007). A review of the outcomes of the recommendations made during pediatric telepsychiatry consultations. *Journal of Telemedicine and Telecare, 13*, 277–281.

Caplan, G., & Caplan, R. (2000). Principles of community psychiatry. *Mental Health Journal, 36*(1), 7–24.

Carpenter-Song, E. A., Schwallie, M. N., & Longhofer, J. (2007). Cultural competence reexamined: Critique and directions for the future. *Psychiatric Services, 58*, 1362–1365.

Collins, C., Hewson, D. L., Munger, R., & Wade, T. T. (2010). *Evolving models of behavioral health integration in primary care. Milbank memorial fund.* <www.integratedprimarycare.com/Milbank%20Integrated%20Care%20Report.pdf> Accessed 02.01.12.

Doherty, W. J., McDaniel, S. H., & Baird, M. A. (1996). Five levels of primary care/behavioral healthcare collaboration. *Behavioral Healthcare Tomorrow, October*, 25–27.

Fortney, J., Pyne, J., Edlund, M., Williams, D., Robinson, D., Mittal, D., et al. (2007). A randomized trial of telemedicine-based collaborative care for depression. *Journal of General Internal Medicine, 22*, 1086–1093.

Fortney, J. C., Maciejewski, M. L., Tripathi, S. P., Deen, T. L., & Pyne, J. M. (2011). A budget impact analysis of telemedicine-based collaborative care for depression. *Medical Care, 49*, 872–880.

Foy, J. M., & Perrin, J. (2010). Enhancing pediatric mental health care: Strategies for preparing a community. *Pediatrics, 125*, S75. doi:10.1542/peds.2010-0788D.

Gallo, J. J., Marino, S., Ford, D., & Anthony, J. C. (1995). Filters on the pathway to mental health care, II. Sociodemographic factors. *Psychological Medicine, 25*, 1149–1160.

Gilbody, S., Bower, P., Fletcher, J., Richards, D., & Sutton, A. J. (2006). Collaborative care for depression: A cumulative meta-analysis and review of longer-term outcomes. *Archives of Internal Medicine, 166*, 2314–2321.

Grubaugh, A. L., Cain, G. D., Elhai, J. D., Patrick, S. L., & Frueh, B. C. (2008). Attitudes toward medical and mental health care delivered via telehealth applications among rural and urban primary care patients. *Journal of Nervous and Mental Disease, 196*, 166–170.

Hauenstein, E., Petterson, S., Rovnyak, V., Merwin, E., Heise, B., & Wagner, D. (2007). Rurality and mental health treatment. *Administration and Policy in Mental Health and Mental Health Services Research, 34*, 255–267.

Hilt, R., McDonell, M. G., Rockhill, C., Golombek, A., & Thompson, J. (2009). The partnership access line: Establishing an empirically based child psychiatry consultation program for Washington State. *Report on Emotional and Behavioral Disorders in Youth, 9*, 9–12.

Hilty, D. M., Nesbitt, T. S., Kuenneth, C. A., Cruz, G. M., & Hales, R. E. (2007). Rural versus suburban primary care needs, utilization, and satisfaction with telepsychiatric consultation. *Journal of Rural Health, 23*, 163–165.

Hilty, D. M., Yellowlees, P. M., Cobb, H. C., Bourgeois, J. A., Neufeld, J. D., & Nesbitt, T. S. (2006). Models of telepsychiatric consultation-liaison service to rural primary care. *Psychosomatics, 47*, 152–157.

Hilty, D. M., Yellowlees, P. M., & Nesbitt, T. S. (2006). Evolution of telepsychiatry to rural sites: Changes over time in types of referral and in primary care providers' knowledge, skills and satisfaction. *General Hospital Psychiatry, 28*, 367–373.

Kessler, R., Stafford, D., & Messier, R. (2009). The problem of integrating behavioral health in the medical home and the questions it leads to. *Journal of Clinical Psychology in Medical Settings, 16*, 4–12. doi:10.1007/s10880-009-9146-y.

Kriechman, A., Salvador, M., & Adelsheim, S. (2010). Expanding the vision: The strengths-based, community-oriented child and adolescent psychiatrist working in schools. *Child and Adolescent Psychiatric Clinics of North America, 19*, 149−162.

Morland, L. A., Greene, C. J., Rosen, C. S., Foy, D., Reilly, P., Shore, J., et al. (2010). Telemedicine for anger management therapy in a rural population of combat veterans with posttraumatic stress disorder: A randomized noninferiority trial. *Journal of Clinical Psychiatry, 71*, 855−863.

Myers, K., Sulzbacher, S., & Melzer, S. M. (2004). Telepsychiatry with children and adolescents: Are patients comparable to those evaluated in usual outpatient care? *Telemedicine Journal and e Health, 10*, 278−285.

Myers, K., Valentine, J., & Melzer, S. (2007). Feasibility, acceptability, and sustainability of telepsychiatry for children and adolescents. *Psychiatric Services, 58*, 1493−1496. doi:10.1176/appi.ps.58.11.1493.

Myers, K., Vander Stoep, A. V., Thompson, K., Zhou, C., & Unitzer, J. (2010). Collaborative care for the treatment of Hispanic children diagnosed with attention-deficit hyperactivity disorder. *General Hospital Psychiatry, 32*, 612−614.

Myers, K. M., Valentine, J. M., & Melzer, S. M. (2008). Child and adolescent telepsychiatry: Utilization and satisfaction. *Telemedicine Journal and e-Health, 14*, 131−137.

Myers, K. M., Vander Stoep, A., McCarty, C. A., Klein, J. B., Palmer, N. B., Geyer, J. R., et al. (2010). Child and adolescent telepsychiatry: Variations in utilization, referral patterns and practice trends. *Journal of Telemed and Telecare, 16*, 128−133.

National Council for Community Behavioral Health Care. *Behavioralhealth/primary care integration and the person-centered healthcare home community.* (2009). <http://www.thenationalcouncil.org/galleries/resources-services%20files/Integration%20and%20Healthcare%20Home.pdf> Accessed 02.01.12.

Neufeld, J. D., Yellowlees, P. M., Hilty, D. M., Cobb, H., & Bourgeois, J. A. (2007). The e-mental health consultation service: Providing enhanced primary-care mental health services through telemedicine. *Psychosomatics, 48*, 135−141.

O'Reilly, R., Bishop, J., Maddox, K., Hutchinson, L., Fisman, M., & Takhar, J. (2007). Is telepsychiatry equivalent to face-to-face psychiatry? Results from a randomized controlled equivalence trial. *Psychiatric Services, 58*, 836−843.

Pignatiello, A., Teshima, J., Boydell, K. M., Minden, D., Vople, T., & Braunberger, P. G. (2011). Child and youth telepsychiatry in rural and remote primary care. *Child and Adolescent Psychiatric Clinics of North America, 20*, 13−28.

Pyne, J. M., Fortney, J. C., Tripathi, S. P., Maciejewski, M. L., Edlund, M. J., & Williams, D. K. (2010). Cost-effectiveness analysis of a rural telemedicine. *Mental Health Services, 47*, 43−49.

Rollman, B. L., Belnap, B. H., Mazumdar, S., Houck, P. R., Zhu, F., Gardner, W., et al. (2005). A randomized trial to improve the quality of treatment for panic and generalized anxiety disorders in primary care. *Archives of General Psychiatry, 62*, 1332−1341.

Ruskin, P. E., Silver-Aylaian, M., Kling, M. A., Reed, S. A., Bradham, D. D., Hebel, J. R., et al. (2004). Treatment outcomes in depression: Comparison of remote treatment through telepsychiatry to in-person treatment. *American Journal of Psychiatry, 161*, 1471−1476.

Sarvet, B., Gold, J., & Straus, J. H. (2011). Bridging the divide between child psychiatry and primary care: The use of telephone consultation within a population-based collaborative system. *Child and Adolescent Psychiatric Clinics of North America, 20*, 41−53.

Shore, J., & Manson, S. (2005). A developmental model for rural telepsychiatry. *Psychiatric Services, 56*, 976−980.

Shore, J., Savin, D., Novins, D., & Manson, S. M. (2006). Cultural aspects of telepsychiatry. *Journal of Telemedicine and Telecare, 12*, 116−121.

Simmons, L. A., & Havens, J. R. (2007). Comorbid substance and mental disorders among rural Americans: Results from the national comorbidity survey. *Journal of Affective Disorders, 99*, 265−271.

Singh, S. P., Arya, D., & Peters, T. (2007). Accuracy of telepsychiatric assessment of new routine outpatient referrals. *BMC Psychiatry, 7*, 55. doi:10.1186/1471-244X-7-55<http://www.biomedcentral.com/1471-244X/7/55>

Strosahl, K. (1998). Integrating behavioral health and primary care services: The primary mental health care model. In A. Blount (Ed.), *Integrated primary care: The future of medical and mental health collaboration* (pp. 139−166). New York, NY: W.W. Norton.

Szeftel, R., Mandelbaum, S., Sulman-Smith, H., Naqvi, S., Szeftel, Z., Coleman, S., et al. (2011). Telepsychiatry for children with developmental disabilities: Applications for patient care and medical education. *Child and Adolescent Psychiatric Clinics of North America, 20*, 95−111.

Telemental Health Standards and Guidelines Working Group. (2009). In B. Grady, K. Myers, E. L. Nelson (Chairs). *Practice guidelines for videoconferencing-based telemental health.* American Telemedicine Association. <http://www.americantelemed.org/files/public/standards/PracticeGuidelinesforVideoconferencing-BasedTeleMentalHealth.pdf>.

The Brown University Child and Adolescent Behavior Letter. (2009). *25*, 5−6. UTMB Health Policy and Legislative Affairs web site: <http://www.utmbhpla.org/oth/Page.asp?PageID=OTH000739> Accessed 23.05.12.

Thielke, S., Vannoy, S., & Unutzer, J. (2007). Integrating mental health and primary care. *Primary Care, 34*, 571−592.

Unützer, J., Schoenbaum, M., Druss, B. G., & Katon, W. J. (2006). Transforming mental health care at the interface with general medicine: Report for the president's commission. *Psychiatric Services, 57*, 37−47.

Van Allen, J., Davis, A. M., & Lassen, S. (2011). The use of telemedicine in pediatric psychology: Research review and current applications. *Child and Adolescent Psychiatric Clinics of North America, 20*, 55−66.

Yellowlees, P. M., Hilty, D. M., Marks, S. L., Neufeld, J., & Bourgeois, J. A. (2008). A retrospective analysis of a child and adolescent e-mental health program. *Journal of American Academy of Child and Adolescent Psychiatry, 47*, 103−107.

Yellowlees, P. M., Odor, A., Parish, M. B., Iosif, A. M., Haught, K., & Hilty, D. (2010). A feasibility study of the use of asynchronous telepsychiatry for psychiatric consultations. *Psychiatric Services, 61*, 838−840.

Yeung, A., Hails, K., Chang, T., Trinh, N., & Fava, M. (2011). A study of the effectiveness of telepsychiatry-based culturally sensitive collaborative treatment of depressed Chinese Americans. *BMC Psychiatry, 11*, 154 <http://www.biomedcentral.com/1471-244X/11/154>

10 Geriatric Telemental Health

Thomas Sheeran[a],*, Jennifer Dealy[a] and Terry Rabinowitz[b]

[a]The Alpert Medical School of Brown University and Rhode Island Hospital, Providence, RI, [b]Departments of Psychiatry, Family Medicine, and Telemedicine, University of Vermont College of Medicine and Fletcher Allen Health Care, Burlington, VT

Introduction

In many ways, using telemedicine to provide mental health services for the elderly may seem like a daunting proposition. Seniors are not conventionally viewed as amenable to either mental health treatment *or* new technology. However, research over the past decade has increasingly been showing that while there are very real usability issues, seniors are receptive to this new form of health service. A number of studies have demonstrated rates of acceptance that are similar to that of other age groups, improvement in mental health outcomes, and in some cases, the added benefit of improvement in other health outcomes (Botsis, Demiris, Pedersen, & Hartvigsen, 2008; Rabinowitz, Murphy et al., 2010; Sheeran et al., 2011). This is encouraging, as there are numerous barriers to quality mental health services for seniors (Conner et al., 2010; Hagebak & Hagebak, 1980; Karlin & Norris, 2006). A significant dearth of geriatric mental health specialists often means that many elderly receive mental health care from their primary care doctors, other health specialists (e.g., cardiologists), or not at all. Even when community mental health services are available, mobility and transportation difficulties may impede seniors' ability to get to these providers (Hagebak & Hagebak, 1980; Lasoski, 1986). Given some of these unique challenges faced by the elderly, telehealth can potentially offer some much-needed solutions to the needs of this growing population.

In this chapter, we describe the literature on the use of telehealth technology for both mental and key nonmental health care for the elderly in a variety of settings. We then present three clinical examples of our experience in conducting telemental health with geriatric populations. Large and fully powered randomized trials on the

---

* Corresponding Author: Thomas Sheeran, The Alpert Medical School of Brown University and Rhode Island Hospital, 593 Eddy Street, Potter 3, Providence, RI 02828. Tel.: +1-401-444-3945, Fax: 1-401-444-3298, E-mail: tsheeran@lifespan.org

Telemental Health. DOI: http://dx.doi.org/10.1016/B978-0-12-416048-4.00010-5

use of videoteleconferencing (VTC) for the provision of clinical services and other applications are limited in geriatric mental health care. Furthermore, applications of other telehealth technologies to the mental health needs of the elderly also are limited, as much of the literature is instead focused on medical conditions. For these reasons, in this chapter, we review telehealth services across a variety of technology platforms and do not limit our discussion to mental health care. Rather, we include telehealth-based technology applications for both medical and mental health care, and highlight those components of use, satisfaction, and outcomes that are most relevant to mental health services for the elderly. We discuss the high, and growing, need for geriatric mental health services, some of the unique challenges that must be addressed in providing these services to this population, and describe the applications of telehealth technologies for geriatric mental health care in community, nursing home, and home care contexts. These technologies include, for example, VTC, remote home telemonitoring, and telephone-based interactive voice response (IVR).

It is important to note that a wide range of terms are used to describe video- and nonvideo-based telehealth technologies for providing health-care services. While there is some agreement in the industry with respect to key terminology, the field is new enough that there remains a lack of clear consensus on many telehealth-related terms. One of the most clear-cut terms is videoteleconferencing, or VTC, which entails real-time, two-way transmission of digitized video images between multiple locations to bring people at physically remote locations together for meetings. Similarly, "telemonitoring" is generally accepted to be the use of remote monitoring devices (audio, video, and physical) to monitor the health status of a patient from a distance, although certain platforms may need to be explained (e.g., IVR, in which respondents record their status over the telephone). Other terms are more ambiguous. For example, telemedicine and telehealth are often used interchangeably, although telemedicine is sometimes associated with direct patient care by a physician, whereas telehealth is viewed as a service that includes broader activities, such as care management, education, and coaching. For the purpose of this chapter, we also include the term telemental health, which we define to be the use of a broad range of technologies to provide mental health services to a population (e.g., VTC for remote psychotherapy and remote monitors that inquire about mood state). If needed, clarification of terms will be provided throughout the chapter.

The Need for Better Geriatric Mental Health Services

According to Loebel, Goldstein, and Kyomen (2011), there is an increasing need for mental health care for elders. This is due in large part to the aging of the baby boomer population and a life expectancy at birth in the United States of 75.2 years for men and 80.4 years for women, compared to 46.3 years for men and 48.3 years for women in 1900 (S. L. Murphy, Jiaquan, & Kochanek, 2012). With this increase in life expectancy is an associated rise in the prevalence of late-life mental illness and an increased need for mental health services. However, there are not enough clinicians with appropriate training to meet these needs (Loebel et al., 2011). Furthermore, although safe and effective treatments are available for many psychiatric conditions in elders, access to these treatments is limited. Mental health problems are associated with disability, functional decline, need for long-term care, poorer quality of life, mortality from comorbid medical conditions or suicide, and increased service utilization and demands on caregivers (Charney et al., 2003).

Psychiatric disorders in elders are often missed, misdiagnosed, or misattributed. More than 80% of more than 1.5 million US nursing-home residents have diagnosable psychiatric disorders, including depression, dementia and associated behavioral complications, delirium, anxiety, sleep impairment, and psychosis (Bartels, Horn et al., 2003; K. M. Murphy et al., 2005; Oliveria et al., 2006; Webber et al., 2005), but only a small proportion of these persons are seen by a mental health specialist (Borson, Liptzin, Nininger, & Rabins, 1987; Smyer, Shea, & Streit, 1994). Nursing homes in the United States are steadily becoming long-term "psychiatric" facilities for elders (Borson et al., 1987; M. J. Burns, Cain, & Husaini, 2001; Dobalian, Tsao, & Radcliff, 2003), particularly with the increasing numbers of assisted-living facilities that now provide care for residents who 20 years ago would have received nursing-home care. As the proportion of residents with mental health problems has increased, there has been recognition that these facilities do not have adequate access to appropriate mental health services, with the greatest unmet needs among small or rural health-care settings (B. J. Burns et al., 1993; Dobalian et al., 2003). Quality concerns about failure to diagnose mental disorders, inappropriate use of psychoactive drugs, physical restraints, inadequate treatment and monitoring, and unnecessary cognitive and functional decline are common among nursing-home residents and their families, regulatory agencies, and the general public (Avorn et al., 1992; Colenda et al., 1999; Evans & Strumpf, 1989; J. Morris et al., 2003; OBRA, 1987).

The health, mobility, and functional challenges that seniors face put them at risk for a number of mental health challenges. This can include, for example, depression, anxiety, loneliness associated with isolation, grief associated with multiple losses and dementia. Furthermore, chronic mental illness, such as bipolar disorder or schizophrenia, requires ongoing management into old age. Chief among these challenges is depression, as this illness is the most prevalent and often cuts across multiple conditions. For example, the early stages of progressive dementia are often associated with depression, as the patient is often aware of his/her lost capacity. According to the World Health Organization, depression is the leading cause of disability as measured by YLDs (years lived with disability) and the fourth leading contributor to the global burden of disease as determined by DALYs (disability adjusted life years: the sum of years of potential life lost due to premature mortality and the years of productive life lost due to disability). Further, not treating these symptoms may lead to significant morbidity or death by suicide (Conwell, Van Orden, & Caine, 2011). Given that older men have the highest suicide rate in the United States, with depression as the most frequently associated risk factor, it is essential for elderly individuals with depression receive access to quality mental health care (Loebel et al., 2011; Yates, Djousse, Kurth, Buring, & Gaziano, 2008).

Barriers to Mental Health Care for the Elderly

Elders face many potential or actual barriers to receiving psychiatric care, including physical or cognitive limitations such as hearing or vision impairment and decreased mobility, prohibitive costs, lack of appropriate sites for care delivery, long distances to travel, medical comorbidity, or provider unwillingness to make appropriate referrals (Loebel et al., 2011). Moreover, there may be cultural, systems, and resource-related barriers present in the elderly patient or the provider (Hagebak & Hagebak, 1980). For example, although psychotherapy for late-life depression is an effective treatment option or adjunct (Gum & Areán, 2004), Areán and colleagues (Alvidrez & Areán, 2002; Areán, Alvidrez, Barrera, Robinson, & Hicks, 2002) found that only 27% of 225 physicians surveyed said they would refer a depressed elder for psychotherapy even though many elders would use psychological services if they were made available to them. Female gender, the belief that psychotherapy is effective for older adults, and physician use of psychosocial techniques were associated with increased willingness to make referrals. Also of concern are the findings of Uncapher and Areán, who queried 215 primary care physicians regarding their willingness to treat older or younger patients with suicidal ideation and found that of the 100 physicians queried about suicidal ideation in older patients, there was less willingness to treat the older suicidal patient (Uncapher & Areán, 2000). These physicians tended to feel that suicidal ideation in an older patient was rational and normal, and the physicians were not optimistic that professional intervention could help these patients.

In addition to provider attitudes, ethnicity, cultural differences, medical comorbidities, and age itself also may present barriers. Despite the high prevalence of late-life mood disorders, Byers, Areán, and Yaffe (2012) found that about 70% of a sample of 348 persons aged 55 years and older with mood or anxiety disorders did not receive psychiatric services. Increased odds of not receiving services were associated with being from a racial or ethnic minority, discomfort with discussing personal problems, being married or cohabitating, and having middle- versus high-income status. Ellis et al. (2009) evaluated the predictors of referral for psycho-oncological care in 326 patients with metastatic gastrointestinal or lung cancer and found that rates of referral progressively declined with each decade of age, with only 22% of those aged 70 years and older referred for care versus 100% of those less than 40 years of age referred.

The differing roles that physicians play in institutional settings may have an indirect impact on geriatric mental health care. Unlike the acute care setting, physicians traditionally have not been active participants in institutional long-term geriatric health care. Their visits and examinations are often brief and cursory, and typically do not include psychiatric components. Although inadequate reimbursement has been cited as a major reason why physicians do not make nursing-home visits, other barriers to providing quality medical care include disinterest in the nursing-home population, difficulty in developing definitive care programs, ineffective interpersonal communication with nursing staff, and lack of training in the needs of the chronically ill-aged person (Colenda et al., 1999). Residents have limited access to physicians, and most access is dependent upon nurses or other professional staff initiating physician input when changes in a resident's condition are observed.

Psychiatric evaluation and treatment are even scarcer in the nursing home (Lombardo & Sherwood, 1992), especially in rural areas (Dobalian et al., 2003; Smyer et al., 1994). When available, 75% of residents referred for psychiatric services are served outside the facility and 53% of facilities have difficulty obtaining any psychiatric services at all (Lombardo & Sherwood, 1992). Most psychiatric treatment in the nursing home is provided by primary care physicians (Lombardo & Sherwood, 1992), with supportive care by licensed and nonlicensed nursing staff, most of whom have little mental health training. Nursing-home physicians identify only 15% of depressed residents, treat only 25% of those identified, but believe they recognize and treat depression well (Banazak, Mullan, Gardiner, & Rajagopalan, 1999; Bartels, Moak, & Dums, 2002) and Directors of Nursing report that nursing-home physicians are a major obstacle to obtaining psychiatric services when they are available (Lombardo & Sherwood, 1992).

Thus, lack of access to on-site psychiatric services is a major barrier to quality mental health care in nursing-home settings. Most psychiatrists prefer to work in private practice and are not trained to handle the multidimensional physical, mental, and social needs of nursing-home residents. Providing "collaborative" consultation and follow-up is also labor intensive and time consuming, often involving not only direct examination of the patient (as in the traditional consultation–liaison model) but also an evaluation of function in the context of the nursing-home environment through discussions with multidisciplinary staff (Bartels Moak, & Dums, 2002). In addition, Directors of Nursing report that psychiatry consultation on nonpharmacological interventions (as well as participation in educating facility staff in assessment and treatment of mental health problems) is inadequate in 75% of nursing homes (Lombardo & Sherwood, 1992).

Nursing-home residents or those in long-term care are not the only elder groups that are underserved with respect to mental health services. There are several potential barriers that may affect access to mental health services for community-dwelling elders, including race and ethnicity, socioeconomic status, geographic location, age, gender, immigrant status, language, sexual orientation, and psychiatric diagnosis (Solway, Estes, Goldberg, & Berry, 2010). Bruce (2002) found that depression goes largely undetected and undertreated among community-dwelling older adults receiving home care services. Weinberger, Mateo, and Sirey (2009) studied perceived barriers to mental health care in 47 subjects (85% women; 30% minority) with a mean age of 82 years and a mean level of depression characterized as "moderate" and found that logistic barriers including cost, transportation, mobility, and insurance were cited most frequently. Attribution about cause of depression was second most frequent with the most frequent attribution of depression being caused by a medical illness, cited by one-third of the subjects.

With respect to race and ethnicity, Conner et al. (2010) identified 50 African-American adults aged 60 years and older with at least mild-to-moderate depression to interview and completed surveys on 37 of these 60. They learned from this group that the black community is not very tolerant of those with a mental illness and that fear of repercussions of having a mental illness and lack of information about mental illness, including availability of treatment and treatment effectiveness, were some of the barriers to seeking treatment. Sorkin, Nguyen, and Ngo-Metzger (2011) compared the prevalence rates of mental distress of more than 20,000 total Chinese, Filipino, South Asian, Japanese, Korean, and Vietnamese adults aged 55 and older to that of non-Hispanic whites and examined subgroup differences in utilization of mental health services. They found that Filipino and Korean Americans were more likely to report symptoms of mental distress than the non-Hispanic whites but were less likely to have seen a primary care provider or to have taken a prescription medication. Japanese Americans were less likely to report symptoms or to make use of mental health services compared to non-Hispanic whites and suggested that these differences might be due to structural barriers, such as a lack of awareness of available services, lack of insurance, and language barriers, which might make it difficult for older adults to get necessary care.

Much of the time in geriatric mental health, service provision not only entails direct care to the patient but also includes consultation to family and the other professionals who work with seniors in a variety of settings. Such settings can include, for example, nursing homes, home care settings, assisted-living facilities, and even senior centers. Although there may be a need, and in some cases even a mandate (e.g., through Medicare), to provide access to specialized mental health providers, most settings find it cost prohibitive or impractical to hire full-time mental health professionals. For example, a common model in nursing homes is to contract with a mental health practice that provides on-site consultations on specific days and times. The nursing home will generate a list of patients to be seen by the geriatric psychiatrist or other mental health professional, who will then evaluate the patient. Although some clinicians (e.g., psychologists and social workers) may provide direct service to the patient on a contractual basis, many times (often in psychiatry) a consultative model is used: the psychiatrist will make recommendations for psychotropic medications to the patient's physician of record in the nursing home, who will then ultimately decide whether to implement the recommendation. As part of this overall model, staff training is often an element of service (e.g., staff inservices on how to identify geriatric depression).

Studies on Geriatric Telemental Health Services

Although telehealth applications for the general population are widespread and numbers are increasing (Hassol et al., 1996; Lipson & Henderson, 1996), less has been accomplished that is specific to elders even though they are a major target group for telemedicine interventions (Afrin, Greenland, Brown, Frankis, & Strange, 2004; Brunk, 2002; Chae et al., 2001; Chan et al., 2005; Corcoran, Hui, & Woo, 2003; Kropf & Grigsby, 1999; Palmas et al., 2006). The majority of telehealth applications for the elderly have focused on medical problems, such as stroke and heart disease, with comparably fewer telemental health applications. Further, Ball (2003) notes that most telemedicine studies targeting elders have consisted of small samples sizes, lacked appropriate controls, and never went beyond the feasibility or pilot stage, although the technology, if successful, would serve an important function, especially for rural elders, in allowing them to receive care in their own homes or communities (Hui, Woo, Hjelm, Zhang, & Tsui, 2001).

Some of the literature on the application of telehealth technology to geriatric mental health care is reviewed below. We focus on the issue of acceptability, which is often misperceived to be universally low among elders, and research on telemental health among some of the most debilitated seniors: those in nursing homes or those who are home bound.

Acceptability of Telemental Health Among the Elderly

Most studies that have evaluated satisfaction with telemental health interventions, or direct services from a clinician to a patient through videoconferencing, have done so only on a global level. Furthermore, most mental health studies have focused on the provision of psychiatric services only. Despite these limited data, there are reasons to be optimistic about the acceptability of telemental health services for the elderly. Among the few studies that have specifically evaluated telemental health care for the elderly, the majority of acceptance rates have been reported as "high," or among those that provide statistics, at 80% or more (Johnston & Jones, 2001; Rabinowitz, Murphy et al., 2010; Sheeran et al., 2011; Turvey, Willyard, Hickman, Klein, & Kukoyi, 2007). A few studies have found significantly lower acceptance rates. For example, Montani et al. (1997) found that only 27% of elderly hospitalized preferred video consultations, due in part to lack of clinician experience with the technology and technical problems. Disparate findings such as these point to the limited data on specific factors that might predict satisfaction and use, although experience and technical reliability are likely predictors. For example, in-home telepsychiatry, particularly for elders who may have stigma with respect to mental health, may create privacy concerns that might not otherwise be present in a psychiatrist's office. Other factors can include the specific type of technology used, participant demographic and clinical characteristics, attitudes and preferences, diseases targeted, clinical purpose (screening, symptom monitoring, and full disease management), and duration of service, to name a few. As discussed below, there is evidence that elders are as accepting of telehealth interventions as other age groups, but comparatively little is known about the scope of that acceptance and use, particularly for mental health care.

Although there is a dearth of research on the elderly's satisfaction with telemental health, there appears to be strong acceptance of the technology among seniors. One of the most mature applications, telestroke care, has consistently demonstrated high acceptance rates among both clinicians and patients (LaMonte et al., 2003; Moskowitz, Chan, Bruns, & Levine, 2011; Schwamm et al., 2004). LaMonte et al. (2003) used videoconferencing to connect emergency room (ER) physicians and their patients to stroke care specialists who would consult with the ER doctor and then perform a full neurological examination with the patient via videoconferencing. Patients, family members, and providers expressed satisfaction with this service. In particular, patients and their family members expressed satisfaction with the "quickness" of specialty emergency care and the "live" picture of the stroke specialist. Similarly, Schwamm et al. (2004) found that 100% of ER physicians agreed that telestroke improved patients' care and 85.7% of patients expressed that the telestroke consultation was "as good as face-to-face consultation." Moskowitz et al. (2011) surveyed providers' attitudes toward telestroke and found that 94.8% of ER physicians and 95.9% of stroke specialists expressed that telestroke would improve diagnosis and treatment, but acknowledged that patient preference for in-person visits may be a barrier to acceptance of this technology.

Similar to the use of videoconferencing in telestroke care, home health care has been using remote telemonitoring of vital signs for some time, again with high rates of satisfaction (Kraai, Luttik, de Jong, Jaarsma, & Hillege, 2011). Kobb, Hoffman, Lodge, and Kline (2003, p. 192) reported the findings of a home telemonitoring systems for veterans and found that 96% of veterans thought the technology "helped them stay healthy," 95% felt "more comfortable having the staff monitor them" and 97% "would recommend the project to other veterans". The high rate of acceptance of home telemonitoring among veterans is encouraging and suggests that they may be amenable to other forms of technology that may improve their health and care, such as videoconferencing. Similarly, 100% of providers felt the intervention improved patients care. Elderly patients with congestive heart failure reported being "comfortable" with in-home interactive telecommunication and more patients were satisfied with teleconsultation than with in-person nurse consultation (Jenkins & McSweeney, 2001). In a qualitative study of cardiac telemonitoring, the majority of elderly users found the technology easy to use, appreciated the convenience of being able to answer questions around their own schedules without leaving their homes, and expressed satisfaction with the information about heart failure that the monitor provided (LaFramboise, Woster, Yager, & Yates, 2009).

Other telemedicine interventions with elderly participants have included telephone monitored chronic heart failure management (Jenkins & McSweeney, 2001), videoconferencing for podiatric examinations (Corcoran et al., 2003), videoconferencing interviews for patients with dementia, which also have been well received (Botsis et al., 2008; Corcoran et al., 2003; Jenkins & McSweeney, 2001; A. G. Lee, Beaver, Jogerst, & Daly, 2003). With seniors in particular, usability is a leading concern, as it is closely related to acceptance and satisfaction. Czaja et al. (2006) found that age is a predictor of computer skill acquisition, but that this effect decreases markedly after controlling for computer self-efficacy, computer anxiety, and cognitive status. While not mental health specific, overall these findings suggest that elders are open to telehealth technology, which suggest opportunities in mental health care.

For mental health applications among the elderly, there is considerably less literature on acceptability and satisfaction, and most studies that include the elderly have often had a mixed population of younger adults as well. The Veterans'

Administration (VA) has conducted a number of studies on telemental health services for posttraumatic stress disorder (PTSD), depression, and other mental health conditions (Fortney et al., 2007; Frueh, 2007; Kobb et al., 2003). For example, Fortney et al. (2007) conducted a large randomized trial of telephone-supported depression care management (DCM) among rural recipients of VA services and found the intervention to be both effective and highly acceptable. Similarly, Frueh et al., (2007) found that telepsychiatry for PTSD was effective and that the majority of participants expressed "strong satisfaction." In a non-VA setting, the Indiana Cancer Pain and Depression (INCPAD) study integrated telephone and web-based patient surveys of pain and depression with nursing-care coordination (Kroenke, Theobald et al., 2009). Of the participants completing the satisfaction surveys, the majority found the technology easy to use (83.1%) and to be helpful or very helpful (72.8%) (Kroenke, Theobald et al., 2009). However, the VA studies have typically consisted of mostly male participants, spanning both young and elderly, while the INCPAD included both genders but also had a mixed-age cohort. Thus, inferences from these studies about female and elderly populations are limited.

The few telemental health studies working solely with a senior population have generally found satisfaction rates to be similar to that of younger groups. For example, Sheeran et al. (2011) found 83% of participants were satisfied or very satisfied with a geriatric telemonitor-supported DCM protocol (as described below). Rabinowitz, Murphy et al. (2010) found that participating residents, their family members, and staff at a rural nursing home expressed satisfaction and acceptance of telepsychiatry consultations via videoconferencing (also described below). Johnston and Jones (2001) evaluated the efficacy of telepsychiatric consultations to residents in a rural nursing home using a VTC system run through a broadband integrated service digital network line that presented the image of the patient on a computer monitor. Investigators found that the patients were satisfied with the technology and especially with the ability to meet with a psychiatrist without having to travel to the clinic.

Studies of telemental health among ethnic minorities have largely included younger age groups, although a few have been conducted with older adults. Yeung et al. (2009) used videoconferencing to conduct follow-up psychiatric visits with Chinese immigrants in a nursing home and to provide support to the patients and their family members, psychoeducation on psychiatric illness, and training to staff on the psychiatric intervention and behavioral modification techniques. Study psychiatrists initially conducted in-person interviews with the participants, who were then followed for two to five sessions using VTC over a T1 line. Participants receiving the intervention, their family members, and participating staff all reported being "highly satisfied" with the intervention. Similarly, Poon, Hui, Dai, Kwok, and Woo (2005) reported that a VTC memory improvement intervention was highly accepted among community-dwelling elderly residents in Hong Kong with cognitive impairment. That study compared a memory improvement intervention via videoconferencing monitors linked through broadband and high-resolution cameras to in-person visits. Patients in both the VTC and in-person groups had improvements in the areas of memory, attention, and language. However, the participants receiving in-person visits had significantly greater improvements in their spatial construction ability, which the study investigators suggested may be attributed to the fact that "this aspect of training often requires physical guidance, which cannot be effectively delivered via VTC" (p. 286). However, 90% of patients in the VTC reported being satisfied with VTC technology.

Overall, the general trend in the literature on telehealth and telemental health for the elderly has been that this population seems to accept the technology as much as younger groups. Indeed, telemental health may be particularly helpful for addressing the isolation that many older adults experience as a result of mobility and transportation limitations. However, a number of caveats and unknowns remain, as these findings only provide a very coarse view of the landscape, since acceptance and satisfaction rates have largely been gross secondary outcomes to effectiveness studies. Little has been collected or reported on specific factors that may impact acceptance. For a population with very unique needs and limitations across many health and functioning domains, this is a serious limitation of the literature to date. With the exception of studies evaluating predictors of computer use among seniors (Czaja et al., 2006), little is known about predictors of mental health service acceptance via telehealth technology. In addition to usability, factors such as technical reliability, portability, required patient behavior changes, attitudes, and preferences are just a few variables that could predict acceptance and use (Whitten & Love, 2005). Notably, there is virtually no data on why *unsatisfied* users may not care for a telemental health intervention. Valuable insight could be garnered by more closely examining the factors that may impact lack of satisfaction with these interventions.

Telepsychiatry in Nursing-Home Settings

To date, there have been relatively few reports of telemental health applications for elders compared to overall telemedicine use in nursing-home settings. Johnston and Jones (2001) reported successful use of telepsychiatry for 71 consultations to rural nursing-home residents over a 2-year period. This study initially used a commercially available videoconferencing program installed on a personal computer with a webcam. After the software proved to be unreliable when communicating across two different telephone service providers, a different system noncomputer-based system was utilized (V-Tel Settop 250). Depression- and dementia-related behavioral conditions were the problems most often treated, and the reported advantages of this modality included rapid response times, flexibility in frequency of consultation, and more efficient use of consultants' time. Similar results were reported by Tang, Chiu, Woo, Hjelm, and Hui (2001) in an analysis of 149 telepsychiatry "visits" to 45 nursing-home residents whose mean age was 84 years, and found the visits to be acceptable to residents and staff and cost-effective. Holden and Dew (2008) reported that both patients and their families were satisfied with one of the first telepsychiatry services designed to provide remote psychiatric care for elders on an inpatient gero-psychiatric unit. They used a firewall-protected, encrypted, high-broadband Polycom system that was compliant with regulations of the Health Insurance Portability and Accountability Act (HIPAA). Hildebrand, Chow, Williams, Nelson, and Wass (2004) reported that neuropsychological testing of older adults was possible using VTC over high-bandwidth connection and Cullum, Weiner, Gehrmann, and Hynan (2006) reported highly similar scores on a battery of neuropsychological tests administered face-to-face versus VTC to older persons with mild cognitive impairment.

Remote Telemonitoring and Geriatric Mental Health Care

The Health Resources and Services Administration (2011) defines telemonitoring as "the process of using audio, video, and other telecommunications and electronic information processing technologies to monitor the health status of a patient from a distance." The American Telemedicine Association defines telemonitoring as the service of collecting and interpreting patient health data using the delivery mechanism of home-to-monitoring-center links (Sheeran et al., 2011). Although the term "monitoring" might imply a rather passive collection and review of data, perhaps one of the most vital components of any home telemonitoring program is the active relationship and care management between the patient and the provider. An effective telemonitoring program creates a conduit for information exchange, connection, and support between the health-care provider and the patient. Given the dearth of research on telemonitoring to support mental health care for elders, we also include some of the literature on medical care, which provides insight on seniors' overall response to the technology.

Remote home telemonitoring developed out of the home care industry to meet the need for better monitoring home care clients at home. The majority of these clients are elderly, postacute, may be frail, and often have multiple medical comorbidities that place them at higher risk for adverse events such as falls or hospitalization (Kraai et al., 2011). Most commonly, illnesses such as heart failure and diabetes have been the focus of home health monitoring, generally because they have indicators of disease status such as blood pressure and blood sugar that should be measured daily.

The types of telemonitoring devices that are available and their capacity to not only capture and transmit health-related data but improve treatment adherence and connect patients to their providers has continued to expand over the past two decades. As far as physical health indices, many monitoring devices now measure patients' blood pressure levels, blood sugar levels, oxygen saturation levels, temperature, and peak flow indexes. Most devices can also be programmed to remind patients to take their medication and to monitor their vitals and to ask patients questions about their physical or mental health. The telemonitor devices can also include videomonitors that allow clinicians to assess and evaluate patients as needed. Automated telemonitor systems do not require the presence of a live, real-time health professional to collect patient data. The information is collected via the input device (telephone, telemonitor device, and computer) and stored and forwarded to a database, which is later reviewed by the provider, typically using software that summarizes biometric data, provides trend data/charts, and flags problematic readings. Telemonitoring platforms can be used for screening, active disease management, long-term follow-up, and relapse prevention.

In recent years, there has been mixed findings with respect to the effectiveness of home monitoring for managing medical illness. A recent randomized clinical trial (RCT) of home monitoring combined with case management in heart failure did not find a significant impact on hospitalization (Chaudhry et al., 2010). Moreover, a large-scale Medicare demonstration project examining disease management found the data inconclusive and did not clearly support the cost-effectiveness of home monitoring (Bott, Kapp, Johnson, & Magno, 2009). In contrast, Jia, Chuang, Wu, Wang, and Chumbler (2009), in an RCT of 774 veterans with diabetes, found that the telehealth treatment group had fewer preventable hospitalizations over a 4-year follow-up period, as well as a lower crude death rate when compared to matched controls not enrolled in telehealth. Several studies have investigated telemonitoring with dementia patients. Smith, Lunde, Hathaway, and Vickers (2007) used telehealth technology to monitor and improve medication adherence in patients with mild dementia living alone. Polycom and Picturetel televideo devices were used over an integrated services digital network (ISDN) connection. Patients who received home monitoring ($n = 8$) had significantly greater medication compliance than participants in the control group ($n = 6$) (Smith et al., 2007). J. H. Lee et al. (2000) evaluated the efficacy of providing treatment via telemedicine, tele-education, and telecounseling for patients with dementia in a nursing home or adult day care center and his/her relatives/caregivers. Study researchers reported that 46% of participants improved.

Several RCTs have evaluated nonautomated telemedicine protocols for collaborative DCM, with the most common service modality being live telephone-supported DCM. In a large VA trial conducted among small clinics without on-site psychiatrists, Fortney et al. (2007) found telemedicine-based (televideo combined with telephone consultation) DCM to be clinically effective and costly, but not so costly as to negate possible adoption. Among a sample of over 600 primary care patients, Simon, Ludman, and Rutter (2009) found that telephone care depression management, consisting of both systematic telephone follow-up and outreach to the patients' treating physicians and an eight-session-structured cognitive—behavioral therapy program conducted by masters-level therapists that focused on behavioral activation, cognitive restructuring, psychoeducation on depression care, and creating a self-care plan, improved the process of care and depression outcomes, at modest cost.

There have been fewer DCM studies using automated telemonitoring. Among feasibility studies, in an evaluation administering the patient health questionnaire-2 item scale (PHQ-2) via IVR home-monitoring system, Turvey, Willyard et al. (2007) found high rates of completion of the items and successful follow-up with the patient health questionnaire-9 items scale (PHQ-9) for patients who screened positive on the PHQ-2. These findings were similar to Ackermann et al. (2005), who evaluated a (live) telephone-based administration of the PHQ-2. Delaney and Apostolidis (2010) found improvement in PHQ-9 scores in a multicomponent heart failure pilot that included education on behavioral activation, although the telemonitor component did not include depression-related items. As described above, the study by Sheeran et al. (2011) of tele-DCM using remote telemonitoring included automated monitoring of depression via the PHQ-2, questions about antidepressant adherence and side effects, and patient education about depression. Patient and nurse care manager satisfaction was high, with preliminary indications of depression improvement.

With respect to measurement validity, results are highly limited and mixed. While many conclude that telemonitor-based assessment is valid, some recommend altering cutoff scores or transforming data to achieve agreement with the assessment standard. In an IVR study by Turvey, Willyard et al. (2007) and Roberts, Sheeran, Turvey, and Rabinowitz (2011), agreement between IVR and paper/pencil PHQ-9 administration was poor for higher levels of symptom severity, suggesting that IVR-administered PHQ-9 may require lower thresholds for caseness. Studies of televideo-based assessments are more common. Grob, Weintraub, Sayles, Raskin, and Ruskin (2001) found high reliability between psychiatric evaluations conducted in-person and via televideo conferencing with 27 nursing-home residents. Psychiatric evaluations included mini-mental status exam, the geriatric depression scale, and the brief psychiatric rating scale. Another study found high agreement between telecognitive televideo and in-person cognitive assessment scores of patients with mild cognitive impairment ($n = 14$) or mild-to-moderate Alzheimer's disease ($n = 19$) (Cullum et al., 2006). However, there was variability between participant's in-person and tele-cognitive assessment scores on the Hopkins Verbal Learning Test, Revised which the authors suggest may reflect that "the personal support of having an examiner in the room may somehow have a beneficial effect on effort/performance on this arguably more challenging task" (Cullum et al., 2006, p. 389).

Suicidality

A key concern with distance-based mental health care is that of suicidality and safety. Elements of suicidality can potentially be addressed using known telephone-based protocols for suicide prevention, such as the practice standards from the National Suicide Prevention Lifeline. A significant complication added by telemonitoring is the asynchronous transmission of data (store-and-forward), which is reviewed at a later time by the clinician. Turvey, Willyard et al. (2007) found no significant complications when using the PHQ-9 suicide risk item in their IVR assessments. However, since patient responses may be reviewed many hours after they are entered, providers run the risk of responding to ideation endorsement after the patient has committed suicide. More work is needed to learn how to respond to this challenge for a population with a high need for suicidality detection and response. At a minimum, patients would need clear education about review and response times, but additional technological and procedural safeguards would almost certainly be required and necessitates further research.

Case Presentations: Three Examples of the Use of Telehealth with Geriatric Populations

Our experiences in nursing home and home health settings are described below. We have found that in telemental health, models similar to same-room care can be implemented. Through collaboration with patients, the nonmental health staff who provide care for them, and even their caretakers and family, mental health services can be provided using a consultative approach. Importantly, leveraging technology in these ways may help to address some of the most important barriers to care, such as access to providers and cost of service delivery.

Telepsychiatry in Nursing-Home Settings

At Fletcher Allen Health Care (FAHC), we (TR) have provided telepsychiatry consultations for rural nursing-home residents since 2002 (Rabinowitz, Brennan, Chumbler, Kobb, & Yellowlees, 2008; Rabinowitz, Murphy et al., 2010; Rabinowitz, Ricci, Caputo, & Murphy, 2004). More than 150 individual patients have been treated through over 400 separate encounters. The program serves a large, almost entirely rural population of Vermont and upstate New York, and provides services to facilities as far as 150 miles away.

Technologically, all telepsychiatry consultations are performed using equipment installed at FAHC, with similar equipment installed at each nursing home. Our current instrumentation comprises state-of-the-art (Polycom, Pleasanton, CA) videoconferencing equipment and large-screen liquid crystal display or cathode ray tube monitors. These systems provide dynamic management of available bandwidth with an extremely low call-failure rate. Many of these units are on wheeled carts that can be easily moved about the hospital and used in any office with appropriate data ports. Transmission is via three basic rate interface ISDN lines transmitting at a bandwidth of 384 kbps. The system's hardware and software are all "standards based" so it has widespread applicability and, together with the use of ISDN, allows users the freedom to place calls to any ISDN-based system, regardless of geographic location or equipment manufacturer. While this implementation uses the older and highly reliable ISDN network, this service can also be provided via Internet protocol (IP) or network-based video to reduce costs and to increase the system's "user friendliness."

All instrumentation has the potential to control the distant site's camera. That is, each has the ability to perform pan-tilt-zoom (PTZ) operations of the distant camera. In addition, all units have picture-in-picture (PIP) functionality. For consultations, the distant sites' PIP and remote PTZ capabilities are disabled as we have found this helps to minimize patient distraction or confusion (especially among those with some degree of cognitive impairment). All telepsychiatry consultations are fully interactive. That is, they include full motion video and audio in both directions for live interactive communication.

All nursing-home telepsychiatry interactions require one or more persons in addition to the patient. There is always a nurse facilitator who may assist with patient history, positioning, orientation, hearing and vision problems, and the occasional instrument malfunction. In addition, we have found it very helpful to have family members present, at least for a portion of the visit, as they have typically provided helpful supplemental information, especially in cases where a patient has chronic or acute cognitive impairment. We also routinely have a member of the social services department to provide important family/background information. We have successfully used amplified headphones for some hearing-impaired patients.

Clinically, telepsychiatry consultations most commonly include assessment and diagnostic evaluation, interviewing of staff and family members to collect additional information, formulating the case and making treatment recommendations (most commonly, psychotropic medications) over the course of a 30–60 min telepsychiatry session. The consultations are facilitated by advance review of patient records, including recent progress notes, the medication record, the medical problem list, and each resident's minimum data set assessment, an instrument that must be completed for each nursing-home resident on admission, quarterly, and whenever an acute change is noted (J. N. Morris et al., 1990, 1997; Rabinowitz, Ricci et al., 2004). As noted above, we did not directly prescribe medications but instead made recommendations to the nursing-home staff (i.e., a receiving nurse), who then passed this information on the physician of record, who implemented (or rejected) the recommendation. In addition to medication consults, we have (less frequently) provided psychotherapy to patients and their family members. Not surprisingly, the primary issues were coping with life changes, losses related to functioning, health, relationships, and independence. In a recent evaluation, we analyzed 278 encounters for 106 patients and estimated potential cost savings of more than $250,000 for physician time, distance savings of 43,000 miles, and more than $3000 saved for fuel (Rabinowitz, Murphy et al., 2010). Our intervention was enthusiastically accepted by virtually all nursing-home residents, family members, and nursing-home personnel, and led to successful patient management.

In addition to these advantages, we have observed unexpected benefits from these consultations. When we started the consultation service, we identified many cases of delirium due to inappropriate medication dose or frequency, medication overuse, polypharmacy, or medication or alcohol withdrawal. Many cases were misdiagnosed as dementia, worsening dementia, or depression. We not only successfully managed delirium by videoconference; in addition, nursing-home staff and consultees became better educated and thus better equipped to prevent, identify, and treat this condition.

Nursing homes may be especially good sites for telemedicine consultations for several reasons:

- The population is relatively stable over time so that residents have the chance to become familiar with the telemedicine team and the technology, leading to greater trust of both.
- Psychiatric emergencies can be managed more quickly, sometimes through urgent telepsychiatry consultations. In addition, if a resident becomes acutely agitated, suicidal, or aggressive during a consultation, numerous support staff can be accessed rapidly for acute containment.
- Telemedicine equipment is not "specialty specific." Therefore, if the equipment was originally purchased for telemental health purposes, it can be easily adapted for other kinds of telemedicine consultations (e.g., teledermatology, teleophthalmology, and telerheumatology). Thus, it is entirely possible to purchase one portable high-quality telemedicine apparatus for an average-sized (e.g., 100-bed) nursing home and to use it for

many different types of telemedicine applications, greatly increasing costs and time saved as well as enabling consultations that might not otherwise be performed.
• Videoconference devices are quite durable: They have few moving parts or short-lived components. Therefore, a typically financially challenged nursing home would be making a wise and cost-effective investment by purchasing this equipment, especially if transmission is accomplished via IP, which adds nothing additional to regular Internet service charges.

We have successfully built an alliance with nursing-home residents using our videoconference approach by paying attention to and responding to the evolving needs of our patients and families, as well as to the needs and recommendations of nursing-home staff. We believe that the nursing-home environment is not unique in this regard. Thus, we provide the following "lessons learned" and actions taken that are likely to improve communication and outcomes when a videoconference approach is used for elders at any venue.

• *Do not underestimate elders' acceptance*
    We observed that many elders not only understood the reasons for using a telemental health rather than a face-to-face approach, they actually appreciated the use of the technology. They asked questions about its effectiveness versus face-to-face consultations, were interested in the instrumentation and how it worked, and appreciated that we spent the time and money to make a videoconference possible. Some of our patients had careers in fields related to telecommunication and were particularly interested in and accepting of our methods.
• *Make family participation the rule rather than the exception*
    We found that family member "buy-in" of our approach was extremely important. They provided helpful background and baseline information, encouraged their loved ones to participate in the videoconference, acted as "surrogate staff" by repeating or restating our questions for patients with hearing or vision impairment, and they helped to explain the technology to patients who were apprehensive or who, because of cognitive impairment, could not fully appreciate the approach.
• *Allow patients and families to use the equipment*
    We always have remote control of the distant site's camera, allowing us to PTZ as needed. For interested patients or families, we have briefly enabled their remote control over our camera, allowing them the opportunity to "drive" the camera, to see how this technology is used and to feel more comfortable with it.
• *Respect and support nursing-home staff*
    We could not perform our consultations without the help of nurses, social workers, and other staff members. There is always a nurse present at the distant site: we meet with her/him before each patient encounter to obtain a new or updated history and to discuss what options might be likely once the visit is completed. We also meet after each encounter to firm up a treatment plan. In addition, the nurse helps with patient positioning, orientation, and "anxiety attenuation," the latter by being a familiar, caring, and competent person, well known to the patient, who can help to allay fears about the new face or faces on the television. The nurse will leave the room if requested or if appropriate to allow some private time for the patient and psychiatrist.

Finally, it is important to comment on the issue of sensory impairment. Vision and hearing impairments are common among elders. Sometimes these deficits made teleconferencing more difficult, but there were very few times when it became impossible to perform a video consultation. We had reasonable success in managing some hearing problems by using amplified headphones. These "one size fits all" prostheses have an adjustable volume control that makes it possible to increase headphone volume without increasing the volume of the television speakers, making it easy to increase residents' input without increasing monitor volume to uncomfortable levels.

So far, we have been less successful in managing vision problems. We try to optimize conditions by ensuring that illumination and contrast at the provider and distant sites are optimized and that image size is sufficient for residents to be able to see the provider. However, some common ophthalmic problems in elders such as macular degeneration or cataracts cannot be greatly improved by these measures alone and still pose a challenge to optimized video consultation. Of course, some easy ways to manage a large proportion of vision and hearing problems include ensuring that: (1) every resident has his/her vision and hearing regularly evaluated, (2) eyeglasses and hearing aids are worn, (3) hearing aids are tuned on, and (4) ears are free of excess wax or other debris.

Tele-DCM for Elderly Rehabilitation Patients

Through collaboration with local nursing-home partners, our group (TS and JD) is currently evaluating an Internet-based VTC protocol for mental health consultation to improve depression treatment and outcomes among nursing-home rehabilitation patients. In an attempt to minimize cost and maximize generalizability, the intervention requires only a high-speed Internet connection and computer with webcam. If necessary, audio is supplemented by using standard conference calling via telephone. The computer's VTC platform is provided by a commercial vendor who has demonstrated adequate data protection and HIPAA compliance, and whose platform has been approved by our group's Institutional Review Board.

The clinical components of the DCM protocol require a nursing-home clinician to be trained in DCM, drawing on the well-established primary and home care models of service. The skill set includes assessing severity depression, monitoring antidepressant adherence and side effects, providing basic depression education to patients and their family members, and professional communication about the patient's depression status (Bruce, 2002). The online VTC component is conducted on a weekly basis and includes, at the nursing home, the nursing-home's depression care manager and if needed, the patient's family. At the remote location are a clinical psychologist (TS) and a geriatric psychiatrist or clinical nurse specialist. The purpose of the VTC is to conduct a virtual case conference, in which the depression care manager provides a status update on patients under her care, reviews patient progress, and discusses ongoing challenges to depression care. If necessary, the patient can be "seen" by the consulting mental health professionals, as the nursing home uses a laptop with integrated webcam for this service and the equipment can easily be brought directly to the patient's room. Although in its early stages of implementation, this protocol has been exceedingly well received and has had minimal technical challenges.

Telemonitor-Based Depression Care Management in Home Care

We (TS and TR) recently published a successful pilot that used home health agencies' routine remote home-monitoring equipment to provide DCM. Home health monitors have been developed by a number of private vendors in the home health industry, which are intended to be used by patients in their home on a daily basis to collect and transmit a number of vital signs to the home health agencies' telehealth nurses. The devices consist of a central device, approximately the size of a desktop radio, with an interactive screen and three to four large buttons. The device has peripherals that measure weight, blood sugar, heart rate, etc. These devices are part of an integrated disease management program at the home care agency and used to measure medical indicators associated with the patient's primary illnesses. They are used daily: using a chime, synthetic voice through speakers (for some devices), and/or touch screen, patients are prompted to measure weight, blood pressure, pulse, etc. Through an interactive screen, these monitors also can "ask" patients simple questions about their health and health-care needs, and can provide basic education about illness, treatment, health, and wellness. These interactive screens also provide an opportunity to ask patients about their depression.

The DCM model assigns a key professional staff member (e.g., nurse and social worker) to the role of depression care manager. This individual coordinates depression care among the patient, the physician and when needed, a mental health specialist. As noted above, key components include symptom assessment, treatment evaluation, patient education, and professional communication. For this pilot, all relevant protocol elements were created in English and in Spanish, including telemonitor items and telehealth nursing materials (e.g., PHQ-9 and antidepressant management guidelines) (Kroenke & Spitzer, 2002; Kroenke, Spitzer, & Williams, 2003). When available, we used established Spanish version measures (e.g., Spanish PHQ-9).

The telemonitors were programmed to briefly assess depression using the two-item PHQ-2, inquire about medication adherence (e.g., "have you been taking your medicine for depression as your doctor has prescribed?"), side effects (e.g., "is your antidepressant medicine causing any unpleasant side effects or other problems?"), and to provide simple education about depression and treatment adherence (e.g., "you should start to feel better within 2–4 weeks of starting your medicine. If you don't, tell your doctor or nurse"). The questions were developed to use the same format that home telemonitors typically use for other disease management and were intended to address each of the key domains while imposing as little burden as possible on patients. While a VTC component was not a part of this intervention, telehealth nurses routinely contacted patients via telephone as part of the protocol. It is not clear that a VTC component would have enhanced this intervention and a study on this could be important for better understanding the potential benefits/drawbacks, and perhaps more importantly, clarifying the feasibility and technical challenges that may be encountered when attempting to include a VTC component with homebound elders.

Overall, acceptance rates of the protocol were high with the vast majority of clinicians and patients reporting high rates of satisfaction with the intervention (Sheeran et al., 2011). Indeed, a number of patients requested to keep the telemonitors when the study ended. Furthermore, among a subset of patients meeting diagnostic criteria for major depression, the mean depression severity was in the "Markedly Severe" range at baseline and in the "Mild" range at follow-up. Thus, there are preliminary indications that using telemonitoring to provide depression care for homebound elders is both highly acceptable and may improve clinical outcomes.

Conclusions

Increasing the visibility and priority of exemplary telemental health programs and the voices of local, state, and national coalitions and grassroots are imperative. Solway et al. (2010) assert, "Significant policy opportunities exist to improve access to mental health services for older adults by overcoming barriers in transportation and outreach and recruitment and training. Improving mental health-care access must be targeted to address these barriers and be respectful of the significant diversity that that exists among and between groups that most experience these barriers." Using a telemedicine approach to address some of these barriers and issues is likely to lead to a greater proportion of elders with psychiatric conditions appropriately diagnosed and treated.

Overall, we believe that telemental health applications for elders have the potential to have a significant positive impact on older persons' mental and overall health, quality of life, and health outcomes. The technology can be used in diverse populations including community-dwelling elders, those in acute care or rehabilitation hospitals, nursing-home residents, and persons in continuing care retirement communities or assisted living. More high-quality research is needed to unequivocally demonstrate telemental health's potential for elders (Rabinowitz et al., 2008), but the evidence so far suggests that it works and can bring mental health care to those who might not otherwise receive it and in addition, can save time and money.

Acknowledgment

The authors express their appreciation to Elijah A. Peterson for his assistance in the preparation of this chapter.

References

Ackermann, R. T., Rosenman, M. B., Downs, S. M., Holmes, A. M., Katz, B. P., Li, J., et al. (2005). Telephonic case-finding of major depression in a Medicaid chronic disease management program for diabetes and heart failure. *General Hospital Psychiatry, 27,* 338–343.

Afrin, L., Greenland, J., Brown, A., Frankis, M., & Strange, C. (Eds.), (2004). *Telemedicine-based access to second opinions for the elderly* Amsterdam: IOS Press.

Alvidrez, J., & Areán, P. A. (2002). Physician willingness to refer older depressed patients for psychotherapy. *International Journal of Psychiatry in Medicine, 32,* 21−35.

Areán, P. A., Alvidrez, J., Barrera, A., Robinson, G. S., & Hicks, S. (2002). Would older medical patients use psychological services? *Gerontologist, 42,* 392−398.

Avorn, J., Soumerai, S. B., Everitt, D. E., Ross-Degnan, D., Beers, M. H., & Sherman, D., et al. (1992). A randomized trial of a program to reduce the use of psychoactive drugs in nursing homes. *New England Journal of Medicine, 327,* 168−173.

Ball, C. (2003). Telemedicine and old age psychiatry. In R. Wooton, P. Yellowlees, & P. McLaren (Eds.), *Telepsychiatry and e-mental health* (pp. 183−196). London: Royal Society of Medicine Press.

Banazak, D. A., Mullan, P. B., Gardiner, J. C., & Rajagopalan, S. (1999). Practice guidelines and late-life depression assessment in long-term care. *Journal of General Internal Medicine, 14,* 438−440.

Bartels, S. J., Horn, S. D., Smout, R. J., Dums, A. R., Flaherty, E., Jones, J. K., et al. (2003). Agitation and depression in frail nursing home elderly patients with dementia: Treatment characteristics and service use. *American Journal of Geriatric Psychiatry, 11,* 231−238.

Bartels, S. J., Moak, G. S., & Dums, A. R. (2002). Models of mental health services in nursing homes: A review of the literature. *Psychiatric Services, 53,* 1390−1396.

Borson, S., Liptzin, B., Nininger, J., & Rabins, P. (1987). Psychiatry and the nursing home. *American Journal of Psychiatry, 144,* 1412−1418.

Botsis, T., Demiris, G., Pedersen, S., & Hartvigsen, G. (2008). Home telecare technologies for the elderly. *Journal of Telemedicine and Telecare, 14,* 333−337.

Bott, D. M., Kapp, M. C., Johnson, L. B., & Magno, L. M. (2009). Disease management for chronically ill beneficiaries in traditional Medicare. *Health Affairs, 28,* 86−98.

Bruce, M. L. (2002). Psychosocial risk factors for depressive disorders in late life. *Biological Psychiatry, 52,* 175−184.

Brunk, D. (2002). Telemedicine is effective in reaching rural elderly: Pilot study of nutrition counseling. *Family Practice News, 32,* 30.

Burns, B. J., Wagner, H. R., Taube, J. E., Magaziner, J., Permutt, T., & Landerman, L. R. (1993). Mental health service use by the elderly in nursing homes. *American Journal of Public Health, 83,* 331−337.

Burns, M. J., Cain, V. A., & Husaini, B. A. (2001). Depression, service utilization, and treatment costs among medicare elderly: Gender differences. *Home Health Care Services Quarterly, 19,* 35−44.

Byers, A. L., Areán, P. A., & Yaffe, K. (2012). Low use of mental health services among older americans with mood and anxiety disorders. *Psychiatric Services, 63,* 66−72.

Chae, Y. M., Heon Lee, J., Hee, Ho, S., Ja Kim, H., Hong Jun, K., & Uk Won, J. (2001). Patient satisfaction with telemedicine in home health services for the elderly. *International Journal of Medical Informatics, 61,* 167−173.

Chan, W. M., Woo, J., Hui, E., Lau, W. W., Lai, J. C., & Lee, D. (2005). A community model for care of elderly people with diabetes via telemedicine. *Applied Nursing Research, 18,* 77−81.

Charney, D. S., Reynolds, C. F., 3rd, Lewis, L., Lebowitz, B. D., Sunderland, T., Alexopoulos, G. S., et al. (2003). Depression and bipolar support alliance consensus statement on the unmet needs in diagnosis and treatment of mood disorders in late life. *Archives of General Psychiatry*, *60*, 664−672.

Chaudhry, S. I., Mattera, J. A., Curtis, J. P., Spertus, J. A., Herrin, J., Lin, Z., et al. (2010). Telemonitoring in patients with heart failure. *The New England Journal of Medicine*, *363*, 2301−2309.

Colenda, C. C., Streim, J., Greene, J. A., Meyers, N., Beckwith, E., & Rabins, P. (1999). The impact of OBRA'87 on psychiatric services in nursing homes. Joint testimony of the American Psychiatric Association and the American Association for Geriatric Psychiatry. *American Journal of Geriatric Psychiatry*, *7*, 12−17.

Conner, K. O., Copeland, V. C., Grote, N. K., Koeske, G., Rosen, D., Reynolds, C. F., 3rd, et al. (2010). Mental health treatment seeking among older adults with depression: The impact of stigma and race. *American Journal of Geriatric Psychiatry*, *18*, 531−543.

Conwell, Y., Van Orden, K., & Caine, E. D. (2011). Suicide in older adults. *Psychiatric Clinics of North America*, *34*, 451−468, ix.

Corcoran, H., Hui, E., & Woo, J. (2003). The acceptability of telemedicine for podiatric intervention in a residential home for the elderly. *Journal of Telemedicine and Telecare*, *9*, 146−149.

Cullum, C. M., Weiner, M. F., Gehrmann, H. R., & Hynan, L. S. (2006). Feasibility of telecognitive assessment in dementia. *Assessment*, *13*, 385−390.

Czaja, S. J., Charness, N., Fisk, A. D., Hertzog, C., Nair, S. N., Rogers, W. A., et al. (2006). Factors predicting the use of technology: Findings from the Center for Research and Education on Aging and Technology Enhancement (CREATE). *Psychology and Aging*, *21*, 333−352.

Delaney, C., & Apostolidis, B. (2010). Pilot testing of a multicomponent home care intervention for older adults with heart failure: An academic clinical partnership. *Journal of Cardiovascular Nursing*, *25*, E27−40.

Dobalian, A., Tsao, J. C., & Radcliff, T. A. (2003). Diagnosed mental and physical health conditions in the United States nursing home population: Differences between urban and rural facilities. *Journal of Rural Health*, *19*, 477−483.

Ellis, J., Lin, J., Walsh, A., Lo, C., Shepherd, F. A., Moore, M., et al. (2009). Predictors of referral for specialized psychosocial oncology care in patients with metastatic cancer: The contributions of age, distress, and marital status. *Journal of Clinical Oncology*, *27*, 699−705.

Evans, L. K., & Strumpf, N. E. (1989). Tying down the elderly. A review of the literature on physical restraint. *Journal of the American Geriatrics Society*, *37*, 65−74.

Fortney, J. C., Pyne, J. M., Edlund, M. J., Williams, D. K., Robinson, D. E., Mittal, D., et al. (2007). A randomized trial of telemedicine-based collaborative care for depression. *Journal of General Internal Medicine*, *22*, 1086−1093.

Frueh, B. C., Monnier, J., Yim, E., Grubaugh, A. L., Hamner, M. B., & Knapp, R. G. (2007). A randomized trial of telepsychiatry for post-traumatic stress disorder. *J Telemed Telecare*, *13*, 142−147.

Grob, P., Weintraub, D., Sayles, D., Raskin, A., & Ruskin, P. (2001). Psychiatric assessment of a nursing home population using audiovisual telecommunication. *Journal of Geriatric Psychiatry and Neurology*, *14*, 63−65.

Gum, A., & Areán, P. A. (2004). Current status of psychotherapy for mental disorders in the elderly. *Current Psychiatry Reports*, *6*, 32−38.

Hagebak, J. E., & Hagebak, B. R. (1980). Serving the mental health needs of the elderly: The case for removing barriers and improving service integration. *Community Mental Health Journal*, *16*, 263−275.

Hassol, A., Gaumer, G., Grigsby, J., Mintzer, C. L., Puskin, D. S., & Brunswick, M. (1996). Rural telemedicine: A national snapshot. *Telemedicine Journal*, *2*, 43−48.

Health Resources and Services Administration. (2011). *HRSA Rural Health: Glossary and Acronyms*. Retrieved 10/30/2011, from < http://www.hrsa.gov/ruralhealth/about/telehealth/glossary.html > .

Hildebrand, R., Chow, H., Williams, C., Nelson, M., & Wass, P. (2004). Feasibility of neuropsychological testing of older adults via videoconference: Implications for assessing the capacity for independent living. *Journal of Telemedicine and Telecare*, *10*, 130−134.

Holden, D., & Dew, E. (2008). Telemedicine in a rural gero-psychiatric inpatient unit: Comparison of perception/satisfaction to onsite psychiatric care. *Telemedicine Journal and E-Health*, *14*, 381−384.

Hui, E., Woo, J., Hjelm, M., Zhang, Y. T., & Tsui, H. T. (2001). Telemedicine: A pilot study in nursing home residents. *Gerontology*, *47*, 82−87.

Jenkins, R. L., & McSweeney, M. (2001). Assessing elderly patients with congestive heart failure via in-home interactive telecommunication. *Journal of Gerontological Nursing*, *27*, 21−27.

Jia, H., Chuang, H. C., Wu, S. S., Wang, X., & Chumbler, N. R. (2009). Long-term effect of home telehealth services on preventable hospitalization use. *Journal of Rehabilitation Resarch and Development*, *46*, 557−566.

Johnston, D., & Jones, B. N. (2001). Telepsychiatry consultations to a rural nursing facility: A 2-year experience. *Journal of Geriatric Psychiatry and Neurology*, *14*, 72−75.

Karlin, B., & Norris, M. (2006). Public mental health care utilization by older adults. *Administration and Policy in Mental Health and Mental Health Services Research*, *33*, 730−736.

Kobb, R., Hoffman, N., Lodge, R., & Kline, S. (2003). Enhancing elder chronic care through technology and care coordination: Report from a pilot. *Telemedicine Journal and e-Health*, *9*, 189−195.

Kraai, I. H., Luttik, M. L., de Jong, R. M., Jaarsma, T., & Hillege, H. L. (2011). Heart failure patients monitored with telemedicine: Patient satisfaction, a review of the literature. *Journal of Cardiac Failure*, *17*, 684−690.

Kroenke, K., & Spitzer, R. L. (2002). The PHQ-9: A new depression diagnostic and severity measure. *Psychiatric Annals*, *32*, 1−7.

Kroenke, K., Spitzer, R. L., & Williams, J. B. (2003). The patient health questionnaire-2: Validity of a two-item depression screener. *Medical Care*, *41*, 1284−1292.

Kroenke, K., Theobald, D., Norton, K., Sanders, R., Schlundt, S., McCalley, S., et al. (2009). The Indiana Cancer Pain and Depression (INCPAD) trial design of a telecare management intervention for cancer-related symptoms and baseline characteristics of study participants. *General Hospital Psychiatry*, *31*, 240−253.

Kropf, N. P., & Grigsby, R. K. (1999). Telemedicine for older adults. *Home Health Care Services Quarterly*, *17*, 1−11.

LaFramboise, L. M., Woster, J., Yager, A., & Yates, B. C. (2009). A technological life buoy: Patient perceptions of the health buddy. *Journal of Cardiovascular Nursing*, *24*, 216−224.

LaMonte, M. P., Bahouth, M. N., Hu, P., Pathan, M. Y., Yarbrough, K. L., Gunawardane, R., et al. (2003). Telemedicine for acute stroke. *Stroke*, *34*, 725−728.

Lasoski, M. C. (1986). Reasons for low utilization of mental health services by the elderly. *Clinical Gerontologist*, *5*, 1−18.

Lee, A. G., Beaver, H. A., Jogerst, G., & Daly, J. M. (2003). Screening elderly patients in an outpatient ophthalmology clinic for dementia, depression, and functional impairment. *Ophthalmology*, *110*, 651−657 (discussion 657)

Lee, J. H., Kim, J. H., Jhoo, J. H., Lee, K. U., Kim, K. W., Lee, D. Y., et al. (2000). A telemedicine system as a care modality for dementia patients in Korea. *Alzheimer Disease and Associated Disorders*, *14*, 94−101.

Lipson, L. R., & Henderson, T. M. (1996). State initiatives to promote telemedicine. *Telemedicine Journal*, *2*, 109−121.

Loebel, J. P., Goldstein, M. Z., & Kyomen, H. H. (2011). The geritaric psychiatrist. In M. E. Agronin, & G. J. Maletta (Eds.), *Principles and practice of geriatric psychiatry* (2nd ed., pp. 37−42). Philadelphia, PA: Lippincott Williams & Wilkins.

Lombardo, N. E., & Sherwood, S. (1992). *The 1992 national telephone survey of nursing home administrators and directors of nursing*. Boston, MA: Research and Training Institute, Hebrew Rehabilitation Center for Aged.

Montani, C., Billaud, N., Tyrrell, J., Fluchaire, I., Malterre, C., Lauvernay, N., et al. (1997). Psychological impact of a remote psychometric consultation with hospitalized elderly people. *Journal of Telemedicine and Telecare*, *3*, 140−145.

Morris, J., Moore, T., Jones, R., Mor, V., Angelelli, J., Berg, K., et al. (2003). *Validation of long-term and post-acute care quality indicators*. Baltimore, MD: Center for Medicare and Medicaid Services.

Morris, J. N., Hawes, C., Fries, B. E., Phillips, C. D., Mor, V., Katz, S., et al. (1990). Designing the national resident assessment instrument for nursing homes. *Gerontologist*, *30*, 293−307.

Morris, J. N., Nonemaker, S., Murphy, K. M., Hawes, C., Fries, B. E., Mor, V., et al. (1997). A commitment to change: Revision of HCFA's RAI. *Journal of the American Geriatrics Society*, *45*, 1011−1016.

Moskowitz, A., Chan, Y. -F. Y., Bruns, J., & Levine, S. R. (2011). Emergency physician and stroke specialist beliefs and expectations regarding telestroke. *Stroke*, *41*, 805−809.

Murphy, K. M., Rabinowitz, T., Nonemaker, S., Morris, J. N., Morrison, M. H., Grigonis, A. M., et al. (2005). An initiative to improve depression recognition and management in long-stay nursing home residents. *Clinical Gerontologist*, *28*, 95−109.

Murphy, S. L., Jiaquan, X., & Kochanek, K. D. (2012). *Deaths: Preliminary data for 2010. National vital statistics reports*. Hyatttsville, MD: National Center for Health Statistics.

National Suicide Prevention Lifeline (NSPL). Suicide Risk Assessment Standards (2007, April 17). Retrieved August, 13, 2012, from < http://www.http://suicidepreventionlifeline. org/CrisisCenters/PracticeStandards.aspx > .

OBRA. (1987). *Omnibus budget reconciliation act of 1987. Public law 100-203. Subtitle C: Nursing home reform*. Signed by President Reagan. Washington, DC.

Oliveria, S. A., Liperoti, R., L'Italien, G., Pugner, K., Safferman, A., Carson, W., et al. (2006). Adverse events among nursing home residents with Alzheimer's disease and psychosis. *Pharmacoepidemiology and Drug Safety*, *15*, 763−774.

Palmas, W., Teresi, J., Morin, P., Wolff, L. T., Field, L., Eimicke, J. P., et al. (2006). Recruitment and enrollment of rural and urban medically underserved elderly into a randomized trial of telemedicine case management for diabetes care. *Telemedicine Journal and e-Health*, *12*, 601−607.

Poon, P., Hui, E., Dai, D., Kwok, T., & Woo, J. (2005). Cognitive intervention for community-dwelling older persons with memory problems: Telemedicine versus face-to-face treatment. *International Journal of Geriatric Psychiatry*, *20*, 285−286.

Rabinowitz, T., Brennan, D. M., Chumbler, N. R., Kobb, R., & Yellowlees, P. (2008). New directions for telemental health research. *Telemedicine Journal and e-Health, 14*, 972–976.

Rabinowitz, T., Murphy, K. M., Amour, J. L., Ricci, M. A., Caputo, M. P., & Newhouse, P. A. (2010). Benefits of a telepsychiatry consultation service for rural nursing home residents. *Telemedicine Journal and e-Health, 16*, 34–40.

Rabinowitz, T., Ricci, M. A., Caputo, M. P., & Murphy, K. M. (2004). Minimum data set facilitates telepsychiatry consultations for nursing home residents. *Telemedicine Journal and e-Health, 10:S*, 46.

Roberts, L., Sheeran, T., Turvey, C., & Rabinowitz, T. (2011). Depression tele-care for elderly patients at home: Successes and challenges. Symposium presented at the American Telemedicine Association International Meeting & Exposition, Tampa, FL.

Schwamm, L. H., Rosenthal, E. S., Hirshberg, A., Schaefer, P. W., Little, E. A., Kvedar, J. C., et al. (2004). Virtual telestroke support for the emergency department evaluation of acute stroke. *Academic Emergency Medicine, 11*, 1193–1197.

Sheeran, T., Rabinowitz, T., Lotterman, J., Reilly, C. F., Brown, S., Donehower, P., et al. (2011). Feasibility and impact of telemonitor-based depression care management for geriatric homecare patients. *Telemedicine Journal and e-Health, 17*, 620–626.

Simon, G. E., Ludman, E. J., & Rutter, C. M. (2009). Incremental benefit and cost of telephone care management and telephone psychotherapy for depression in primary care. *Archives of General Psychiatry, 66*, 1081–1089.

Smith, G. E., Lunde, A. M., Hathaway, J. C., & Vickers, K. S. (2007). Telehealth home monitoring of solitary persons with mild dementia. *American Journal of Alzheimer's Disease and Other Dementias, 22*, 20–26.

Smyer, M. A., Shea, D. G., & Streit, A. (1994). The provision and use of mental health services in nursing homes: Results from the National Medical Expenditure Survey. *American Journal of Public Health, 84*, 284–287.

Solway, E., Estes, C. L., Goldberg, S., & Berry, J. (2010). Access barriers to mental health services for older adults from diverse populations: Perspectives of leaders in mental health and aging. *Journal of Aging and Social Policy, 22*, 360–378.

Sorkin, D. H., Nguyen, H., & Ngo-Metzger, Q. (2011). Assessing the mental health needs and barriers to care among a diverse sample of Asian American older adults. *Journal of General Internal Medicine, 26*, 595–602.

Tang, W. K., Chiu, H., Woo, J., Hjelm, M., & Hui, E. (2001). Telepsychiatry in psychogeriatric service: A pilot study. *International Journal of Geriatric Psychiatry, 16*, 88–93.

Turvey, C. L., Willyard, D., Hickman, D. H., Klein, D. M., & Kukoyi, O. (2007). Telehealth screen for depression in a chronic illness care management program. *Telemedicine Journal and e-Health, 13*, 51–56.

Uncapher, H., & Areán, P. A. (2000). Physicians are less willing to treat suicidal ideation in older patients. *Journal of the American Geriatrics Society, 48*, 188–192.

Webber, A. P., Martin, J. L., Harker, J. O., Josephson, K. R., Rubenstein, L. Z., Alessi, C. A., et al. (2005). Depression in older patients admitted for postacute nursing home rehabilitation. *Journal of the American Geriatrics Society, 53*, 1017–1022.

Weinberger, M. I., Mateo, C., & Sirey, J. A. (2009). Perceived barriers to mental health care and goal setting among depressed, community-dwelling older adults. *Journal of Patient Preference and Adherence, 3*, 145–149.

Whitten, P., & Love, B. (2005). Patient and provider satisfaction with the use of telemedicine: Overview and rationale for cautious enthusiasm. *Journal of Postgraduate Medicine, 51*, 294–300.

World Health Organization. Depression. 2012. <http://www.who.int/mental_health/management/depression/definition/en/> Accessed 25.05.12.

Yates, L. B., Djousse, L., Kurth, T., Buring, J. E., & Gaziano, J. M. (2008). Exceptional longevity in men: Modifiable factors associated with survival and function to age 90 years. *Archives of Internal Medicine, 168*, 284–290.

Yeung, A., Johnson, D. P., Trinh, N. H., Weng, W. C., Kvedar, J., & Fava, M. (2009). Feasibility and effectiveness of telepsychiatry services for Chinese immigrants in a nursing home. *Telemedicine Journal and e-Health, 15*, 336–341.

11 Child and Adolescent Telemental Health

*L. Lee Carlisle**

Department of Psychiatry and Behavioral Sciences, Division of Child
and Adolescent Psychiatry, University of Washington
School of Medicine, Seattle, WA

Introduction

Access to mental health care for children is problematic, a primary reason being
the shortage of expert child-trained mental health specialists, particularly child and
adolescent psychiatrists. For children in underserved communities, such as rural
areas, small towns, or even inner cities, the problem is magnified because, in addition to the general shortage, there is a severe maldistribution of child psychiatrists
favoring metropolitan regions. And, despite a long-term awareness of these issues
and developing models to address the shortages (Hilt, 2011; Katon, Richardson
et al., 2010; Myers, Palmer, & Geyer, 2011), every indication is that both trends
will continue and many of the country's youth will not have adequate access
to mental health care. Given the mandates put forth by the federal government
(New Freedom Commission on Mental Health, 2003) as well as national organizations (Spooner & Gotlieb, 2004) for a more equable distribution of mental health
care for children and the pending health care reform proposed by the Obama
administration, how then is this care to be delivered to so many of the country's
underserved youth? It is clear that traditional methods and models have not and
will not be able to meet this challenge and, therefore, it is also clear that alternative
methods of health care delivery will need to be developed and implemented in
order to achieve the ideal of improved mental health care access to rural and impoverished youth. One solution that addresses both forks of the child and adolescent
mental health workforce issues—low supply and maldistribution—has been poised
and ready for several years now, waiting on the tarmac. Child and adolescent
telemental health is no longer a goal for the future. Barriers which, in the past,
made large-scale implementation of child and adolescent telemental health

* Corresponding Author: L. Lee Carlisle, Department of Psychiatry and Behavioral Sciences, Division of
Child and Adolescent Psychiatry, University of Washington School of Medicine, Seattle, WA. Tel.:
+1-253-756-2679, Fax: +1-253-761-7518, E-mail:Lynda.carlisle@seattlechildrens.org

Telemental Health. DOI: http://dx.doi.org/10.1016/B978-0-12-416048-4.00011-7

impractical have either fallen by the wayside or become manageable. Clearance is granted. It is time for child and adolescent telemental health to take off.

Literature Review

While this chapter covers child and adolescent mental health generally, most of the published literature and programs developed across the country have focused on telepsychiatry. Therefore, most of this chapter addresses telepsychiatry specifically. When the broader discipline of children's mental health is addressed, the term telemental health is used.

Ten years ago, technical and economic issues were still major hurdles impeding a more generalized use of telemental health. Over the past decade, however, wired cities, rapid growth of the Internet, and the development of new, improved, and more affordable technology have considerably reduced these barriers (Yellowlees & Nafiz, 2010). The Federal Communications Commission has recently issued its plan to extend broadband into the remaining unserviced areas (Moe, 2011). Yet, in regard specifically to child telemental health, there are still speed bumps on the road. Primary among these is the development of an evidence base supporting the effectiveness of telemental health as a service delivery model with youth and second ensuring sound, evidence-based practice by telemental health providers. This section will highlight some of the most pertinent studies relating to child and adolescent telemental health, as summarized in Table 11.1.

The quality and quantity of literature concerning telemental health for children continues to grow, yet it still lacks the large, controlled, and replicable studies needed to establish the sound treatment criteria that evidence-based medicine requires. Most research to date has been descriptive, documenting that telemental health with children and adolescents is feasible in diverse settings (Boydell, Volpe, & Pignatello, 2010; Greenberg, Boydell, & Volpe, 2006; Myers, Valentine, & Melzer, 2007) and acceptable to referring physicians (Hilty, Yellowlees, Cobb, Neufeld, & Bourgeois, 2006; Nesbitt, Marcin, Daschbach, & Cole 2005), parents (Elford, White, Bowering et al., 2000; Elford, White, St. John et al., 2001; Myers, Sulzbacher, & Melzer, 2004; Myers, Valentine, & Melzer, 2008), and even youth (Myers, Valentine, Melzer, & Morgenthaler, 2006). Few studies, however, have focused on treatment outcomes comparing videoconferencing sessions with the more traditional face-to-face encounters. A recent review by Diamond and Bloch (2010) focused on this issue, concluding that, while the data justifying telepsychiatry is weak, there are no data to suggest that this process contributes to negative outcomes.

Developmental and Clinical Considerations

Applications of telepsychiatry with youth have been described across most developmental and diagnostic categories. Children as young as 3 years old have been evaluated and treated (Elford, White, Bowering et al., 2000; Myers, Sulzbacher, & Melzer, 2004). School-aged children comprise the modal age group (Broder,

Table 11.1 Selected Literature: Child Telemental Health

	Type of Study[a]	Title	#	Findings/Conclusions
Elford, White, Bowering et al. (2000)	RTC	A randomized, controlled trial of child psychiatric assessments conducted using videoconferencing	25	High concordance (96%) between telepsychiatrist and in-person psychiatrist regarding diagnoses and recommendations
Nelson et al. (2003)	RTC	Treating childhood depression over videoconferencing	28	Comparable reduction of children's depressive symptoms in response to therapy delivered in-person or through videoteleconferencing
Diamond and Bloch (2010)	RW	Telepsychiatry assessments of child or adolescent behavior disorders: a review of evidence and issues	–	Concluded that, while there are significant weaknesses in the research justifying child telemental health, there is no data that suggest the process leads to negative outcomes
Yellowlees et al. (2008)	PP	A retrospective analysis of a child and adolescent telemental health program	41	Telepsychiatry associated with improved symptoms at 3 months: boys improved oppositional scores and girls improved mood scores
Myers, Vander Stoep, McCarty et al. (2010)	DS	Child and adolescent telepsychiatry: variations in utilization, referral patterns, and practice trends	701	Referrals from 191 PCPs (1–89 referrals per PCP), representative diagnostic profile, different practice styles by telepsychiatrists
Myers, Sulzbacher, and Melzer (2004)	DS	Telepsychiatry with children and adolescents: Are patients comparable to those evaluated in usual outpatient care?	368	Comparison of patients in telepsychiatry and outpatient clinics showed no differences in diagnoses, demographics, payer status
Myers, Valentine, Melzer, and Morganthaler (2006)	DS	Telepsychiatry with incarcerated youth	115	79.8% of youth receiving telepsychiatry services at rural juvenile corrections in Washington rated overall satisfaction with

(Continued)

Table 11.1 (Continued)

	Type of Study[a]	Title	#	Findings/Conclusions
				telepsychiatry as "very good" or "outstanding"
Myers, Valentine, and Melzer (2007)	DS	Feasibility, acceptability, and sustainability of telepsychiatry with children and adolescents	62	High level of satisfaction with telepsychiatry among PCPs; pediatricians more satisfied than family physicians
Fox, Connor, McCullers, and Waters (2008)	PP	Effect of behavioral health and specialty care telemedicine program on goal attainment for youth in juvenile detention	190	Increases in number of goals for each youth and in the proportion of youth who achieved goals
Stain et al. (2011)	C	The feasibility of videoconferencing for neuropsychological assessments of rural youth experiencing early psychosis	11	Pilot study shoed excellent correlation between face-to-face evaluations and those done via videoconferencing; in addition, they found high levels of patient acceptance for the remote testing

PCPs, primary care physicians.
[a]C, controlled; RTC, randomized controlled; RW, review; DS, descriptive; PP, pre–post study design.

Manson, Boydell, & Teshima, 2004; Hockey, Yellowlees, & Murphy, 2004; Myers, Sulzbacher, & Melzer, 2004; Nelson, Barnard, & Cain, 2003; Stain et al., 2011) with attention-deficit hyperactivity disorder (ADHD), the most commonly treated disorder. Most diagnostic groups, however, have been treated (Myers, Sulzbacher, & Melzer, 2004; Myers, Valentine, & Melzer, 2007). Developmentally impaired children may not be able to provide their own perspectives, but school's records, their parents', and telepsychiatrist's observations can readily facilitate treatment planning. Uncooperative children pose special challenges, yet, with appropriate assistance at the patient site, this can be effectively treated. Overall, the appropriateness of a youth for telepsychiatry should be individualized to developmental considerations, parents' preferences, available supports at the patient site, and the telepsychiatrist's resourcefulness. Adolescents are generally easy to engage in telepsychiatry sessions and like having time apart from their parent to discuss concerns with the telepsychiatrist alone. The age of consent for agreeing to health care services varies by states. Just as in usual in-person care, adolescents may need to provide their written consent for teletreatment in addition to consent for treatment in general.

In a randomized investigation of 23 youth evaluated through telepsychiatry and in-person sessions, 96% of the diagnoses and treatment recommendations were comparable as was family satisfaction (Elford, White, Bowering et al., 2000). This sample is small but suggests reliability of diagnoses made with children through videoconferencing. More recently, Stain et al. (2011) in a small ($N = 11$) controlled study evaluating psychosis in patients 14−27 years of age found excellent correlation between face-to-face evaluations and those done via videoconferencing. This study was conducted at a bandwidth of 384 kb/s supporting the use of moderate level bandwidth and resolution to detect salient features of the history and mental status examination on initial evaluation when conducted through videoconferencing. In addition, they found high levels of patient acceptance for the remote testing. Though this was a small, pilot study, the results are still encouraging.

Two outcome studies support the effectiveness of treatment provided through telemental health. In an equivalency trial, 28 depressed children 8−12 years old were randomized to telemental health or in-person treatment using cognitive behavioral therapy (CBT) (Nelson et al., 2003). The telemental health intervention was conducted at low bandwidth of 128 kb/s. The two groups showed comparable improvements over 8 weeks. The sample was small and the length of treatment rather short; but, there were no differences in dropouts, missed sessions, or other utilization variables. This study suggests that treatment can be successfully conducted through telemental health and that low bandwidth may be adequate for this application. Low bandwidth would make such interventions feasible for organizations that cannot afford higher end equipment and bandwidth. In another study, retrospective assessment of outcomes with a convenience sample of 41 youth found improvements in the Affect and Oppositional Domains of the Child Behavior Checklist (CBCL) 3 months after initial telepsychiatric consultation (Yellowlees, Hilty, Marks, Neufeld, & Bourgeois, 2008). These youths were part of a larger telemental health service and received a single consultative session or short-term interventions. As the CBCL is a broad measure of childhood psychopathology, changes in its dimensional scales cannot generally be appreciated over the short term. Thus, detection of improvements in these two domains is impressive and suggests effectiveness of telemental health for providing interventions.

ADHD has been one of the most widely studied disorders of childhood using telemental health (Palmer et al., 2010). There have been three published research articles on the topic of ADHD and telemental health. In an 18-month study in Washington State, 369 youth age 3−19 years were evaluated and treated, 210 youth in person at a traditional outpatient psychiatric clinic and 159 through telepsychiatry. The groups were comparable in age, gender, diagnoses, and payer status. The diagnostic profile was similar across groups and ADHD was the most common diagnosis in both settings (Myers, Sulzbacher, & Melzer, 2004). An evaluation of this telepsychiatry clinic 7 years later continued to show that ADHD was the most commonly treated clinical disorder (Myers, Vander Stoep, McCarty et al., 2010). ADHD was also found to be the most common diagnosis (36%) for youth referred to a telepsychiatry clinic in 10 rural settings in Northern California (Yellowlees et al., 2008).

At the Seattle Children's Research Institute, a large randomized controlled clinical trial to assess the efficacy of telemental health in treating ADHD is being funded by National Institute of Mental Health and is at the halfway mark. While full results of the randomized clinical trial are not yet available, preliminary findings are encouraging. The study is enrolling children with complex cases of ADHD, most of who have not responded to prior interventions. The participants include 250 children ages 5.5–12 years of age who are randomized to one of two intervention groups. One group receives a one-time consultation by a telepsychiatrist with follow-up treatment recommendations provided to the primary care provider. The other group receives six sessions of combined telepsychiatric care and parent behavioral training. This active intervention group receives evidence-based treatment and/or consensus-based guideline care for medication management with psychoeducation on the neurobiological model of ADHD and parent training on raising a child with ADHD. Preliminary data from this study indicate that families in the intervention group have a high rate of completion of offered sessions (avg. = 5.5/6.0) (Grover, Rockhill, Kim, Swardstrom, Vander Stoep, & Myers, 2011). The telepsychiatrists provided clinical sessions per protocol with 81% fidelity. Medication treatment by consensus guidelines was provided with 69% fidelity and when the telepsychiatrists deviated from protocol they provided clinically appropriate justification 82% of the time (Rockhill et al., 2011). To date, pre/postintervention results indicate that children considerably improve their overall ADHD symptomatology by approximately 40% as compared with prior treatment in their communities (Grover et al., 2011).

The good, the bad, and the unknown, then, of child telemental health research and experience can be summed up as follows. Good news: patients (Boydell et al., 2010; Myers, Valentine, & Melzer, 2008) and referring physicians (Cloutier, Cappelli, Glennie, & Keresztes, 2008; Myers, Valentine, & Melzer, 2007) consistently report high levels of satisfaction with care rendered through telemental health; early research suggests that child and adolescent telemental health should be comparable to face-to-face treatment, and there are no data to suggest that it contributes to negative outcomes (Diamond & Bloch, 2010). It has even been suggested that for some children and adolescents, telepsychiatry may be superior to traditional face-to-face consultation as a method of psychiatric assessment (Hilty, Yellowlees, Sonik, Derlet, & Hendren, 2009; Pakyurek, Yellowlees, & Hilty, 2010). On the downside, however, child and adolescent telemental health lacks evidence-based criteria on which to base treatment and outcome studies are sorely needed.

The Practice of Child and Adolescent Telemental Health

Models of Care and Clinical Practice: Primary Care

Several models have been described for the provision of telemental health services in the primary care setting (see Chapters 9 and 16). These models have been examined sparsely in child and adolescent telemental health but should be readily adaptable to youth. Integrating mental health into primary care medicine is not a new idea or process. However, in the context of telemedicine, it takes on new significance and opportunities. Telemental health should not be thought of as a technology simply to be inserted into traditional models of health care delivery. Its full potential will only be achieved when new methods and models of care are developed to take advantage of telemedicine's unique capabilities (Speedie, Ferguson, Sanders, & Doarn, 2008). For example, the American Academy of Pediatrics has made several recommendations regarding the integration of mental health care into pediatric practice (American Academy of Pediatrics, 2009) and telemedicine figured prominently among them. Traditional models of care are dependent upon face-to-face interaction with patients, scheduled or episodic care, and the locations of physician and patient. Telemental health has the potential to remove these dependencies and thus improve care while at the same time lowering the cost for all parties involved.

Dobbins et al. (2011) have described the "Consultation Conference" built on Caplan's model of Consultee-Centered Consultation (Caplan & Caplan, 2000). In this model, a group of primary care providers present cases via videoconferencing to a child telepsychiatrist who serves as both expert and mediator of a group discussion. The primary care providers gain proficiency in managing patients, thereby functionally expanding the consultative role of the child psychiatrist and bringing it to the location where needed. This model strengthens the hand of the primary care provider who becomes increasingly more comfortable providing mental health care. This model, the telemental health consultation conference, allows a range of options for service delivery. For example, consultation from a telepsychiatrist may be provided to a group of primary care providers at a single major medical center site with high definition/high bandwidth but may also provide consultation to multiple providers at multiple different sites who are connected from their desktop computers through a "bridge" to the telepsychiatrist's site (Arora et al., 2011).

Another model utilizing telemedicine, which has been successful for several years, in the treatment of adults with chronic medical or psychiatric disorders, is called "colocated collaborative care." This model provides consultation to a primary care provider from a psychiatrist who is on site to consult to the primary care provider and to provide direct patient evaluation for the most complex patients. This model has allowed up to 75% of referred patients to receive all of their psychiatric care within the primary care clinic, thereby conserving scarce specialty services for the most complex patients (Pomerantz et al., 2010), a process that has also been referred to as "stepped collaborative care" (Katon, Von Korff et al., 1999). In another collaborative care model, a care manager located at the clinic with the primary care providers serves as a liaison between the primary care provider and the psychiatrist who is located at a distant site. The psychiatrist consults to the primary care provider through the care manager in weekly telephone consultation. The care manager may be a nurse, social worker, or even a bachelor level therapist depending on the system's resource. A system is crafted to collect appropriate clinical data from patients, to optimize their use of medication and psychosocial interventions, and to track their timely follow-up appointments. The use of a care manager allows services to be incorporated into the primary care setting; it also makes such services financially feasible. This model of care has been examined for the treatment of depression in adolescents using a nurse care manager (Richardson, McCauley, & Katon, 2009) and ADHD in Hispanic children ages 6−12 years old using social workers as care managers (Myers, Vander Stoep, Thompson, Zhou, & Unützer, 2010). In pre/postoutcomes, both of these models were feasible, well accepted by the families and revealed evidence of effectiveness in pre/postevaluation.

These collaborative care models have not yet incorporated telemental health. Incorporation of telemental health could help to build more personal connection among the primary care provider, care manager, and psychiatrist. In particular, the care manager position is a novel approach that requires training and ongoing support to function optimally. Telemental health can improve trust and team building.

Yet another model has been termed a "stabilization model" which is more like the traditional psychiatric clinic as it involves direct service to patients (Myers, Sulzbacher, & Melzer, 2004; Myers, Vander Stoep, McCarty et al., 2010). In this model, the telepsychiatrist assumes psychiatric care of the patient for a period of time. When patients stabilize, they are referred back to the primary care provider with specific recommendations for ongoing care. Direct telepsychiatric services may be delivered in a variety of locations such as a specific group practice of physicians, a regional medical center to which many different physicians refer, or a free standing specialty clinic. Scheduling may become complicated as more agencies are involved in arranging such appointments.

Models of Care and Clinical Practice: Other Sites of Practice

When child and adolescent telemental health services are provided in settings other than primary care, other models of service delivery will be needed. Further, these models will have to be adapted to the site of service, its resources, and the capabilities of available staff. Child and adolescent telemental health programs are currently situated in a wide variety of locations such as community mental health centers (Cain & Spaulding, 2006), urban day care (Cain & Spaulding, 2006), schools (Alicata, Saltman, & Ulrich, 2006; Harper, 2006), corrections (Myers, Valentine, Melzer, & Morganthaler, 2006), and residential settings (Storck, 2007). A community mental health center in a small town may have high bandwidth and a general psychiatrist or nurse practitioner who writes prescriptions and orders laboratory tests in consultation with a the child and adolescent psychiatrist. Or, a community mental health center in an impoverished frontier community may have access to only low bandwidth and no other psychiatric providers. A child and adolescent telepsychiatrist will need to determine whether it is possible to adequately assess the youth to provide direct care including prescribing or whether a collaborative model with a local physician is best. Correctional settings often have a local physician and nurse to render medical care and may work collaboratively with the telepsychiatrist to provide psychiatric care. Many schools have K12 or videoconferencing capabilities that should ideally allow the development of models of care to serve the children in this naturalistic setting. However, the location of the equipment may not allow sufficient confidentiality or may not provide adequate availability to ensure predictability in scheduling care. Creativity by the child and adolescent telepsychiatrist is an important characteristic in developing a feasible telepsychiatry practice that serves the needs of all stakeholders.

The times are definitely a-changing. While universities and other major medical centers continue to be at the forefront of providing child and adolescent telemental health services to distant communities, their territory has been infiltrated by commercial interests and private practitioners. Many companies in an urban setting contract with a community clinic in a rural or underserved area and a telepsychiatrist in another site to provide care. There are not yet any data on how well these triadic relationships function or the care delivered. These arrangements may be particularly common or helpful for federally qualified health centers which receive special funding to obtain such specialty services for their patients (Michael, Lardiere, Jones, & Perez, 2010). Telepsychiatry also offers the potential to practice from the private office, even a home office. Practitioners who, for a variety of reasons, might not be able to leave their usual practice setting can extend their reach to new populations through videoconferencing, thus increasing the variety of their practice without compromising productivity—and effectively expanding or redistributing the workforce (Glueck, 2011). This trend is likely to continue growing given its appeal to multiple stakeholders and entrepreneurial health care providers.

The cryptic "elephant in the room," as noted by Whitten and Holtz (2008), is that more widespread use of telemental health care for children would significantly and fundamentally change both the material conditions and manner of a physicians' practice. For example, offices would need to be set up differently, new equipment purchased, technical help hired, additional training needed—in fact, the structure of our residency programs will need to be altered to include training for competence in telemental health. Nevertheless, it seems inevitable that more equitable mental health care for children and adolescents is taking off and riding upon the broad bandwidths of telemental health. Where it will land, nobody can know for sure. But, if it increases access to competent evidence-based care, it will be a major step to realizing the dream of parity in mental health care for youth.

Optimizing the Virtual Clinical Encounter with Children and Families

The key to successful telepsychiatry with children and adolescents, as with all models and methods of treatment, is effective clinical care. Likewise, just as traditional clinical encounters are influenced factors that affect the face-to-face clinical relationship, telemedicine encounters are influenced by a different set of factors: those affecting the virtual clinical relationship (Onor & Misan, 2005). Many of these factors have been addressed in Chapters 3 and 5. The following addresses factors specifically relevant to conducting telemental health with children and adolescents, while following the practice parameters of the American Academy of Child and Adolescent Psychiatry (2008).

The Interview Room

One of the biggest mistakes in arranging space for telemental health with children is assuming that a small exam room or leftover small office will suffice, or that a conference room can be usurped. Such spaces do not allow accurate, safe, and satisfying encounters. In addition to providing privacy, the room should be large enough to accommodate the youth and at least one parent, and possibly a clinical staff member (depending on the model of care). Ideally, the room should also accommodate another person, such as a teacher or extended family member. There should be enough space to evaluate the child's motor skills, play, and self-control (American Academy of Child and Adolescent Psychiatry, 1997a, 1997b). If the room is too large, hyperactive children may get overly excited and disrupt the session by running about the room and over and under the furniture. This distracts the parents who may then shift focus to child management issues. A small table allowing the child to draw or play should be included. However, it should not interfere with the clinician's ability to view the child's motor skills, such as fidgeting while playing. The table should allow viewing of the child's drawing so that fine motor skills can be viewed and the child's attentional skills can be appreciated while conversing with the parent. If the patient site is in a medical clinic, the interview room may need to be cleared of fragile equipment that could distract or be potentially dangerous to the child if overturned or pulled off the walls. The usual physician swirling stool is a prime example of something both distracting and potentially dangerous. Choosing a low stimulation room is best.

Toys and Activities

It is important to have toys available for young children. It is even more important to have ones that are appropriate. Noisy toys must be avoided. The microphones are quite sensitive and tend to amplify extraneous sounds, which interferes with verbal communication. Even toys that "only" click or clank or pop occasionally and do not cause much concern under normal circumstances can markedly degrade the audio portion of the session. Proactive parents who wish to bring toys to entertain their children must be told at the time the appointment is scheduled to bring ones that are quiet. The reasons may not be intuitive but if explained to them, the parents are generally quiet happy to adhere to the request. Even seemingly benign toys such as Legos can be too noisy as the child rustles through a box looking for the right piece if he/she is too close to the microphone.

Toys with small pieces that must be picked up before the next session may cause delays in transition to the next patient and needlessly decrease efficiency. The cleanup process is an inconvenience to the staff at the clinic as well. Primary colored foam blocks, K-nex, books with Velcro detachable items, markers, and paper are excellent choices. Electronic toys are extremely distracting and absorb the child's attention, as a rule, should be avoided. The one exception to this rule: if the parents need time to talk with the telepsychiatrist or therapist and the child is beginning to distract them, a video game such as Nintendo DS with *sound off* and *a plug in* (in case the battery runs down) can be used if all else fails. The key is to know when to bring it out, which is *only after all essential data has been obtained from the child.*

The Triadic Virtual Relationship

The interpersonal dimensions of establishing the virtual relationship during telemental health care have been addressed in Chapter 3. These include emphasized screen presence, adjusting verbal communication to compensate for auditory lag, gesturing to facilitate communication, and lack of access to the naturally occurring nuances of communication present when sitting in the same-room with an individual. The child and adolescent telepsychiatrist must further attend to establishing and maintaining a relationship with two, and occasionally more, individuals (except in cases of older adolescents who may, at least for parts of the session, be in the room alone). It is important for teletherapists to understand and employ techniques which will allow them to quickly establish rapport with the patient. For all but the most disruptive or delayed youth, rapport building can be facilitated by giving them a close-up on the full monitor screen, i.e., showing them themselves on television. For systems that cannot show a full screen display, then showing youth their image in the "picture-in-picture" box on the screen is also a good ice breaker, even if not as dramatic. For many youth, the best rapport builder is to teach them, with their parents' assistance, how to manipulate the camera to obtain close-ups of themselves and their parents, or to scan the telepsychiatrist's room. Most youth also enjoy making the telepsychiatrist go away at the end of the session by disconnecting with the remote control. However, any such use of the equipment requires an active parent who can place boundaries upon the child's use of the remote control, including taking it back from an oppositional child who tries to control the encounter electronically. Apart from the electronics of the encounter, care must be taken to avoid falling into a pattern of overemphasizing the relationship with either the parent or the youth or inadvertently setting up a struggle between them.

Camera placement is crucial, both to establishing a therapeutic relationship and assessing its quality, particularly in relation to eye contact. Participants will naturally want to look at the monitor, not at the camera while communicating. By the same token, the patient will sense eye contact from the telepsychiatrist only when the latter is looking into the camera—or, to put it another way, in order to give the patient eye contact while also observing the patient's presentation, one must alternate gaze between the monitor, or image of the patient, and the camera. Additionally, the telepsychiatrist may have to take notes or check the computer for clinical information. Thus, telepsychiatrists need to remember to shift their gaze from monitor to camera in order to provide sufficient eye contact to optimize relatedness. With children and adolescents, eye contact is an important developmental consideration, especially when assessing anxiety, depression, psychosis, autism spectrum disorders, and attachment disorders. A camera mounted above monitor will cause the child to appear to be looking downward, perhaps suggesting depression or anxiety. Conversely, a camera placed below the monitor will make the child appear to be looking upward, conveying the possibility of autism spectrum disorders. These views might falsely convey difficulties in relatedness and/or impede rapport building. Eye contact is one of the few aspects of the mental status examination that is subject to assessment error during videoconferencing sessions. Ideally, telepsychiatrists would always query parents about the child's eye contact so as to accurately assess relatedness—even when the difficulty seems obvious. Furthermore, asking about eye contact can often lead to more relevant clinical data, such as to the child's development and internal experiences, e.g., whether poor eye contact reflects social anxiety or paranoid thinking.

As opposed to engaging a child, especially younger children, in play during a traditional session where everyone is in the same-room, rapport building can be more of a challenge with videoconferencing. Nonetheless, with practice and the right approach, it is ultimately quite doable. One helpful rapport-building process is to have the child show the telepsychiatrist a toy or bring a picture he/she has drawn up to the camera for a closer look. Some children do this spontaneously, demonstrating well-developed attention and relatedness skills. Sometimes children like to have their drawings faxed to the telepsychiatrist. Having a fax machine in the telepsychiatrist's room allows immediate feedback for the child, but faxing a copy after the session is acceptable to most children. Using demonstrative, animated gestures to augment communication during videoconferencing also improves rapport. This style may not come naturally for all but can be developed with practice. It may be particularly helpful for tired or less animated parents. Raising children with mental illness can lead to sleep deprivation and parents, on occasion, may even begin to nod off during a session. If one is accustomed to public speaking, the same interactive skills that engage the audience by showing interest in how the message is received also works in the videoconference setting. For example, when discussing medication adherence one might ask how it works best in their home. Looking to the parents and child as experts in their own home will increase engagement. Another technique that helps to keep the child and family engaged is to vary the tone and volume of one's voice. Easy to understand handouts are useful both during the session, to focus attention, and for later reference in implementing care at home. Handouts with some entertaining graphics may engage older children in the educational endeavor.

Other Dynamics

For children and adolescents, this triadic virtual relationship may be diffused over other individuals. Often, for convenience and/or due to the high cost of day care, siblings attend the sessions. Because of the particular importance that sibling relationships hold in child and adolescent psychiatry, their presence during a videoconferencing session may, at times, be quite beneficial. It can also be an excellent opportunity for pychoeducation of siblings, who may see the patient as receiving special favors or avoiding consequences due to their mental illness. And occasionally, for lower functioning patients, siblings will become caregivers as they grow into adulthood and survive the parents. Knowledge and understanding of the interactions between siblings, which can be stressors for both parties, can be appreciated during a videoconferencing session. Extended family members, as well, often provide valuable insights that may aid in facilitating assessment and treatment. Further, because the family is being treated at a familiar community setting and the session is woven into their usual daily routine, they are likely to be more relaxed and forthcoming than if they had to travel a long distance to a major, and unfamiliar, medical center. Such comfort may contribute to a realistic or naturalistic appreciation of the dynamics. The pan and zoom capabilities of the camera allow the telepsychiatrists to follow the siblings' interactions and affective responses during a session. High bandwidth is most appropriate and least distracting to families so that they are more likely to convey poignant issues and interactions.

Collateral Information and Collaboration

Teachers' input is recommended for most youths, especially those from culturally diverse groups. Additionally, school-based and clinic-based videoconferencing sessions have the potential to provide more information than is usually provided in written educational materials. For children with ADHD or disruptive behavioral disorders, teacher input is essential for diagnosis. Teacher input is also invaluable for treatment planning, including development of an individual educational plan (IEP) or accommodations. In addition, teacher input via videoconferencing provides a medium for team building with the psychiatrist. It is important to assess what systems the school has for providing such services. For example, more rural areas may not have broadband access and may rely on videophones or plain old telephone systems (POTS). Others have systems with high-bandwidth and high-definition monitors, but they are permanently located in the principal's office and do not afford sufficient privacy. Thus, some schools may be ideal to provide consultation to school personnel through videoconferencing, but direct care to students will require the telepsychiatrist to understand the school setup and milieu. For immigrant families, or families from other culturally diverse backgrounds, the schools may provide an ideal setting to obtain direct services. They are accustomed to sending their children to school and dealing with professional staff, there is no stigma attached to visiting the school, and teachers are generally respected and trusted so that they can serve as effective intermediaries with the family and telepsychiatrist.

The Clinical Session

Clinical care provided through telepsychiatry should be consistent with the AACAP's practice parameters. The Practice Parameter for the Psychiatric Assessment of Children and Adolescents (American Academy of Child and Adolescent Psychiatry, 1997a) recommends that some time be spent interviewing the youth alone. Older children with good impulse control, adequate verbal skills, and the ability to separate can be interviewed alone. For younger, developmentally impaired, or impulsive youth, traditional play sessions may be challenging and require a modified approach. The child can be observed interacting with staff in a structured or free play session, and some limited play with the child may be possible over the telemonitor, e.g., by drawing pictures and then discussing themes or by developing play scenarios with puppets.

In the patient room, ideally (though one does not always have this luxury), there should be a therapist or clinic staff person well versed in the needs of the telepsychiatry patient—e.g., performing vital signs, assisting in the room if there is a technical issue, dealing with a disruptive child whom the parent is unable to manage, or triaging to an emergency room or crisis services if the child or family member is suicidal. For parents with a distressing history to relate to the telepsychiatrist, one that is potentially harmful or otherwise inappropriate for the child to hear, it is useful to have staff who are able take the child out of the room for a brief period of time and allow an open, frank discussion. If one does not have this support in the clinic, the family can be advised to return next session with a safe adult who can take the child to the waiting room for part of the session. It is also helpful for someone at the remote site to provide rating scales for the youth and parents, and to make sure they are available to the telepsychiatrist in a timely manner in order to assist them in making an accurate diagnosis and/or assessing the effectiveness of treatment interventions. However, in reality, telemental health sessions often occur during other busy clinics or with limited staff or in other adverse conditions. Thus, the expert telepsychiatrist learns how to manage the remote site and family through a virtual relationship and sometimes, sessions have to be prematurely terminated. It is crucial to have a telephone in the patient's room so that if technical difficulties arise, the telepsychiatrist can contact the family in the room without inconveniencing staff in a busy clinic.

Treatment in Child and Adolescent Telemental Health

Pharmacotherapy

Medication treatment in telepsychiatry is described in Chapter 16 and is briefly reviewed here in relation to children and adolescence.

Pharmacotherapy is the most commonly requested telepsychiatry service and should comply with existing practice parameters (American Academy of Child and Adolescent Psychiatry, 2009). The approach to medication management will depend to some extent on the system in which the telepsychiatrist is working. Medication may be prescribed directly by the telepsychiatrist, by a collaborating nurse practitioner, or by the referring primary care physician. Whichever approach is used, clear procedures should be communicated regarding the method for obtaining initial prescriptions, refills, and for managing complications between sessions. Some modifications or complications are anticipated in child and adolescent telepsychiatry. Children often need to take medications at schools, day care, or other after-school facilities. This may require a second prescription. Generally, parents can just split a prescription into two bottles, one for home and one for the other site. However, sometimes a school requires its own bottle labeled by the pharmacy. This will require special arrangements with the pharmacy. Schools and other organizations may not be fully compliant in administering medication to the child during the school day. Careful collaboration with the school may then be needed to ensure good care. Stimulant medications prescribed for ADHD will need special procedures as these medications are designated by the Drug Enforcement agency as Schedule II drugs and automatic refills are not possible. Patients will need prescriptions for each month's supply. Thus, coordination among the patient, primary care physician, and telepsychiatrist needs to be carefully established. If a system is not worked out ahead of time, chaos and delays can easily arise.

Monitoring for adverse medication effects can readily be accomplished through videoconferencing. Tics, even mild ones, can be readily detected with moderate bandwidths of 256 kbits/s. The Abnormal Involuntary Movement Scale (AIMS) can easily be done for children on atypical antipsychotics by observing their movements as they enter the room and then having them sit in a chair in full view and taking them through the steps of the short, but crucial, exam. A web site is available to demonstrate the AIMS through videoconferencing (www.nrbh.org). Or, if they are already seated, then have the child walk for the provider after the exam. As always, asking the parents and child about any abnormal movements, especially tongue movements, through education about possible side effects makes them a crucial partner in the process. If a child is on an alpha agonist such as guanfacine for aggression or ADHD, orthostatic blood pressure and pulse should be determined. This, obviously, will need to be done by a person on the other end. With automated blood pressure monitors and multicuff systems now standard in most clinics, this can easily be performed by someone with minimal medical training at the beginning of the session—and the information is invaluable as one adjusts the guanfacine.

Perhaps the most important prescribing issue in telepsychiatry for children and adolescents is that many do not want to take medications, which they perceive as making them different from their peers. From a practical standpoint, this issue can often be handled by using, when available, long acting preparations and thereby avoiding the stigma of taking medication at school. The bigger task, however, is determining how to optimize the virtual relationship so as to overcome this barrier with the child. As the child and psychiatrist are not in the same-room, nuances of interpersonal communication cannot be relied upon to bring the child to adherence. This is a time for the telepsychiatrist, parent, and child to bring some concrete behavioral modification approaches and practical negotiation skills to bear on the situation. A positive consequence of such an approach is that it may be an opportunity to teach the parent and child some new effective communication skills.

Psychotherapy

Chapters 15 and 19 address the status of teletherapy. There has been only one study published on psychotherapy with youth through videoconferencing (Nelson et al.,

2003). However, several empirical studies have been published regarding the effectiveness of online CBT in adolescents and children that show modest success and promise for videoconferencing. A review article revealed eight studies of four Internet-based CBT programs for anxiety and depression in children and adolescents. Three studies were randomized controlled trials (RCTs), two with BRAVE-ONLINE in children ages 7–14 and the third MoodGYM in ages 13–17 ($N = 1477$). Each of the RCT studies showed a modest reduction in symptoms postintervention. The first two studies were clinic based with support from clinicians and the third was school based. Overall, six of the eight studies showed postintervention reduction in anxiety and/or depression (Calear & Christensen, 2010). The "Sadness Program," an Internet-based clinician-assisted computerized CBT, was studied ($n = 45$) in an RCT of CBT versus wait-list. The study used the Beck Depression Inventory and the Patient Health Questionnaire (9 item) and found that the program reduced depressive symptoms from pretreatment to posttreatment to a statistically significant degree (Perini, Titov, & Andrews, 2009). This appears to be an area ready for further study in telemental health. For the studies that utilized therapist support by phone or online, the conclusion was that therapist support improved outcomes (Calear & Christensen, 2010; Perini et al., 2009). These studies suggest a role for such therapist support through videoconferencing, either directly to the teen's home computer or at the local health clinic or mental health center. Such an approach would integrate new electronic patient-initiated treatment with more traditional aspects of psychotherapy such as rapport, guidance, encouragement to complete treatment modules, and individualized adaptation of therapy modules when needed. As such teletherapy sessions could be adjunctive to the online modules, they could be relatively infrequent to contain costs and other inconveniences, but sufficiently available for times when teens are in crisis.

Care Between Sessions

Families receiving ongoing services will need guidelines about interim care. Nonscheduled care is helpful to patients and communities, but difficult to arrange. If offered, patients should be informed of how to access such services. If not, then alternatives should be identified, especially for crises. Some telepsychiatrists recommend e-mail contact (Hilty, Yellowlees, Cobb et al., 2006). Procedures for interim care emphasize the importance of integrating telepsychiatry into a system of care so that other components can be accessed according to the youth's needs, the family's resources, and to reduce confusion for families and burden for clinicians (American Academy of Child and Adolescent Psychiatry, 2007).

Telepsychiatry in a Youth's System of Care

Many children and adolescents referred to telepsychiatry will be designated as seriously emotionally disabled by their schools and/or by the public mental health system providing services to them and their families. States vary in the systems of care provided to these children. Child and adolescent telepsychiatry services will then depend in part on other services available in the child's system of care. Limited telepsychiatry interventions, such as diagnostic and pharmacologic services, might be needed in a community providing a comprehensive system of care but may not be not possible in a less-well-developed system. Alternatively, less-well-developed systems might rely on the telepsychiatrist for more services. In particular, many children served in the public sector have other family members, particularly a parent, also in need of care. The child and adolescent telepsychiatrist may then provide additional services such as psychotherapy or parent behavioral training and may provide services to multiple family members.

Child and adolescent psychiatrists may also be asked to provide staff education. Many rural communities do not have access to child-trained therapists or case managers. Adult-trained staff covers all clients' needs. With increasing emphasis on providing evidence-based mental health care, new models of service delivery and training of staff in remote areas are needed.

The child and adolescent telepsychiatrist may then provide opportunities to increase the skills of local therapists who are not trained to work with children as well as staff who might need continuing education. Similarly, consultation with teachers and other professionals serving families may be incorporated into the child psychiatrist's position. The telepsychiatrist can readily collaborate in the child's care by virtually meeting on demand with local team members, such as school personnel.

Telemental Health in the Juvenile Justice System

The juvenile justice system (JJS) is a prime example of how telemental health can facilitate and often improve mental health care for a group of underserved youth. Due to conflicting circumstances of patient needs, legal mandates, moral and ethical concerns, and/or logistical issues, traditional on-site psychiatric care in JJS is at times a difficult, even untenable, proposition. Four states—Tennesee, New Mexico, Louisiana, and Washington—struggling to provide adequate psychiatric care for their incarcerated youth instituted telemental health to better meet the needs of this population. (Kaliebe, Heneghan, & Kim, 2011).

In New Mexico, a statewide telemental health teleconferencing system, in place since 2005, includes juvenile detention centers, juvenile parole and probation offices, and, as of 2010, group homes used as reintegration centers. The New Mexico JJS state requirement that psychiatric patients be seen monthly was difficult to meet when providers had to be on site for the appointment. Child psychiatrists were difficult to retain and costly, especially when appointments were canceled at the last minute—a common occurrence in such settings (e.g., lockdowns). The implementation of telemental health care, a system that includes juvenile detention centers, juvenile parole and probation offices, and, as of 2010, group homes used as reintegration centers have greatly improved the timeliness and availability of care. In addition, for some patients, the same telepsychiatrist is available to provide a continuity of care after the youth is released to a group home or reintegration center.

In 2000, the Louisiana JJS, under legal pressure from the US Department of Justice to provide adequate mental health services, contracted with the Louisiana State University Health Sciences Center (LSUHSH) to provide telemental health services. This system employed a variety of telemental health providers. A nursing staff accompanies the youth to each session to provide continuity of care after the telemental health sessions. Similar to the New Mexico program, there is a capacity for continuity with the parole office as many youth have difficulty finding timely community-based follow-up care.

In 2001, also under legal pressure, Tennessee instituted a teleconferencing system to provide mental health care for the youth in their five correctional centers. Though the program was variably accepted by the sites, overall, major benefits were described including improved care, increased timeliness of care, improved accuracy of diagnosis, reduced emergency room psychiatric visits, and reduced use of psychotropic medications—a longtime concern for youth in JJS and especially for minority youth who are overrepresented (Alegria, Vallas, & Pumariega, 2010). Stated difficulties varied among the sites and related to issues of providing appropriate space for privacy without compromising supervision. Some barriers were related to lack of interest by the institution that was thought to be complicated by deficits in the process of introduction of the new program and its benefits.

In Washington State, the JJS is termed the Juvenile Rehabilitation Administration (JRA). When the JRA's goal to provide mental health services on-site at JRA facilities was logistically difficult at one site, a minimum-security facility over 200 miles from Seattle, they contracted with Seattle Children's Hospital for telepsychiatry services. Over 29 months, 115 youth were treated with a total of 275 telepsychiatry sessions (Myers, Valentine, Melzer, & Morganthaler, 2006). Youth were very satisfied with their care. The major complaint was lack of privacy. Staff responded to this by changing the model, so only the nurse practitioner attended the sessions. The telepsychiatrist's major concern was the need for considerable between sessions care. This issue underscores the need to carefully craft a system that appropriately integrates the telepsychiatrist's skills and availability while training local staff to tend to nonpsychiatric mental health needs.

Cultural Competence

Cultural concerns have been covered in other sections of the text. The following is a brief overview of additional issues to consider when focusing on children and adolescents. Given the United States' rapidly changing demographics—it is predicted that by 2030 Euro-Americans will no longer be a majority among children under age 18 (US Census, 2009)—cultural competence for child psychiatry could be greatly enhanced by telemental health. In the current draft of practice parameters for Cultural Competence for the American Academy of Child and Adolescent Psychiatry (presented in the member forum on October 21, 2011, at the Joint Meeting of the CACAP and AACAP in Toronto, Canada), principles were posited in draft form that support the use of creative ways to improve the mental health in our increasingly multiracial, multicultural society. Creative ways are clearly consistent with the advances of telemental health as telepsychiatry has already been used successfully with minority youth, such as African-Americans (Cain & Spaulding, 2006), Hispanics (Adelsheim, 2008; Harper, 2006), American Indians (Savin, Garry, Zuccaro, & Novins, 2006), and Hawaiians (Alicata et al., 2006).

Principles were proposed to address inclusion of family members as well as key members of traditional extended families in all aspects of treatment. In collectivist cultures, extended family involvement may be the only way to address psychiatric issues in contrast to individualist cultures where immediate relatives or, in the case of adolescent patients, the individual may be all that is necessary. The inclusion of extended family and nonblood "relatives" who possess an equivalent emotional bond (fictive kin) (Chatters, Taylor, & Jayakody, 1994) have been shown to be essential in attaining the collateral input necessary for an accurate diagnosis and treatment plan. For culturally diverse patients, it is important that clinicians ascertain whom the patient considers family and determine if this is a source of stress or support for them (Myers, 2004). Because it is provided in community-based sites that multiple family members, both biologic and/or fictive, can easily access, telemental health may better facilitate care for culturally diverse populations than would more traditional methods of care. Youth in these families will likely be comfortable with the technology, but elders or immigrant parents may need some convincing or modification of approach to help them engage fully in the distant assessment and treatment. No data are yet available to guide service delivery in this regard.

Another proposal is to provide care in the language in which the child and family are fluent, which is difficult to accomplish in remote, underserved areas and inner-city community clinics where resources are limited. However, if the care is provided via telepsychiatry housed in an urban medical center, there is likely better access to interpreter services. Yet another proposed principal that lends itself to telemedicine is to provide treatment in a familiar setting within the community. Diverse children and families have shown a strong preference to receive care in ethnically specific community clinics (Akutsu, Castillo, & Snowden, 2007; Dean, Jaycox, Langley, Kataoka, & Stein, 2008) or school-based services (Kataoka et al., 2003).

For multicultural youth, especially those living in areas underserved by mental health—which is quite common—delivering care in their local environment will enhance the overall experience and increase access for this growing population. To provide culturally competent care for mentally ill, culturally complex youth and families, telemental health is one way to meet the challenge of serving the ever growing needs of our changing youth population. When providing care remotely, one can more likely respect the preferences of the child and family, but the important improvements of telepsychiatry is having the capacity to bring the treatment to a location comfortable to the family and allow the opportunity for extended family members to attend without the hardship of traveling to an urban area for this specialized care.

Moving Forward

As child and adolescent telepsychiatry is not yet integrated into the mainstream of mental health care, it is important that practitioners collect clinical outcome data to document the effectiveness and quality of their care. Outcomes may be measured with broadband scales, disorder-specific scales, symptom-based scales, and functional assessments. Assessments should include both the parent's assessment of their child and the child's self-report. Quality utilization indicators should be specific to the patient's community and stakeholders in the youth's system of care, such as treating clinicians, schools, therapists, funding agencies, community representatives, and families.

Summary and Conclusions

The times are definitely a-changing. Universities and other mega medical centers are no longer sole bastions for child telemental health programs: they have infiltrated private practice—a trend that is likely to continue growing (Glueck, 2011), as noted in Chapter 7. Patients and families have readily accepted child and adolescent telepsychiatry, and programs are now situated in a wide variety of locations including community medical centers (Myers, Sulzbacher, & Melzer, 2004), community mental health centers (Cain & Spaulding, 2006), urban day care centers (Cain & Spaulding, 2006), rural schools (Alicata et al., 2006; Harper, 2006; Pakyurek et al., 2010), corrections facilities (Myers, Valentine, Melzer, & Morganthaler, 2006), and residential settings (Storck, 2007). Telepsychiatry also offers the potential to practice from home. Practitioners who, for a variety of reasons, might want to work from home can maintain their practice, thus increasing the productivity of existing psychiatrists and effectively expanding the workforce (Myers, Vander Stoep, McCarty et al., 2010).

    And yet, despite the optimistic outlook outlined above, there are still major obstacles to the growth of telepsychiatry into a major player within the child and adolescent psychiatric community. A major obstacle, as in other areas of telepsychiatry, is reimbursement. As programs continue to grow and provide outcome data on the effectiveness of their services, reimbursement will improve. A more difficult obstacle is child and adolescent psychiatrists' reluctance to adopt this approach to care. While telepsychiatry offers the opportunity to redistribute the workforce and increase access in underserved areas, there are, as yet, still insufficient child and adolescent psychiatrists to serve even easy to access urban and suburban areas. A new breed of child and adolescent psychiatrist, interested in reaching underserved populations and who embraces technological approaches to mental health care, will be needed.

    The future of child and adolescent telepsychiatry lies in solid research. Outcome studies are now needed to demonstrate that child and adolescent telepsychiatry is comparable to in-person psychiatric care and superior to care rendered in primary care. With efficacy demonstrated, it will be important to examine optimal models of telepsychiatry care to youth. Efficacy studies are also needed to show whether telepsychiatry can be used to disseminate evidence-based treatments and to train clinicians in remote communities. While awaiting efficacy studies, telepsychiatric care should adhere to evidence-based guidelines and best practices as summarized in the practice parameters of the AACAP.

A major barrier has been the lack of availability of telemental health in the most needy, most remote, communities. The Federal Communications Commission has recently issued its plan to extend broadband into remaining unserviced areas (Moe, 2011). Another potential barrier, addressed by Whitten and Holtz (2008), is a cryptic "elephant in the room"—the reality that a more widespread use of telemental health care for children would significantly and fundamentally change both the material conditions and manner of physicians' practice. Nevertheless, it seems inevitable that mental health care for children and adolescents is about to take off and ride upon the broad bandwidths of telemental health. Where it will land, nobody can know for sure, but in all likelihood it will be a better place than we are presently.

References

Adelsheim, S. (2008). Telepsychiatry with rural school-based health centers in New Mexico. Clinical perspectives, presented at the *55th annual meeting of the American academy of child and adolescent psychiatry*. Chicago, IL.

Akutsu, P. D., Castillo, E. D., & Snowden, L. R. (2007). Differential referral patterns to ethnic-specific and mainstream mental health programs for four Asian American groups. *American Journal of Orthopsychiatry, 77*, 95–103.

Alegria, M., Vallas, M., & Pumariega, A. (2010). Racial and ethnic disparities in pediatric mental health. *Child and Adolescent Psychiatric Clinics of North America, 19*, 759–774.

Alicata, D., Saltman, D., & Ulrich, D. (2006). Child and adolescent telepsychiatry in rural Hawaii. Abstract 5172:1.17-2. Clinical perspectives, presented at the *53rd annual meeting of the American academy of child and adolescent psychiatry*. San Diego, CA.

American Academy of Child and Adolescent Psychiatry (1997a). Practice parameters for the psychiatric assessment of children and adolescents. *Journal of American Academy of Child and Adolescent Psychiatry, 36*(10 Suppl.), 4S–20S.

American Academy of Child and Adolescent Psychiatry (1997b). Practice parameters for the psychiatric assessment of infants and toddlers (0–36 months). *Journal of American Academy of Child Adolescent Psychiatry, 36*(10 Suppl.), 21S–36S.

American Academy of Child and Adolescent Psychiatry (2007). Practice parameter on child and adolescent mental health care in community systems of care. *Journal of the American Academy of Child and Adolescent Psychiatry, 46*, 284–299.

American Academy of Child and Adolescent Psychiatry (2008). Practice parameter for child and adolescent telepsychiatry. *Journal of American Academy of Child and Adolescent Psychiatry, 47*, 1468–1483.

American Academy of Child and Adolescent Psychiatry (2009). Practice parameter on the use of psychotropic medications in children and adolescents. *Journal of American Academy of Child and Adolescent Psychiatry, 48*, 961–973.

American Academy of Pediatrics (2009). The future of pediatrics: Mental health competencies for pediatric primary care. Committee on psychosocial aspects of child and family health and task force on mental health. *Pediatrics, 124*, 410−421.

Arora, S., Kalishman, S., Dion, D., Som, D., Thornton, K., Bankhurst, A., et al. (2011). Partnering urban academic medical centers and rural primary care clinicians to provide complex chronic disease care. *Health Affairs, 30*, 1176−1184.

Boydell, K., Volpe, T., & Pignatello, A. (2010). A qualitative study of young people's perspectives on receiving psychiatric services via televideo. *Journal of the Canadian Academy of Child Adolescent Psychiatry, 19*, 5−11.

Broder, E., Manson, E., Boydell, K., & Teshima, J. (2004). Use of telepsychiatry for child psychiatric issues: First 500 cases. *Canadian Journal of Psychiatry Bulletin, 36*, 11−15.

Cain, S., & Spaulding, R. (2006). Telepsychiatry: Lessons from two models of care. Abstract 5172:1.17-2. Clinical perspectives, presented at the *53rd annual meeting of the American academy of child and adolescent psychiatry*. San Diego, CA.

Calear, A. L., & Christensen, H. (2010). Review of Internet-based prevention and treatment programs for anxiety and depression in children and adolescents. *Medical Journal of Australia, 192*. (11)Suppl. 12−14

Caplan, G., & Caplan, R. (2000). Principles of community psychiatry. *Mental Health Journal, 36*(1), 7−24.

Chatters, L. M., Taylor, R. J., & Jayakody, J. S. (1994). Fictive kinship relationships in Black extended families. *Journal of Comparative Family Studies, 25*, 297−312.

Cloutier, P., Cappelli, M., Glennie, J. E., & Keresztes, C. (2008). Mental health services for children and youth: A survey of physicians' knowledge, attitudes and use of telehealth services. *Journal of Telemedicine and Telecare, 14*, 98−101.

Dean, K. L., Jaycox, L. H., Langley, A. K., Kataoka, S. H., & Stein, B. D. (2008). School-based disaster mental health services: Clinical, policy and community challenges. *Professional Psychology: Research and Practice, 39*, 52−57.

Diamond, J. M., & Bloch, M. (2010). Telepsychiatry assessments of child or adolescent behavior disorders: A review of evidence and issues. *Telemedicine Journal and e-Health, 16*, 712−716.

Dobbins, M. I., Roberts, N., Vicari, S. K., Seale, D., Bogdanich, R., & Record, J. (2011). The consultation conference: A new model of collaboration for child psychiatry and primary care. *Academic Psychiatry, 35*, 260−262.

Elford, R., White, H., Bowering, R., Ghandi, A., Maddiggan, K., St, John, K., et al. (2000). A randomized, controlled trial of child psychiatric assessments conducted using videoconferencing. *Journal of Telemedicine and Telecare, 6*, 73−82.

Elford, R., White, H., St John, K., Maddigan, B., Ghandi, M., & Bowering, R. (2001). A prospective satisfaction study and cost analysis of a pilot child telepsychiatry service in Newfoundland. *Journal of Telemedicine and Telecare, 7*, 73−81.

Fox, K. C., Connor, P., McCullers, E., & Waters, T. (2008). Effect of a behavioural health and specialty care telemedicine programme on goal attainment for youths in juvenile detention. *Journal of Telemedicine and Telecare, 14*, 227−230.

Glueck, D. A. (2011). Telepsychiatry in private practice. *Child and Adolescent Psychiatric Clinics of North America, 20*, 1−11.

Greenberg, N., Boydell, K. M., & Volpe, T. (2006). Paediatric telepsychiatry in Ontario: Caregiver and service provider perspectives. *Journal of Behavioural Health Services Research, 33*, 105−111.

Grover, S. S., Rockhill, C. M., Kim, G. M., Swardstrom M., Vander Stoep, A., & Myers, K. (2011). Improving quality of care for youth with ADHD: Components of successful medication intervention. Abstract 1.23. In: *Scientific proceedings of the 2011 joint annual meeting of the American academy of child and adolescent psychiatry and the Canadian academy of child and adolescent psychiatry*, Vol. XXXVIII. Toronto, ON.

Harper, R. A. (2006). Telepsychiatry consultation to schools and mobile clinics in rural Texas. Abstract 5172:1.17-2. Clinical perspectives, presented at the *53rd annual meeting of the American academy of child and adolescent psychiatry*. San Diego, CA.

Hilt, R. (2011). This issue: Assessment of pediatric mental health. *Pediatric Annals*, *40*, 472–474.

Hilty, D. M., Yellowlees, P. M., Cobb, H. C., Neufeld, J. D., & Bourgeois, J. A. (2006). Use of secure e-mail and telephone: Psychiatric consultations to accelerate rural health service delivery. *Telemedicine Journal and e-Health*, *12*, 490–495.

Hilty, D. M., Yellowlees, P. M., Sonik, P., Derlet, M., & Hendren, R. L. (2009). Rural child and adolescent telepsychiatry: Successes and struggles. *Pediatric Annals*, *38*, 228–232.

Hockey, A. D., Yellowlees, P. M., & Murphy, S. (2004). Evaluation of a pilot second-opinion child telepsychiatry service. *Journal of Telemedicine and Telecare*, *10* (Suppl. 1), 48–50.

Kaliebe, K. E., Heneghan, J., & Kim, T. J. (2011). Telepsychiatry in juvenile justice settings. *Child and Adolescent Psychiatric Clinics of North America*, *20*, 113–123.

Kataoka, S., Stein, B., Jaycox, L., Wong, M., Escudero, P., Tu, W., et al. (2003). A school-based mental health program for traumatized Latino immigrant children. *Journal of the American Academy of Child and Adolescent Psychiatry*, *42*, 311–318.

Katon, W., Richardson, L., Russo, J., McCarty, C. A., Rockhill, C., McCauley, E., et al. (2010). Depressive symptoms in adolescence: The association with multiple health risk behaviors. *General Hospital Psychiatry*, *32*, 233–239.

Katon, W., Von Korff, M., Lin, E., Simon, G., Walker, E., Unützer, J., et al. (1999). Stepped collaborative care for primary care patients with persistent symptoms of depression a randomized trial. *Archives of General Psychiatry*, *56*, 1109–1115.

Michael, R., Lardiere, M. R., Jones, E., & Perez, M. (2010). *National association of community health centers. Assessment of behavioral health services in federally qualified health centers.* <http://www.fqhcmd.com/uploads/4/7/3/5/4735489/nachc_2010_assessment_of_behavioral_health_services_in_fqhcs_1_14_11_final.pdf/> Accessed 14.01.12.

Moe, J. (2011). FCC approves plan to expand broadband and wireless to rural areas. *Marketplace from American Public Media*<http://marketplace.publicradio.org/display/web/2011/10/28/tech-report-fcc-approves-plan-to-expand-broadband-and-wireless-rural-areas/> (October 28, 2011) Accessed 29.11.11.

Myers, G. E. (2004). Addressing the effects of culture on the boundary-keeping practices of psychiatry residents educated outside of the United States. *Academic Psychiatry*, *28*, 47–55.

Myers, K. M., Sulzbacher, S., & Melzer, S. M. (2004). Telepsychiatry with children and adolescents: are patients comparable to those evaluated in usual outpatient care? *Telemedicine Journal and e-Health*, *10*, 278–285.

Myers, K. M., Valentine, J. M., & Melzer, S. M. (2007). Feasibility, acceptability, and sustainability of telepsychiatry with children and adolescents. *Psychiatric Services*, *58*, 1493–1496.

Myers, K. M., Valentine, J. M., & Melzer, S. M. (2008). Child and adolescent telepsychiatry: Utilization and satisfaction. *Telemedicine Journal and e-Health*, *14*, 131–137.

Myers, K. M., Valentine, J. M., Melzer, S. M., & Morganthaler, R. (2006). Telepsychiatry with incarcerated youth. *Journal of Adolescent Health*, *38*, 643–648.

Myers, K. M., Vander Stoep, A., McCarty, C. A., Klein, J. B., Palmer, N. B., Geyer, J. R., et al. (2010). Child and adolescent telepsychiatry: Variations in utilization referral patterns and practice trends. *Journal of Telemedicine and Telecare, 16,* 128−133.

Myers, K. M., Vander Stoep, A., Thompson, K., Zhou, C., & Unützer, J. (2010). Collaborative care for the treatment of Hispanic children diagnosed with ADHD. *General Hospital Psychiatry, 32,* 612−614.

Myers, K. M., Palmer, N. B., & Geyer, J. R. (2011). Research in child and adolescent telemental health. *Child and Adolescent Psychiatric Clinics of North America, 20,* 155−171.

Nelson, E. L., Barnard, M., & Cain, S. (2003). Treating childhood depression over videoconferencing. *Telemedicine Journal and e-Health, 9,* 49−55.

Nesbitt, T. S., Marcin, J. P., Daschbach, M. M., & Cole, S. L. (2005). Perceptions of local health care quality in 7 rural communities with telemedicine. *Journal of Rural Health, 21,* 79−85.

Achieving the promise: Transforming mental health care in America. (2003). Rockville, MD: New Freedom Commission on Mental Health, DHHS Pub. No. SMA-03-3832.

Onor, M. S., & Misan, M. D. (2005). The clinical interview and the doctor−patient relationship in telemedicine. *Telemedicine Journal and e-Health, 11,* 102−105.

Pakyurek, M., Yellowlees, P., & Hilty, D. (2010). The child and adolescent telepsychiatry consultation: Can it be a more effective clinical process for certain patient than conventional practice? *Telemedicine Journal and e-Health, 16,* 289−292.

Palmer, N. B., Myers, K. M., Vander Stoep, A., McCarthy, C. A., Geyer, J. R., & DeSalvo, A. (2010). Attention-deficit/hyperactivity disorder and telemental health. *Current Psychiatry Reports, 12,* 409−417.

Perini, S., Titov, N., & Andrews, G. (2009). Clinician-assisted Internet-based treatment is effective for depression: Randomized controlled trial. *Australian and New Zealand Journal of Psychiatry, 43,* 571−578.

Pomerantz, A. S., Shiner, B., Watts, B. V., Detzer, M. J., Kutter, C., Street, B., et al. (2010). The White River model of colocated collaborative care: A platform for mental and behavioral health care in the medical home. *Journal on Families, Systems, & Health, 28,* 114−129.

Richardson, L., McCauley, E., & Katon, W. (2009). Collaborative care for adolescent depression: A pilot study. *General Hospital Psychiatry, 31,* 36−45.

Rockhill, C. M., Grover, S. S., Kim, G. M., Waldron, L., Yranela, C., Swardstrom, M., et al. (2011). Adherence to consensus-based guidelines in telepsychiatry. Abstract 5.12. In: *Scientific proceedings of the 2011 joint annual meeting of the American academy of child and adolescent psychiatry and the Canadian academy of child and adolescent psychiatry,* Vol. XXXVIII. Toronto, ON.

Savin, D., Garry, M. T., Zuccaro, P., & Novins, D. (2006). Telepsychiatry for treating rural American Indian youth. *Journal of the American Academy of Child and Adolescent Psychiatry, 45,* 484−488.

Speedie, S. M., Ferguson, S. A., Sanders, J., & Doarn, M. B (2008). The promise of new care delivery models. *Telemedicine Journal and e-Health, 14,* 964−967.

Spooner, A. S., & Gotlieb, E. M. (2004). Telemedicine: Pediatric applications. *Pediatrics, 113,* 639−643.

Stain, H. J., Payne, K., Thienel, R., Michie, P., Carr, V., & Kelly, B. (2011). The feasibility of videoconferencing for neuropsychological assessments of rural youth experiencing early psychosis. *Journal of Telemedicine and Telecare, 17,* 328−331.

Storck, M. (2007). Bringing the community to the state hospital through teleconferencing. Clinical perspectives, presented at the *54th annual meeting of the American academy of child and adolescent psychiatry*. Boston, MA.

US Census. United States population projections: 2000 to 2050. (2009) <http://www.census. gov/population/www/projections/analytical-document09.pdf/> Accessed 22.06.11.

Whitten, P., & Holtz, B. (2008). Provider utilization of telemedicine: The elephant in the room. *Telemedicine Journal and e-Health, 14*, 995–997.

Yellowlees, P., & Nafiz, N. (2010). The psychiatrist–patient relationship of the future: Anytime, anywhere? *Harvard Review of Psychiatry, 18*, 96–102.

Yellowlees, P. M., Hilty, D. M., Marks, S. L., Neufeld, J., & Bourgeois, J. A. (2008). A retrospective analysis of a child and adolescent telemental health program. *Journal of the American Academy of Child and Adolescent Psychiatry, 47*, 103–107.

12 Rural Veterans and Telemental Health Service Delivery

Leslie Morland* and Karen Kloezeman

National Center for PTSD—Pacific Island Division, Department of
Veterans Affairs Pacific Island Health Care System, Honolulu, HI

Introduction

The delivery of health care services to rural veteran populations has been a challenge for the Department of Veterans Affairs (VA) across war eras. A critical barrier to care for many rural veterans is limited access to specialty care (Weeks, Wallace, Wang, Lee, & Kazis, 2006), particularly for the large number of returning Operation Enduring Freedom/Operation Iraqi Freedom (OEF/OIF) veterans living in rural and remote areas (Westermeyer, Canive, Thuras, Chesness, & Thompson, 2002). The delivery of specialty mental health services via telemental health (TMH) has become increasingly important for increasing access to care for rural veteran populations. Studies are currently being conducted on the use of TMH modalities to deliver mental health interventions to veterans; however, there is a need for further investigations of specialized psychological interventions and veteran populations. This chapter will address the mental health needs of rural veterans and then discuss the role of TMH in increasing their access to care. Our specific program of TMH research for posttraumatic stress disorder (PTSD) and related lessons learned will be discussed. The methodological and clinical considerations, cost-effectiveness, and challenges associated with the TMH delivery modality in the VA are presented.

Rural Veteran Population

Currently, 3.3 million (approximately 40%) of the 8 million VA health care system users in the United States (U.S.) reside in rural areas (U.S. Department of Veterans Affairs, 2012). This number is expected to rise in light of recent research showing

* Corresponding Author: Leslie A. Morland, National Center for PTSD—Pacific Islands Division, Department of Veterans Affairs Pacific Islands Health Care System, 3375 Koapaka Street, Suite I-560, Honolulu, HI 96819. Tel.: + 808-566-1934, Fax: +808-566-1885, E-mail: Leslie.Morland@va.gov

Telemental Health. DOI: http://dx.doi.org/10.1016/B978-0-12-416048-4.00012-9

that the number of OEF/OIF soldiers recruited from rural areas has grown relative to the number recruited from urban areas (Kane, 2006); thus, many soldiers of the current war are likely to return to rural areas after separating from the military. Across the U.S., the proportion of veterans living in rural areas varies according to the region of the country. The VA health care system has divided the U.S. into 21 regional health care networks, or Veterans Integrated Service Networks, and established its own classification system to distinguish between urban and rural areas. The VA's system categorizes geographic areas into *urban, rural,* and *highly rural.* When this system is used to classify veterans, 59%, 39%, and 2% have been categorized as residing in urban, rural, and highly rural areas, respectively. In addition, 45% of the community-based outpatient clinics (CBOCs) of the VA were found to be located in rural areas (Hartman, 2007). The VA and other health care providers are faced with numerous challenges when delivering health services to veterans dispersed across wide, sparsely populated geographic areas.

Studies of VA populations suggest there are notable differences between rural veterans and those residing in urban settings. For example, in a sample of homeless veterans ($N = 3595$), significant differences were reported in personal, medical, and health care utilization characteristics between homeless veterans residing in nonmetropolitan and metropolitan areas (Gordon, Haas, Luther, Hilton, & Goldstein, 2010). Specifically, nonmetropolitan homeless veterans were more likely to be white, have served in the Persian Gulf or pre-Vietnam era, have recent employment history, and receive public financial assistance. In addition, utilization of VA health care services was predicted by metropolitan status, such that metropolitan homeless veterans were more likely (OR = 1.36, $P = 0.0008$) than their nonmetropolitan counterparts to have used VA care in the 6 months prior to the study. Furthermore, black nonmetropolitan homeless veterans were less likely to use VA services than their white counterparts (OR = 0.77, $P = 0.023$). Another study investigating mental health case management in the VA compared the sociodemographic characteristics of 5221 rural and urban veterans with mental illness and found that rural veterans were significantly older, evidenced higher rates of unemployment, and had fewer years of education (Mohamed, Neale, & Rosenheck, 2009). These findings suggest that rural veterans wait longer to obtain mental health treatment, face greater psychosocial stressors, and have fewer personal resources for coping or overcoming these stressors. In addition, rural veterans in this study were more likely to be Caucasian, disabled, receive VA benefits, and have a person designated to manage their funds.

Mental Health Disorders in Veterans

Veterans frequently experience physical and mental health disorders after active duty and exposure to combat situations. Mental health disorders commonly reported among veterans include PTSD, depression, anxiety disorder, adjustment disorder, and substance use disorders (Seal, Berenthal, Miner, Sen, & Marmar, 2007). In particular, PTSD has been estimated to be prevalent in approximately 15% of Vietnam veterans (Dohrenwend et al., 2006) and in 10 − 20% of returning OEF/OIF military veterans (Hoge, Castro et al., 2004; Thomas et al., 2010). Research conducted with veterans with mental illness have evidenced that these individuals also experience a number of additional co-occurring deleterious conditions. Veterans are at a high risk for suicide (Kaplan, Huguet, McFarland, & Newsom, 2007) and display high rates of substance and alcohol use (Wagner et al., 2007). Combat exposure has been related to substantial morbidity in terms of PTSD, depression, substance abuse, and social and occupational impairments (Prigerson, Maciejewski, & Rosenheck, 2002). Furthermore, veterans with PTSD are at an increased risk for comorbid psychiatric conditions, as PTSD has been associated with higher rates of physical problems (Grieger et al., 2006; Schnurr & Spiro, 1999), mortality (Johnson, Fontana, Lubin, Corn, & Rosenheck, 2004), suicide (Kang & Bullman, 2008), functional impairment (Frueh, Turner, Beidel, & Cahill, 2001; Thorp & Stein, 2005; Thorp & Stein, 2008), and dysregulated anger and hostility (Chemtob, Hamada, Roitblat, & Muraoka, 1994; Jakupcak et al., 2007) in veteran populations.

Studies with OEF/OIF military personnel and veterans suggest that soldiers who were deployed to Iraq are at higher risk for developing mental health difficulties, likely because of their increased exposure to combat situations relative to soldiers deployed to other locations (e.g., Afghanistan). A survey of returning OEF/OIF soldiers indicated that 71−86% of these veterans were involved in firefight during their deployment to Iraq (Hoge, Castro et al., 2004). This study also screened OEF/OIF soldiers for symptoms of depression, generalized anxiety, and PTSD and found that Marines returning from Iraq were significantly more likely to report symptoms of these mental health problems than military personnel before deployment or those returning from deployment to Afghanistan. A population-based descriptive study of soldiers returning from Iraq, Afghanistan, and other locations demonstrated that 19.1%, 11.3%, and 8.5% of these veterans, respectively, reported mental health problems postdeployment (Hoge, Auchterlonie, & Milliken, 2006). Furthermore, younger OEF/OIF military personnel (i. e., 18−24 years of age) have shown a higher risk for PTSD and other mental health diagnoses than returning soldiers aged 40 years or older (Seal, Berenthal et al., 2007). An increasingly pertinent topic under investigation in studies conducted with VA populations is the high incidence of traumatic brain injury (TBI) (Hoge, McGurk et al., 2008; Tanielian & Jaycox, 2008) and comorbidity between TBI and associated psychiatric conditions (Carlson et al., 2010) evidenced in returning OEF/OIF veterans. Given the high prevalence rate of mental health disorders and related problems in veteran populations and the generation of OEF/OIF veterans that will be matriculating into the VA system in the coming years, it is important for research to address current concerns about access to effective mental health services in the VA for both returning OEF/OIF soldiers and veterans of previous war eras.

Rural−Urban Health Disparities in Veterans

Studies on differences in prevalence rates of mental health disorders between urban and rural veterans have demonstrated mixed results. An investigation conducted with survey data of 748,216 veterans found that rural veterans were less likely than urban veterans to have mental health disorders; however, rural veterans had a higher prevalence of physical diseases and lower physical and mental quality of life (Weeks, Wallace et al.,

2006). Additionally, those rural veterans with mental illness were more likely to experience a greater disease burden and incur greater health care costs (Wallace, Weeks, Wang, Lee, & Kazis, 2006). Similarly, a comparison of rural, urban, and suburban veterans found that rural veterans had poorer health-related quality of life and more physical health comorbidities than their urban and suburban counterparts even after controlling for sociodemographic factors (i.e., age, gender, employment status, race) (Weeks, Kazis et al., 2004); however, this study also indicated that rural veterans had fewer mental health comorbidities. While it is difficult to identify potential explanations for this pattern of findings without further research, it is clear that veterans from all geographic areas have a high need for services to address a wide variety of physical and mental health care concerns.

In summary, estimates of the number of veterans residing in rural areas vary somewhat depending on the geographic area classification system used, but converge to indicate that they represent a small but important proportion of the total US veteran population that will continue to grow as soldiers from the current war era return. Deployed veterans, particularly those serving in high-conflict areas such as Iraq, are at high risk of developing psychiatric disorders. Findings on rural–urban disparities in physical and mental health disease prevalences are mixed but suggest that rural veterans with mental illness suffer a greater disease burden relative to their urban and suburban counterparts. Thus, the need to provide them with quality mental health treatment will be high. Understanding current patterns of service utilization and barriers to accessing care at the VA is the first step toward identifying ways to improve service delivery to rural veterans.

Access to Care

Residents of rural areas have evidenced significant disparities in access to health care and specialized services when comparisons are conducted between rural and urban populations (President's New Freedom Commission on Mental Health, 2004; Beachler, Holloman, & Herman, 2003). In the U.S., many individuals with mental health disorders, especially those residing in rural communities and racial minorities, do not receive adequate treatment after being diagnosed with these conditions (Wang et al., 2005). Given the recent evidence that many OEF/OIF veterans will be returning to rural communities, the underutilization of mental health care among rural populations is a particularly relevant problem for the VA. Furthermore, rural veterans have less access to specialized mental health care and often rely on receiving services and screening for mental health disorders through a primary care medical setting (Seal, Berenthal et al., 2007).

VA Health Care Service Utilization

Medical Health Service Use Determinants

There is a large body of research on the utilization of general medical and primary care among VA populations (Payne et al., 2005), including veterans with psychiatric illnesses (Chwastiak, Rosenheck, & Kazis, 2008) and physical health problems (Elhai, Richardson, & Pedlar, 2007). A full review of the literature based on the determinants of utilization of medical health care is beyond the scope of this chapter; however, it is notable that veterans with mental health disorders have evidenced higher rates of medical health care utilization. The relationship between the presence and severity of mental health disorder and higher rates of primary care utilization has been a fairly robust finding (Calhoun, Bosworth, Grambow, Dudley, & Beckham, 2002). Cohen et al. (2009) found that among 249,440 returning Iraq and Afghanistan veterans, those with a mental health diagnosis other than PTSD had 55% higher medical service use compared to those with no mental health diagnosis. For veterans with PTSD, medical service utilization rates were even higher—a startling 91% higher than those with no mental health difficulties. High rates of physical health care service use appears to be particularly associated with PTSD and thus far has not been accounted for solely by the presence of a mental disturbance or comorbidity alone (Schnurr, Friedman, Sengupta, Jankowski, & Holmes, 2000). Younger veterans (i.e., less than 52 years of age) with PTSD have been shown to utilize significantly more health services than their peer counterparts without PTSD (Calhoun et al., 2002). Symptoms of PTSD have also been related to greater use of medical services in older veterans (Schnurr & Spiro, 1999).

Mental Health Treatment Utilization Determinants

Given their relatively greater need for services, an important area of research is the examination of potential predictors of VA mental health service utilization in the veteran population. Studies of the relationship between predictive factors and VA mental health utilization have yielded few consistent trends, with the exception of war era. Specifically, OEF/OIF veterans appear to be accessing treatment services at much higher rates than Vietnam-era veterans. Seal, Maguen et al. (2010) found that 35.7% of a sample of 238,098 OEF/OIF veterans received at least one new mental health diagnosis during the study window. Within this subsample, 66.9% visited a VA mental health clinic at least one time in the year following diagnosis. Similarly, a nationally representative sample of 1965 OEF/OIF veterans found that of those with probable PTSD or depression, 53% reported seeking professional services for a mental health concern (in a VA or non-VA clinic) within the past year (Tanielian & Jaycox, 2008). In an active duty sample of 222,620 OIF personnel, 35% reported accessing mental health services in the 12 months following their return from deployment (Hoge Auchterlonie & Milliken, 2006). In comparison, a nationally representative sample of 1198 Vietnam veterans found that only 7.5% reported they had ever used VA mental health services (Kulka et al., 1990).

The relationships between demographic factors (i.e., age, income, education) and mental health service utilization by veterans have been studied in a number of investigations. Research findings on the relationship between age and utilization of VA health care services have been mixed, with research indicating no relationship and other studies finding positive or inverse relationships between utilization and age among veterans. Payne et al. (2005) indicated that younger veterans utilized more VA mental health services; however, older veterans were more likely to have recently seen a doctor for a medical condition. These investigators also found evidence that increased mental health service utilization was associated with having a service connected disability, poorer self-rated mental health status, and multiple mental health disorders.

Similar to the findings of research on determinants of health service utilization among veterans, studies investigating mental health treatment in the VA have found that veterans with PTSD were more likely to have used VA mental health services than veterans without PTSD (Rosenheck & Fontana, 1995). Furthermore, the severity of PTSD symptomatology has been associated with increased mental health service use (Calhoun et al., 2002). An archival study of 87 male combat veterans with combat-related PTSD found no association between predictors involving demographic variables, illness/need (i.e., severity of PTSD symptoms) and enabling resource variables (i.e., income and distance to the VA), and con-sumption of PTSD-related or primary care health services (Elhai, Reeves, & Frueh, 2004). These findings suggest that veterans with PTSD make up a fairly distinct subgroup within the larger veteran population, with their own specific needs in regards to health care treatment and utilization.

Research investigating the relationship between racial group status and use of mental health services in veteran populations has resulted in mixed findings. Studies with veterans have revealed no association between racial group status and mental health care utilization (Frueh, Elhai, Monnier, Hamner, & Knapp, 2004). However, Rosenheck and Fontana (1994) provided evidence that veterans of ethno-cultural minorities were less likely to use mental health services than other ethnici-ties. In an archival study of predictors of VA mental health and medical service use in veterans with combat-related PTSD, Caucasian racial status predicted prescrip-tion of psychiatric medications (Elhai, Reeves, Frueh et al., 2004). Another study found that African-American veterans evidenced higher rates of medical ser-vice use, while those identified as Native Hawaiian or Japanese American accessed VA health care at lower-than-expected rates as compared to Caucasian veterans (Schnurr et al., 2000). African-American ethnicity has also been related to increased likelihood of accessing inpatient mental health (Rosenheck & Fontana, 1994) and substance abuse treatment (Rosenheck & Fontana, 1996).

Mental Health Treatment Utilization by Rural Veterans

Research has indicated that rural veterans have less frequent contact with health care professionals and participate in fewer recovery-oriented services than urban veterans. Thus, the utilization of mental health care by rural veterans is relevant topic for the VA. An investigation of assertive community treatment delivered to a rural VA population with mental illness demonstrated that although rural veterans had less contact with mental health professionals than their urban counterparts, these encounters were more likely to take place in the community, rather than a medical center setting. These rural veterans were also found to primarily receive services from an individual case manager rather than from a team of treatment pro-viders (Mohamed et al., 2009). A study conducted with a sample of older,

Medicare-eligible veterans living in rural New England showed that these veterans were more likely to seek services, particularly inpatient and specialty services, at private sector clinics rather than at CBOCs (Weeks, Mahar, & Wright, 2005). Research with rural veteran populations also indicates that specialized mental health services are being underutilized, despite the increased availability of PTSD interventions throughout the VA and the high prevalence of PTSD and associated impairment in this population. Seal, Maguen et al. (2010) found that less than 10% of veterans returning from Iraq and Afghanistan with a mental health diagnoses received minimally adequate psychological care.

As studies of mental health care utilization in the VA clearly highlight, veterans who suffer from PTSD have an increased need for access to both general and specialty physical and mental health care services. Nevertheless, research suggests that veterans living in rural locations may be disadvantaged when it comes to accessing appropriate care. In a study of 214,791 veterans newly diagnosed with depression, anxiety, and PTSD, those living in rural locations were significantly less likely to receive therapy and had a more limited dose relative to their urban counterparts (Cully, Jameson, Phillips, Kunik, & Fortney, 2010). However, this is not a uniform finding, as Elhai, Baugher, Quevillian, Sauvageot, and Frueh (2004) found no differences between rural and urban veterans with combat-related PTSD ($n = 100$) on PTSD symptoms or service utilization. The differing results of these two studies may be due to differences in study methodology or the small sample size in the latter study. Findings that veterans residing in rural areas experience increased mental and physical disease prevalence is further complicated by barriers that exist in access to health care in these regions.

Barriers to Access to Care

Veterans face critical barriers to accessing medical and specialty mental health care. The barriers to veterans seeking mental health care have been broadly categorized into geographically-based obstacles, which are associated with physical and personal environmental constraints, and veteran-based obstacles, which center on a veteran's tendency to avoid perceived stigma associated with mental health treatment (Hoge, Castro et al., 2004). Another categorization of barriers in access to care among military populations was suggested by a nationally representative survey of 1965 OEF/OIF veterans (Tanielian & Jaycox, 2008). Veterans ($n = 752$) were asked about barriers to care if they screened positive for a "possible need for services" (i.e., at least mild depression and subthreshold PTSD). The identified barriers were grouped into three areas: (a) logistical (i.e., difficult to get time off work), (b) institutional/cultural, and (c) beliefs/preferences for treatment. The barriers to care that were most often reported were in the institutional/cultural category (i.e., fear it would harm career, fear of being denied a security clearance in the future, coworkers would have less confidence in me), while logistical barriers were the least frequently reported. Identified barriers that were beliefs or preferences for treatment included ideas that medications would have too many side effects, family or friends would be more helpful than a professional, and a person should handle problems on their own.

Geographic and Logistical Obstacles

Many veterans residing in rural areas find it difficult to reach VA programs due to barriers associated with both logistics (i.e., time to travel to appointments) and cost (i.e., transportation costs), which significantly lower service acquisition rates. Rural veterans have added barriers related to fewer provider and specialty service options, greater distances to travel to receive services, and increased transportation needs (Hoge, Castro et al., 2004). The relationship between VA health care utilization and the amount of time spent traveling or the distance that a veteran travels to the clinic to receive these services has been studied in a number of research endeavors. A study of OEF/OIF veterans found that living more than 50 miles away from a VA facility was significantly associated with failure to attend at least one mental health follow-up visit in the first year after a veteran was newly diagnosed with PTSD (Seal, Maguen et al., 2010). Although the majority of OEF/OIF veterans (85%) with any new mental health diagnosis lived within 25 miles of a VA facility and only 2% lived more than 50 miles away, providing access to care for this small but important minority is a foremost challenge for the VA.

Stigma

Recent military returnees perceive strong stigma against the disclosure of psychiatric symptoms. Many active duty and veteran samples have reported underutilization of mental health services due to concerns about the shame and stigma associated with seeking treatment for mental health problems. Within the military culture, "succumbing" to PTSD may be perceived by those with the disorder as a failure, a weakness, and as evidence of an innate deficiency of strength (Friedman, Schnurr, Sengupta, Holmes, & Ashcraft, 2004). In fact, Hoge, Castro et al. (2004) found that 65% of those meeting criteria for a mental health disorder endorsed "I would be seen as weak" and 59% endorsed "Members of my unit might have less confidence in me" as reasons they did not seek treatment. An attitude of "wanting to solve my own problems" is a motive identified in many studies to describe failure to acquire services (Kulka et al., 1990). A study conducted with Caucasian and African-American OIF National Guardsmen indicated that a majority of the veterans in their study endorsed the beliefs that they "ought to handle it on my own" or "didn't want to believe I had a problem" as reasons for not seeking mental health treatment (Stecker, Fortney, Hamilton, & Ajzen, 2007). Additionally, fear that documentation in the medical record of a mental health problem might have an adverse effect on the advancement of military or nonmilitary careers is also a barrier to seeking psychological treatment within the Department of Defense (DoD) and VA settings.

Attrition from the Military

Another barrier that veterans face when seeking health care in the VA is attrition from military service, which is strongly correlated with mental disorders. High rates of attrition from the military have been evidenced in studies conducted with veterans with mental health disorders. Approximately 45–50% of all service members that were hospitalized for a mental disorder separated from military service within 6 months, in comparison with only 12% of those hospitalized for any other illness category (Hoge, Lesikar et al., 2002; Hoge, Toboni et al., 2005). These veterans may be involuntarily separated from service for a variety of reasons, such as medical disability, legal problems, and misconduct. Once veterans leave the military, the provision of adequate health care services in rural areas becomes especially problematic due to decreased access to care and shortages in health care professionals outside of the VA system.

Attrition from Mental Health Treatment

Many veterans who initiate psychotherapies drop out of psychological treatment before attending an adequate number of sessions for the treatment to be effective (Hoge, 2011). High rates of treatment dropout (i.e., up to 30%) have been evidenced among veterans in effectiveness trials of prolonged exposure (PE) for PTSD (Tuerk et al., 2011; Yoder et al., 2012). Investigations involving mental health screening and utilization in the VA showed that even among the more than 40% of PTSD-positive veterans who reported an interest in receiving help, only one in ten actually procured services (Hoge, Auchterlonie, & Milliken, 2006). Seal, Maguen et al. (2010) found that 27% of treatment-seeking veterans in their sample attended nine or more sessions in the past year, but only 9.5% had received a sufficient dose of "sustained treatment" (i.e., at least nine sessions in 15 weeks), which was used as a proxy for the probable administration of an evidence-based protocol, such as PE for PTSD (Foa, Hembree, & Rothbaum, 2007). Furthermore, while rates of initial access of VA mental health services have increased fivefold (or more) since the Vietnam conflict, rates of receiving "adequate" care (i.e., a sustained dose of mental health treatment) remain very low. In the Tanielian and Jaycox (2008) study, only 18% of respondents seeking mental health services received "minimally adequate" therapy, which was defined as eight or more sessions, at least 30 minutes in length, with a mental health professional in the past 12 months. Thus, while efforts by the DoD and the VA to increase access to and utilization of VA mental health care appear to be succeeding in raising rates of initial encounters into the system, these efforts have been less successful at keeping veterans engaged in prolonged treatment.

Women Veterans

Much of the research to date on veteran health has focused on male veterans; however, women veterans are one of the fastest growing groups of new patients across the VA system. Some reports suggest that female veterans who seek out VA services are almost twice as likely to report mental health concerns to their VA providers as their male counterparts (Katz, Bloor, Cojucar, & Draper, 2007), suggesting a need to increase the knowledge base on access to care for these veterans and study the unique barriers to care for female veterans. Women veterans may experience significant impairment, given evidence that women do worse both physically and mentally after major traumatic events independent of the severity and mechanism of the trauma (Holbrook & Hoyt, 2004). Furthermore, women veterans have been shown to experience higher rates of interpersonal violence than civilian women (Dichter, Cerulli, & Bossarte, 2011), therefore increasing the chances that women veterans will be exposed to traumatic events. As with men in rural communities, women in rural communities receive less specialty mental health treatment than those living in metropolitan areas (Hauenstein et al., 2006). There is also growing literature on gender differences in access to medical care, which suggests that women and men report differences in their utilization and experiences of the health care system (Brittle & Bird, 2007). Among women in the general population, noted barriers to accessing care include issues such as caregiving responsibilities and lack of time, with younger women who are parents and attend work or school reporting "extreme role overload" and a need for health care providers to see them promptly, provide services efficiently, and be willing to provide information or prescriptions over the phone (Scholle et al., 2000). Exploration of potential barriers to the use of VA care indicate that lack of information about the VA, perceptions of the inferiority of VA care, and reported inconvenience of VA care are deterrents to VA use for many women veterans (Washington, Yano, Simon, & Sun, 2006). Additional barriers to care include the availability of needed services, especially women-specific services, and factors related to the logistics of receiving care at the VA, such as the waiting time to obtain care and issues related to continuity of care (Vogt et al., 2006).

These barriers, as well as others that may be unique to an individual veteran's situation, combine to present a hurdle that some veterans must overcome in order to access and subsequently benefit from effective physical and mental health care. In order to help address such barriers and fulfill their commitment to provide all veterans access to evidence-based interventions, the DoD and VA advocate using nonconventional modes of service delivery, such as using telecommunications, to help deliver mental health treatments.

Limitations in the Access to Care Literature

The influx of OEF/OIF veterans returning to the U.S. from deployment and their subsequent need to acquire VA mental health care services highlight the need for research on the determinants of the utilization of VA mental health services among veterans. The current research literature on mental health treatment utilization among veterans has led to discrepant findings; therefore, basing conclusions on the results of these studies is problematic. No doubt, methodology and operationalization of study variables can account for some discrepancy in findings. These difficulties may be due to the lack of specific and consistent operational definitions for outcome measures of mental health treatment utilization. Studies vary in the parameters for these outcomes, such that some studies define minimally adequate care in terms of length and intensity of psychological treatment interventions, while other research determines this criterion based on use of, and response to, psychiatric medications.

Studies show that veterans deployed during the current war era and veterans who served in the Vietnam War differ in their rates of VA services utilization. Further exploration of the differences in predictors of utilization in veterans from both war eras is warranted, as research concerning these specific variables can inform service providers about how to deliver the most effective mental health treatment across age groups. Seal, Maguen et al. (2010) speculate that war-era differences in mental health care utilization may be due to several factors, including sampling and methodology differences, different rates of combat exposure, DoD and VA efforts to increase early screening and identification of at-risk service members (e.g., mandatory screening after deployment), increased accessibility to effective mental health services (e.g., free service-related health care for 5 years after service separation, opening specialty mental health care clinics, embedding mental health providers in primary care settings, mandated access to evidence-based psychotherapy for all veterans with PTSD), and decreased related stigma (e.g., increased education and awareness, normalizing trauma-related stress). However, the relative impact of these hypothesized factors has yet to be empirically examined.

Studies have been conducted with Vietnam veterans of Caucasian, African-American, Hispanic, American Indian, Native Hawaiian, and Japanese American ancestry in order to investigate minority status as a risk factor for increased PTSD symptomatology; however, the inclusion of a larger number of racial minorities in research on access to care is warranted. A recent analysis of data of the 2004 and 2005 military recruits indicated that while the number of Caucasian military is proportional to their representation in the U.S. population (recruitment-to-population ratio of 0.97), Native Hawaiian/other Pacific Islander recruits were the most overrepresented (recruitment-to-population ratio of 7.49) and Asian recruits were the most underrepresented (recruitment-to-population ratio of 0.69) across ethnic groups in the U.S. (Kane, 2006). Additional investigations of ethnic differences in barriers to access to care in the VA would contribute to a greater understanding of how to best treat mental health disorders in veterans from ethnic minorities.

Another limitation in the access to care literature is the lack of inclusion of veterans for whom barriers in access to care prevent them from utilizing VA health care services. Though a few studies use nationally representative samples, most of the current research in this area relies on data from treatment-seeking VA populations; therefore, the true population of interest is not represented in the literature. There is also a lack of data on non-VA health services use; therefore, it is not possible to determine the extent of mental health care that is sought and received by veterans outside of the VA. The factors that facilitate veterans to utilize VA health care also need to be assessed in order to identify strengths in the VA health care system.

Finally, there is also demonstrated need for research on the best approaches to increasing access to specialty mental health care services. Some investigators have noted that these interventions can be effectively delivered through primary health care systems (Pols & Oak, 2007) or via innovative delivery modalities, such as clinical videoteleconferencing (CVT).

TMH and the Department of Veterans Affairs

In the past two decades, tremendous developments have been made in the range, availability, and ease-of-access to different forms of telecommunications technology. This "digital revolution" has given rise to a new field, known as "telehealth," that examines applications of this technology in medical and mental health settings. Telehealth may be defined as the use of electronic communications and information technologies to provide and support health care when distance separates the provider from the patient (Field, 1996). Telehealth that is specific to mental health, or TMH, includes the provision of psychological services, cognitive testing, and general psychiatry over a telecommunications modality. CVT is one example of a telehealth modality that has become increasingly available in a wide variety of institutions and service systems for diverse purposes, such as reaching underserved and difficult-to-access populations (e.g., prisoners, rural inhabitants) or increasing the convenience of health services for those with mobility concerns that may be due to illness, injury, or lack of transportation. With CVT technology, a patient/provider encounter is interactive and takes place in real time through a television monitor. Typically, the specialty provider is located at the larger medical facility and the patient is located at the more rural or remote site. CVT allows for synchronous face-to-face communication over the telemonitor between patient and provider.

Research with returning OEF/OIF populations suggests that there is a new generation of military troops with high levels of mental health disorders (Goldzweig, Balekian, Rolon, Yano, & Shekelle, 2006). Thus, it is critical that we increase access to established evidence-based treatment (EBT) for returning troops who live in rural or remote areas. In 2008, the VA mandated that all veterans and active duty Reserve and National Guard be provided with access to specialized quality mental health care, such as EBT for PTSD, regardless of their geographic location (U.S. Department of Veterans Affairs, 2008). In order to meet this mandate and reach veterans who face barriers to traditional in-person service delivery, the VA has developed several initiatives in recent years that prioritize the role of CVT as a potential solution to the persistent problem of access to care that often exits in remote areas of the U.S.

CVT offers a number of advantages over traditional treatment approaches (Glueckauf, Whitton, & Nickelson, 2002; Jerome & Zaylor, 2000; Perednia & Allen, 1995). One central benefit is lower cost without sacrificing the quality of care (Morland, Frueh, Pierce, & Miyahira, 2003). Patients participating in CVT treatments have also benefited in terms of decreases in costs of transportation, travel time, and missed work (Bose, McLaren, Riley, & Mohammedali, 2001; Elford et al., 2000; Trott & Blignault, 1998). In addition, CVT enhances access to treatment for veterans with serious injuries or scheduling difficulties due to work, school, or childcare responsibilities. CVT technology is rapidly becoming available at lower costs, allowing it to be implemented at a greater number of sites, and thereby increasing system coverage areas to the point that TMH is becoming a viable "standard" alternative service delivery modality for a significant proportion of veterans (Dunn et al., 2000).

The importance of TMH technology, such as CVT, as a means for meeting the VA and DoD goal to provide quality care to military populations was affirmed before the Subcommittee on Health, Committee on Veteran's Affairs, U.S. House of Representatives, on May 18, 2005. At this hearing, Dr. Adam Darkins, Chief Consultant to Care Coordination, affirmed the VA's commitment to use telemedicine to address urgent patient care needs and to increase access to care for rural veterans. He identified TMH care services as one of five priority areas for future development by the VA. Recent testimony before the same subcommittee has further emphasized the need for providing increased access to care for rural veterans. Clinicians across the VA have begun to utilize CVT services as a mode to deliver specialized psychological treatments to rural populations.

Due to the influx of TMH programs nationwide across the VA, as well as the growing need for specialty programs, it is crucial that we evaluate the clinical effectiveness of this mode of service delivery. Research has focused on a range of factors in order to determine the clinical effectiveness of the CVT modality.

Clinical Effectiveness of Psychotherapies Delivered via CVT

CVT has good initial research supporting the general feasibility of CVT applications (Cowain, 2001; Deitsch, Frueh, & Santos, 2000; Frueh, Monnier et al., 2007; Mannion, Fahy, Duffy, Broderick, & Gethins, 1998; Ruskin et al., 1998) and has been successfully demonstrated in rural areas across the nation (F. W. Brown, 1998; Ermer, 1999; Grady & Clayton, 2002; Magaletta, Fagan, & Ax, 1998; Nesbitt, Hilty, Kuenneth, & Siefkin, 2000). Furthermore, CVT has demonstrated feasibility with a broad range of difficult-to-treat patient populations, such as the elderly (Poon, Hui, Dai, Kwok, & Woo, 2005), patients with thought disorders (Zarate et al., 1997), and avoidant/reluctant patients (Brodey, Claypoole, Motto, Arias, & Goss, 2000; Haslam & McLaren, 2000; Zaylor, Whitten, & Kingsley, 2000). Data further indicate that rural medical patients who have never used CVT technology are willing to receive mental health care via this medium if it would improve access to care (Grubaugh, Cain, Elhai, Patrick, & Frueh, 2008). Rigorous outcome studies comparing the CVT modality to traditional service delivery methods are limited, but those that have been conducted provide preliminary support for the use of CVT (R. Brown et al., 1999; Frueh, Monnier et al., 2007; McLaren, Ahlbom, Riley, Mohammedali, & Denis, 2002; Morland, Greene, Rosen et al., 2010; Zaylor et al., 2000). Research has demonstrated high levels of patient and clinician satisfaction with, and general reliability of, CVT applications (Frueh, Deitsch et al., 2000) as well as feasibility of group therapy via a CVT modality (Morland, Hynes, Mackintosh, Resick, & Chard, 2011; Morland, Pierce, & Wong, 2005).

Considerations Associated with CVT Delivery

Therapist Fidelity and Competence

Given that one of the primary goals of using CVT in the VA system is to increase access to specialized mental health services for difficulties such as PTSD, anger, and depression, which include the use of specific, complex, manualized protocols, one potential concern is whether the modality will impact therapist adherence and fidelity to these manualized treatments. Morland, Greene, Grubbs et al. (2011) compared therapist adherence to a manualized evidence-based protocol for anger management in a randomized clinical trial (RCT) of in-person ($n = 64$) versus CVT ($n = 61$) delivery with a sample of 125 rural male combat veterans with PTSD. Five therapists who were experienced with manualized cognitive–behavioral therapy (CBT) protocols but inexperienced with the CVT modality prior to the study delivered the treatment. Overall, therapist adherence was excellent ($M = 96\%$, $SD = 1\%$), with no significant effects found for therapist, modality, domain of ratings (didactic content vs process aspects), or any combination thereof, suggesting that the change in modality did not affect the therapist's ability to maintain treatment fidelity (Ruskin et al., 2004). Another study investigated therapist competence (i.e., developing rapport and conveying empathy) and adherence (i.e., structuring sessions and providing feedback) to a manualized cognitive–behavioral group psychotherapy targeting social skills delivered to veterans with PTSD in-person and via the CVT modality (Frueh, Monnier et al., 2007). Results indicated that therapist competence and adherence were similar in the two delivery modalities. In fact, veterans rated the therapist as "good to excellent" on rapport/empathy in both the in-person and the CVT conditions. These studies suggest that specialized mental health interventions can be competently delivered via CVT.

Attitudes Toward CVT Service Delivery

The utility of CVT for both mental health and general health care rests not only with the therapists and the systems they operate in but also with the willingness of veterans and providers to accept treatment over this modality. At least one study has examined this directly by surveying 190 primary care patients regarding their degree of comfort with CVT delivery of medical and mental health services (Grubaugh et al., 2008). Given that one of the primary aims of CVT is to increase access to care for those living in remote areas, these investigators compared the responses of rural ($n = 112$) and urban ($n = 78$) residents and found no significant differences in attitudes toward CVT delivery of medical and/or psychiatric services. Both groups displayed a comparable preference for in-person treatment but a moderate amount of confidence in the alternative modality of CVT. Groups were also similar in their concerns with the technology, with approximately two-thirds endorsing the statement that "CVT [telehealth] is not as effective as face-to-face [delivery]." This suggests that patients are moderately receptive to the possibility of receiving services over new, novel telehealth modalities, but may benefit from receiving additional information regarding their safety and feasibility in order to enhance their confidence in them.

Impact of CVT on Group Process

A small number of studies, including a study conducted with inmates (Morgan, Patrick, & Magaletta, 2008), have examined group processes (e.g., treatment engagement, therapeutic alliance) in CVT conditions with nonveteran populations and generally found no significant differences on key elements (i.e., client satisfaction, perceptions of therapeutic relationship) of treatment between the CVT and in-person delivery modalities. RCTs of group interventions delivered via CVT with veterans have reported high degrees of patient and clinician satisfaction (Deitsch et al., 2000; Morland, Pierce, & Wong, 2005) and comparable rates of attendance (Morland, Pierce, & Wong, 2005; Shore & Manson, 2005) and information retention (Morland, Pierce, & Wong, 2005). A study comparing a CBT skills group for veterans with PTSD delivered via CVT versus in-person found no significant between-group differences on session attendance, attrition, treatment credibility, and treatment satisfaction; however, there were significant between-group differences on homework compliance, with those receiving in-person treatment completing significantly more than the CVT group (Frueh et al., 2007). Additionally, veterans in the in-person condition reported significantly more comfort in speaking with their therapist posttreatment than those in the CVT group. The authors noted that these results should be interpreted cautiously, due to the low sample size for conditions and the presence of potential confounds (e.g., disability-seeking status). In a pilot cohort of a PTSD intervention delivered via CVT, the use of CVT did not appear to negatively impact veterans' confidence in treatment outcomes or satisfaction with received services (Morland, Greene, Grubbs, et al., 2011). Participants in both conditions reported high levels of treatment credibility, satisfaction with care, and homework adherence.

In a larger clinical trial, Grady and Clayton (2002) randomized 112 male combat veterans with PTSD and moderate-to-severe anger problems to receive 12 weeks of a group cognitive–behavioral treatment for anger either in-person or via CVT. Results on group process outcomes found the two conditions comparable on most process variables, including treatment satisfaction, treatment credibility, group cohesion, session attendance, homework completion, and treatment dropout rates. However, those in the CVT group displayed a nonsignificant trend toward lower levels of alliance with the therapist, and that therapist alliance was associated with outcomes at the individual (i.e., stronger alliance was associated with greater improvement), but not at the group level (Greene et al., 2010). Studies have also suggested that comfort and alliance with the therapist may be somewhat lower with CVT-administered treatment, but that these subtle differences in group process did not negatively impact clinical outcomes or patient tolerance and acceptance of the modality (Frueh, Monnier et al., 2007; Greene et al., 2010). However, it does suggest that clinicians administering therapy via CVT may potentially need to take extra measures to ensure that therapeutic alliance is established and maintained.

Cost-Effectiveness of CVT

The issue of cost-effectiveness is central to discussions of continued implementation of TMH approaches. Initial attempts to address the question of cost-effectiveness have suggested that TMH programs can be less expensive for patients, reducing travel time, travel costs, and time off from work (Mielonen, Ohinmaa,

Moring, & Isohanni, 2002; Simpson, Doze, Urness, Hailey, & Jacobs, 2001). However, researchers caution that cost analyses may be dependent upon workload (Harley, 2006; Persaud et al., 2005), the regional demand for services (Werner, 2001), and the presence of a high-speed wide-area network (Dunn et al., 2000). Literature in this area is limited and has been criticized for not considering a myriad of key costs (Monnier, Knapp, & Frueh, 2003), and some have argued that a TMH program must first demonstrate its effectiveness before cost analysis outcomes can be considered accurate (Kennedy, 2005).

PTSD has been found to be one of the most costly psychiatric conditions (Greenberg et al., 1999; Kessler, 2000; Solomon & Davidson, 1997); therefore, projects investigating the cost of delivering psychological treatments to veterans with PTSD are particularly warranted. Studies within the VA have demonstrated that telemedicine can be applied in a cost-effective manner (Fortney, Maciejewski, Warren, & Burgess, 2005) and that access to care can be increased without driving up overall costs. Economic modeling is often used to compare the costs of a new treatment or service protocol to the cost of existing treatment delivery systems (if any) and/or the cost of providing no treatment, which in turn informs medical or mental health policy decisions. One study (Ruskin et al., 2004) found CVT and in-person psychiatric treatment for depression equivalent in health care cost across modalities. Given that mental health treatment over CVT is an emerging area of study, few studies have yet looked at the relative cost-effectiveness of this service delivery modality.

Technology Used to Provide CVT

The connectivity used in CVT could be an important factor in determining outcomes and whether veterans perceive their care as comparable to care provided in-person. Higher bandwidth through dedicated T1 lines is assumed to best approximate an in-person visit. Therefore, most VA sites use bandwidth over 368 kbits/s for individual session which is then increased for group sessions. A combination of high-definition large flat-screen monitors and desktop systems are used according to the CVT application and resources in the rural community. To date, the choice of technology has not been evaluated as a major factor in the feasibility or success of CVT.

Challenges Associated with CVT Delivery

Although TMH effectively increases access to specialty care for veterans facing significant barriers, limitations do exist when delivering mental health services over a CVT modality. Frequently reported challenges of conducting CVT have included limited access to treatment room space and high-speed Internet at small rural clinics, managing logistics (i.e., escorting veterans to the group treatment room, sending and receiving treatment and homework materials via fax, distributing outcome measures), and difficulties audiotaping sessions for subsequent clinical supervision, which is often a training requirement for certification in EBTs such as PE and cognitive processing therapy (CPT). To date, there has been little formal discussion in the literature of the challenges associated with CVT delivery and how to address them. However, our research group, the National Center for PTSD— Pacific Island Division (NCPTSD, PID) at the VA Pacific Island Health Care System, recently published the practice implications of and possible solutions to these challenges based on our extensive experiences conducting treatment studies using CVT technology.

As a result of our extensive experience with using CVT in these studies, we have found the need to somewhat modify EBT delivery to better suit this modality. First, it is important for novice CVT therapists to be aware that sessions will likely require additional planning time as compared to in-person delivery to ensure things run smoothly (e.g., audiotaping equipment is ready, CVT line is scheduled, staff at both sites are aware of appointment). Second, the need for a strong collaborative relationship between service delivery sites (e.g., the large medical center and rural CBOC) is vital to the successful resolution of space and logistical challenges, as assistance from staff at the remote location is needed to ensure the CVT technology is working properly, escort the veteran to the treatment space, and facilitate the exchange of completed homework assignments between the veterans and the therapist (e.g., via fax machines or scanner if possible). Third, based on our experience, we found having two co-therapists per group to deliver a manualized protocol for PTSD (i.e., CPT) was important, particularly in the CVT condition. Specifically, the therapist found it difficult to be fully attentive to the needs of all of the participants while also collecting and reviewing the homework sheets, answering questions, and moving briskly through the ambitious content agenda without the help of a second therapist.

In addition to the logistical challenges, our research team also encountered challenges that were more specific to our unique treatment population that resulted in modification to the CBT intervention protocol used in this study. For example, we found that many of the rural participants varied drastically in their baseline understanding of PTSD and basic cognitive—behavioral concepts due to limited prior experience with mental health services. In order to address this variability and increase each veteran's ability to benefit from treatment, we added an individual 2 hour pretreatment orientation session to our protocol to review general psychoeducation and CBT concepts. In addition, we also found it necessary to follow the CPT manual's suggestions for modifying worksheets to make them easier to follow for some veterans. This study is still under way, therefore final results are pending. However, outcomes for the initial pilot cohort (Morland, Hynes et al., 2011), in combination with the results of our prior RCT on clinical outcomes (Morland, Greene, Rosen et al., 2010), group process outcomes (Greene et al., 2010), and treatment fidelity (Morland, Greene, Grubbs et al., 2011) of a group anger management treatment delivered via CVT, suggest that while these minor modifications improved the ease of delivery of CPT over CVT, they do not alter or undermine the effectiveness of the intended EBT protocol. Thus, while the modifications discussed here are specific to CPT and the characteristics of the treatment population, they illustrate that experienced clinicians can adapt structured protocols to fit the unique needs of the modality and of the target population without compromising the integrity of the intervention.

Limitations in the CVT Literature

The current research literature on mental health delivered via TMH demonstrates the extensive needs that might be met through this treatment modality; however, despite the applicability of CVT for increasing access to care, there are several marked limitations in the current research.

The most salient limitation is the lack of prospective RCTs of CVT applications. Rigorously designed research studies that include prospective, randomized evaluations of clinical, process, and cost outcomes for TMH interventions are still needed (Monnier et al., 2003). Future research must also more closely examine factors related to the overall clinical effectiveness of delivering treatments over CVT. Outcomes of particular interest include clinical outcome variables (e.g., measures of general illness severity and disorder specific symptoms), process outcome variables (e.g., general satisfaction and acceptance, client perception of treatment, therapeutic alliance, treatment adherence, session attendance, attrition, treatment credibility/expectancy. For example, since some clients are able to more easily establish a therapeutic alliance remotely than others, future research may examine client factors potentially associated with stronger therapeutic alliance and/or cohesion with group treatment members when services are delivered via CVT. Furthermore, research conducted in the VA on CVT has failed to include women veterans as participants in their studies. Given the large number of returning OEF/OIF women veterans, investigations on the clinical and process outcomes and unique considerations associated with delivering interventions to this population would be an important contribution to research on CVT. Research focused in these areas is needed to determine if and to what degree TMH services should be developed and maintained, with whom, and under what circumstances. Lastly, in addition to overall clinical effectiveness, the question of treatment costs remains relatively unanswered. Future research that incorporates comprehensive cost analyses within effective TMH treatment approaches is needed to provide satisfactory answers.

Future Directions

Currently, there are several studies under way, funded through both the VA and the DOD, that specifically address clinical and cost aspects of proving care over a CVT modality. For example, our research group, the NCPTSD, PID, is located in the VA Health Care System that provides services to military populations in a large geographic area, including the Hawaiian Islands, Guam, Saipan, the Northern Mariana Islands, and American Samoa. Given that 4.6 million square miles of water separates these islands, the high proportion of veterans diagnosed with PTSD in this VA (approximately 33%), and that the need for alternative service delivery modalities is particularly great in this health care system, this geographic region is particularly well suited to studies of the CVT modality. We currently have two federally funded RCTs under way examining the clinical, process, and cost outcomes of delivering CPT to male and female veterans with military-related PTSD via the

CVT modality. Findings from these studies will contribute to the much needed literature regarding clinical and cost-effectiveness of the CVT modality.

Thus far, studies of CVT have primarily looked at service delivery from one VA health care office to another, but future research should also investigate the safety, feasibility, and acceptability of in-home delivery. When CVT is used in a manner that is truly equivalent to in-person treatment (i.e., used in an office-based setting), the strongest advantage with CVT technology also becomes its primary constraint. Namely, the practitioner is constrained to seeing the veteran in a formal therapeutic setting and is reliant on him/her to be an accurate reporter of his/her environment outside the office (e.g., home life, quality of interpersonal relationships, occupational functioning). Social ecological models of behavior suggest that many contextual and individual factors are likely to influence veterans' response to PTSD treatment following war trauma; therefore, considering them when planning and delivering therapeutic interventions for PTSD might increase the potency of the treatment. Thus, CVT delivered in-home would allow the clinician to observe the veteran in his/her social ecology in order to identify person- and environment-specific factors that could play a vital role in treatment planning, engagement, and response (Tuerk, Grubaugh, Hamner, & Foa, 2009). Obstacles to protocol adherence existing in the veteran's environment can be observed and resolved. Home-based treatment may also help to overcome barriers to service utilization, such as the logistical barriers of travel and stigma, and has been associated with lower dropout rates than traditional care (Henggeler, Pickrel, Brondino, & Crouch, 1996; Rybarczyk, Lopez, Benson, Alsten, & Stepanski, 2002). Given the benefits that exist with the in-home delivery of CVT, future research investigating this delivery modality would be a substantial contribution to the field of TMH.

Conclusions

Since 2002, the VA has systematically implemented a program to provide real-time CVT between mental health providers and veterans. In the past decade, over 45,000 patients have successfully participated in more than 125,000 clinical encounters via the CVT modality. CVT service delivery in the VA is now one of the mainstays of delivering mental health care. This technology movement supports several national initiatives focused on increasing access to evidence-based psychotherapy for a range of diagnostic presentations. The VA has also recently implemented a mandate that all veterans with PTSD have access to EBTs wherever they obtain care in the VHA (U.S. Department of Veterans Affairs, 2008). In support of this effort, the VA recently launched a nationwide dissemination initiative ("rollout") of these EBTs for PTSD over a CVT modality. This rollout includes further developing the infrastructure to support broad utilization of CVT as well as providing national trainings. The broad acceptance of this modality across the VA, as well as the exciting research supporting the clinical and potential cost benefits, will allow the VA to access to an otherwise underserved population. Psychotherapy provided via CVT may enhance utilization of treatment for veterans who face access barriers such as geographic distance, transportation, medical limitations, or work responsibilities.

Future research directions will eventually allow the VA to harness the benefits from technologies, such as home-based CVT, mobile devices, and smart phone applications, in order to treat veterans regardless of their geographic location. CVT technology and new smart phone mobile applications, which allow real-time face-to-face interaction, hold the promise of improving access to care and supporting a true "patient-centered" approach. Home-based psychotherapy over a CVT modality may additionally enhance treatment acceptance and adherence, reduce stigma, increase trust, and reduce early termination (Hicken & Plowhead, 2010). Although home-based CVT treatment delivery poses some unique challenges, there is preliminary evidence that it can be used safely and effectively to improve symptoms (Hicken & Plowhead, 2010; Luxton, Sirotin, & Mishkind, 2010). Although future research is still needed in order to better understand the clinical effectiveness of providing protocols over CVT and the unique challenges or required modifications when providing EBTs over a CVT modality, this is clearly the direction the field is headed. With the increased focus on a "patient-centered model" in the VA, the necessity of technology will only intensify as a primary mechanism to increase access and utilization of mental health services for veterans across the nation.

References

Beachler, M., Holloman, C., & Herman, J. (2003). Southern rural access program: An overview. *Journal of Rural Health, 19*, 301–307.

Bose, U., McLaren, P., Riley, A., & Mohammedali, A. (2001). The use of telepsychiatry in the brief counseling of non-psychotic patients from an inner-London general practice. *Journal of Telemedicine and Telecare, 7*, 8–10.

Brittle, C., & Bird, C. A. (2007). *Literature review on effective sex- and gender-based systems/models of care.* Arlington, VA: Uncommon Insights, LLC.

Brodey, B. B., Claypoole, K. H., Motto, J., Arias, R. G., & Goss, R. (2000). Satisfaction of forensic psychiatric patients with remote telepsychiatric evaluation. *Psychiatric Services, 51*, 1305–1307.

Brown, F. W. (1998). Rural telepsychiatry. *Psychiatric Services, 49*, 963–964.

Brown, R., Pain, K., Berwald, C., Hirschi, P., Delehanty, R., & Miller, H. (1999). Distance education and caregiver support groups: Comparison of traditional and telephone groups. *Journal of Head Trauma Rehabilitation, 14*, 257–268.

Calhoun, P. S., Bosworth, H. B., Grambow, S. C., Dudley, T. K., & Beckham, J. C. (2002). Medical service utilization by veterans seeking help for posttraumatic stress disorder. *American Journal of Psychiatry, 159*, 2081–2086.

Carlson, K. F., Nelson, D., Orazem, R. J., Nugent, S., Cifu, D. X., & Sayer, N. A. (2010). Psychiatric diagnoses among Iraq and Afghanistan war veterans screened for deployment-related traumatic brain injury. *Journal of Traumatic Stress, 23*, 17–24.

Chemtob, C. M., Hamada, R. S., Roitblat, H. L., & Muraoka, M. Y. (1994). Anger, impulsivity, and anger control in combat-related posttraumatic stress disorder. *Journal of Consulting and Clinical Psychology, 62*, 827–832.

Chwastiak, L. A., Rosenheck, R. A., & Kazis, L. E. (2008). Utilization of primay care by veterans with psychiatric illness in the National Department of Veterans Affairs health care system. *Journal of General Internal Medicine, 23,* 1835–1840.

Cohen, B. E., Gima, K., Berthenthal, D., Kim, S., Marmar, C. R., & Seal, K. H. (2009). Mental health diagnoses and utilization of VA non-mental health medical services among returning Iraq and Afghanistan veterans. *Journal of General Internal Medicine, 25,* 18–24.

Cowain, T. (2001). Cognitive–behavioural therapy via videoconferencing to a rural area. *Australian and New Zealand Journal of Psychiatry, 35,* 62–64.

Cully, J. A., Jameson, J. P., Phillips, L. L., Kunik, M. E., & Fortney, J. C. (2010). Use of psychotherapy by rural and urban veterans. *Journal of Rural Health, 26,* 225–233.

Deitsch, S. E., Frueh, B. C., & Santos, A. B. (2000). Telepsychiatry for post-traumatic stress disorder. *Journal of Telemedicine and Telecare, 6,* 184–186.

Dichter, M. E., Cerulli, C., & Bossarte, R. M. (2011). Intimate partner violence victimization among women veterans and associated heart health risks. *Women's Health Issues, 21,* S190–S194.

Dohrenwend, B. P., Turner, B., Turse, N. A., Adams, B. G., Koenen, K. C., & Marshall, R. (2006). The psychological risks of Vietnam for U.S. veterans: A revisit with new data and methods. *Science, 313,* 979–982.

Dunn, B. E., Choi, H., Almagro, U. A., Recla, D. L., Krupinski, E. A., & Weinstein, R. S. (2000). Telepathology networking in VISN-12 of the veterans health administration. *Telemedicine Journal and e-Health, 6,* 349–354.

Elford, R., White, H., Bowering, R., Ghandi, A., Maddiggan, B., & St. John, K. (2000). A randomized, controlled trial of child psychiatric assessments conducted using videoconferencing. *Journal of Telemedicine and Telecare, 6,* 73–82.

Elhai, J. D., Baugher, S. N., Quevillian, R. P., Sauvageot, J., & Frueh, B. C. (2004). Psychiatric symptoms and health service utilization in rural and urban combat veterans with posttraumatic stress disorder. *Journal of Nervous and Mental Disease, 192,* 701–704.

Elhai, J. D., Reeves, A. N., & Frueh, B. C. (2004). Predictors of mental health and medical service use in veterans presenting with combat-related posttraumatic stress disorder. *Psychological Services, 1,* 111–119.

Elhai, J. D., Richardson, J. D., & Pedlar, D. J. (2007). Predictors of general medical and psychological treatment use among a national sample of peacekeeping veterans with health problems. *Journal of Anxiety Disorders, 21,* 580–589.

Ermer, D. J. (1999). Experience with a rural telepsychiatry clinic for children and adolescents. *Psychiatric Services, 50,* 260–261.

Field, M. (1996). *Telemental health—A guide to assessing telecommunications in health care.* Washington, DC: National Academy Press.

Foa, E. B., Hembree, E. A., & Rothbaum, B. O. (2007). *Prolonged exposure therapy for PTSD: Emotional processing of traumatic experiences.* New York, NY: Oxford University Press.

Fortney, J. C., Maciejewski, M. L., Warren, J. J., & Burgess, J. F. (2005). Does improving geographic access to VA primary care services impact patients' patterns of utilization and costs? *Inquiry, 42,* 29–42.

Friedman, M. J., Schnurr, P. P., Sengupta, A., Holmes, T., & Ashcraft, M. (2004). The Hawaii Vietnam veterans project: Is minority status a risk factor for posttraumatic stress disorder? *Journal of Nervous and Mental Disease, 192,* 42–50.

Frueh, B. C., Deitsch, S. E., Santos, A. B., Gold, P. B., Johnson, M. R., Meisler, N., et al. (2000). Procedural and methodological issues in telepsychiatry research and program development. *Psychiatric Services, 51,* 1522−1527.

Frueh, B. C., Elhai, J. D., Monnier, J., Hamner, M. B., & Knapp, R. G. (2004). Symptom patterns and service use among African-American and Caucasian veterans with combat-related PTSD. *Psychological Services, 1,* 22−30.

Frueh, B. C., Monnier, J., Grubaugh, A. L., Elhai, J. D., Yim, E., & Knapp, R. (2007). Therapist adherence and competence with manualized cognitive−behavioral therapy for PTSD delivered via videoconferencing technology. *Behavior Modification, 31,* 856−866.

Frueh, B. C., Turner, S. M., Beidel, D. C., & Cahill, S. P. (2001). Assessment of social functioning in combat veterans with PTSD. *Aggression and Violent Behavior, 6,* 79−90.

Glueckauf, R. L., Whitton, J. D., & Nickelson, D. W. (2002). Telehealth: The new frontier in rehabilitation and health care. In M. Scherer (Ed.): *Assistive technology: Matching device and consumer for successful rehabilitation.* (pp. 197−213). Washington, DC: American Psychological Association.

Goldzweig, C. L., Balekian, T. M., Rolon, C., Yano, E. M., & Shekelle, P. G. (2006). The state of women veteran's health research: Results of a systematic literature review. *Journal of General Internal Medicine, 21,* S82−S92.

Gordon, A. J., Haas, G. L., Luther, J. F., Hilton, M. T., & Goldstein, G. (2010). Personal, medical, and healthcare utilization among homeless veterans served by metropolitan and nonmetropolitan veterans facilities. *Psychological Services, 7,* 65−74.

Grady, S. K., & Clayton, S. L. (2002). The role of patient recruitment protocols in telehealth. *Journal of Telemedicine and Telecare, 8,* 87−91.

Greenberg, P. E., Sisitsky, T., Kessler, R. C., Finkelstein, S. N., Berndt, E. R., Davidson, J. R. T., et al. (1999). The economic burden of anxiety disorders in the 1990s. *Journal of Clinical Psychiatry, 60,* 427−435.

Greene, C. J., Morland, L. A., Macdonald, A., Frueh, B. C., Grubbs, K. M., & Rosen, C. S. (2010). How does tele-mental health affect group therapy process? Secondary analysis of a noninferiority trial. *Journal of Consulting and Clinical Psychology, 78,* 746−750.

Grieger, T. A., Cozza, S. J., Ursano, R. J., Hoge, C., Martinez, P. E., Engel, C. C., et al. (2006). Posttraumatic stress disorder and depression in battle-injured soldiers. *American Journal of Psychiatry, 163,* 1777−1783.

Grubaugh, A. L., Cain, G. D., Elhai, J. D., Patrick, S. L., & Frueh, B. C. (2008). Attitudes toward medical and mental health care delivered via telehealth application among rural and urban primary care patients. *Journal of Nervous and Mental Disease, 196,* 166−170.

Harley, J. (2006). Economic evaluation of a tertiary telepsychiatry service to an island. *Journal of Telemedicine and Telecare, 12,* 354−357.

Hartman, R. (2007, July). *Statement of Richard Hartman, Director, VHA Policy Analysis and Forecasting before the Senate Committee on Veterans' Affairs.* Retrieved from the U.S. Department of Veterans Affairs website: http://www.va.gov/OCA/testimony/svac/070721RH.asp

Haslam, R., & McLaren, P. (2000). Interactive television for an urban adult mental health service: The guy's psychiatric intensive care unit telepsychiatry project. *Journal of Telemedicine and Telecare, 6,* S50−S52.

Hauenstein, E. J., Petterson, S., Merwin, E., Rovnyak, V., Heise, B., & Wagner, D. (2006). Rurality, gender, and mental health treatment. *Family and Community Health: The Journal of Health Promotion and Maintenance, 29,* 169−185.

Henggeler, S. W., Pickrel, S. G., Brondino, M. J., & Crouch, J. L. (1996). Eliminating (almost) treatment dropout of substance abusing or dependent delinquents through home-based multisystemic therapy. *American Journal of Psychiatry, 153*, 427–428.

Hicken, B. L., & Plowhead, A. (2010). A model for home-based psychology from the veterans health administration. *Professional Psychology: Research and Practice, 41*, 340–346.

Hoge, C. W. (2011). Interventions for war-related posttraumatic stress disorder: Meeting veterans where they are. *Journal of the American Medical Association, 306*, 549–551.

Hoge, C. W., Auchterlonie, J. L., & Milliken, C. S. (2006). Mental health problems, use of mental health services, and attrition from military service after returning from deployment to Iraq or Afghanistan. *Journal of the American Medical Association, 295*, 1023–1032.

Hoge, C. W., Castro, C. A., Messer, S. C., McGurk, D., Cotting, D. I., & Koffman, R. L. (2004). Combat duty in Iraq and Afghanistan, mental health problems, and barriers to care. *New England Journal of Medicine, 351*, 13–22.

Hoge, C. W., Lesikar, S. E., Guevara, R., Lange, J., Brundage, J. F., Engel., C. C., et al. (2002). Mental disorders among U.S. military personnel in the 1990s: Association with high levels of health care utilization and early military attrition. *American Journal of Psychiatry, 159*, 1576–1583.

Hoge, C. W., McGurk, D., Thomas, J. L., Cox, A. L., Engel, C. C., & Castro, C. A. (2008). Mild traumatic brain injury in U.S. soldiers returning from Iraq. *New England Journal of Medicine, 358*, 453–463.

Hoge, C. W., Toboni, H. E., Messer, S. C., Bell, N., Amoroso, P., & Orman, D. T. (2005). The occupational burden of mental disorders in the U.S. military: Psychiatric hospitalizations, involuntary separations, and disability. *American Journal of Psychiatry, 162*, 585–591.

Holbrook, T. L., & Hoyt, D. B. (2004). The impact of major trauma: Quality-of-life outcomes are worse in women than in men, independent of mechanism and injury severity. *Journal of Trauma, 56*, 284–290.

Jakupcak, M., Conybeare, D., Phelps, L., Hunt, S., Holmes, H. A., Felker, B., et al. (2007). Anger, hostility, and aggression among Iraq and Afghanistan war veterans reporting PTSD and subthreshold PTSD. *Journal of Traumatic Stress, 20*, 945–954.

Jerome, L. W., & Zaylor, C. (2000). Cyberspace: Creating a therapeutic environment for telehealth applications. *Professional Psychology: Research and Practice, 31*, 478–483.

Johnson, D. R., Fontana, A., Lubin, H., Corn, B., & Rosenheck, R. (2004). Long-term course of treatment-seeking Vietnam veterans with posttraumatic stress disorder: Mortality, clinical condition, and life satisfaction. *Journal of Nervous and Mental Disease, 192*, 35–41.

Kane, T. (2006). *Who are the recruits? The demographic characteristics of U.S. military enlistment*. Washington, DC: Heritage Foundation.

Kang, H. K., & Bullman, T. A. (2008). Risk of suicide among U.S. veterans after returning from the Iraq and Afghanistan war zones. *Journal of the American Medical Association, 300*, 652–653.

Kaplan, M. S., Huguet, N., McFarland, B. H., & Newsom, J. T. (2007). Suicide among male veterans: A prospective population-based study. *Journal of Epidemiological Community Health, 61*, 619–624.

Katz, L. S., Bloor, L. E., Cojucar, G., & Draper, T. (2007). Women who served in Iraq seeking mental health services: Relationships between military sexual trauma, symptoms, and readjustment. *Psychological Services, 4*, 239–249.

Kennedy, C. A. (2005). The challenges of economic evaluations of remote technical health interventions. *Clinical and Investigative Medicine*, *61*, 4−12.

Kessler, R. C. (2000). Posttraumatic stress disorder: The burden to the individual and to society. *Journal of Clinical Psychiatry*, *61*, 4−12.

Kulka, R. A., Schlenger, W. E., Fairbank, J. A., Hough, R. L., Jordan, B. K., Marmar, C. R., et al. (1990). *Trauma and the Vietnam War generation: Report of findings from the National Vietnam Veterans Readjustment Study*. New York, NY: Brunner/Mazel.

Luxton, D. D., Sirotin, A. P., & Mishkind, M. C. (2010). Safety of telemental healthcare delivered to clinically unsupervised settings: A systematic review. *Telemedicine Journal and e-Health*, *16*, 705−711.

Magaletta, P. R., Fagan, T. J., & Ax, R. K. (1998). Advancing psychology services through telehealth in the Federal Bureau of Prisons. *Professional Psychology: Research and Practice*, *29*, 543−548.

Mannion, L., Fahy, T. J., Duffy, C., Broderick, M., & Gethins, E. (1998). Telepsychiatry: An island pilot project. *Journal of Telemedicine and Telecare*, *4*, 62−63.

McLaren, P., Ahlbom, J., Riley, A., Mohammedali, A., & Denis, M. (2002). The North Lewisham telepsychiatry project: Beyond the pilot phase. *Journal of Telemedicine and Telecare*, *8*, 98−100.

Mielonen, M. L., Ohinmaa, A., Moring, J., & Isohanni, M. (2002). Videoconferencing in telepsychiatry. *Journal of Technology in Human Services*, *20*, 183−199.

Mohamed, S., Neale, M., & Rosenheck, R. A. (2009). VA intensive mental health case management in urban and rural areas: Veteran characteristics and service delivery. *Psychiatric Services*, *60*, 914−921.

Monnier, J., Knapp, R. G., & Frueh, B. C. (2003). Recent advances in telepsychiatry: An updated review. *Psychiatric Services*, *53*, 1604−1609.

Morgan, R. D., Patrick, A. R., & Magaletta, P. R. (2008). Does the use of telemental health alter the treatment experience? Inmates' perceptions of telemental health versus face-to-face treatment modalities. *Journal of Consulting and Clinical Psychology*, *76*, 158−162.

Morland, L. A., Frueh, B. C., Pierce, K., & Miyahira, S. (2003). PTSD and telemental health: Updates and future directions. *PTSD Clinical Quarterly*, *12*, 1−5.

Morland, L. A., Greene, C. J., Grubbs, K. M., Kloezeman, K., Mackintosh, M., Rosen, C., et al. (2011). Therapist adherence to manualized cognitive−behavioral therapy for anger management delivered to veterans with PTSD via videoteleconferencing. *Journal of Clinical Psychology*, *67*, 629−638.

Morland, L. A., Greene, C. J., Rosen, C. S., Foy, D., Reilly, P., Shore, J., et al. (2010). Telemedicine for anger management therapy in a rural population of combat veterans with posttraumatic stress disorder: A randomized noninferiority trial. *Journal of Clinical Psychiatry*, *71*, 855−863.

Morland, L. A., Hynes, A. K., Mackintosh, M., Resick, P. A., & Chard, K. (2011). Group cognitive processing therapy for PTSD delivered to rural combat veterans via telemental health: Lessons learned from a pilot cohort. *Journal of Traumatic Stress*, *24*, 465−469.

Morland, L. A., Pierce, K., & Wong, M. (2005). Telehealth and PSTD psychoeducation groups in the Pacific Islands: A feasibility study. *Telehealth and Telecare*, *10*, 286−289.

Nesbitt, T. S., Hilty, D. M., Kuenneth, C. A., & Siefkin, A. (2000). Development of a telemedicine program: A review of 1000 videoconferencing consultations. *Western Journal of Medicine*, *173*, 169−174.

Payne, S. M. C., Lee, A., Clark, J. A., Rogers, W. H., Miller, D. R., Skinner, K. M., et al. (2005). Utilization of medical services by veterans health study (VHS) respondents. *Journal of Ambulatory Care Management*, *28*, 125−140.

Perednia, D. A., & Allen, A. (1995). Telemedicine technology and clinical applications. *Journal of the American Medical Association, 273,* 483–488.

Persaud, D. D., Jreige, S., Skedgel, C., Finley, J., Sargeant, J., & Hanlon, N. (2005). An incremental cost analysis of telehealtth in Nova Scotia from a societal perspective. *Journal of Telemedicine and Telecare, 11,* 77–84.

Pols, H., & Oak, S. (2007). War and military mental health: The U.S. psychiatric response in the 20th century. *American Journal of Public Health, 97,* 2132–2142.

Poon, P., Hui, E., Dai, D., Kwok, T., & Woo, J. (2005). Cognitive intervention for community-dwelling older persons with memory problems: Telemedicine versus face-to-face treatment. *International Journal of Geriatric Psychiatry, 20,* 285–286.

President's New Freedom Commission on Mental Health. (2004). *Achieving the promise: Transforming mental health care in America, executive summary* (Publication SMA-03-3832). Retrieved from Substance Abuse and Mental Health Services Administration. < http://store.samhsa.gov/shin/content//SMA03-3831/SMA03-3831.pdf >.

Prigerson, H. G., Maciejewski, P. K., & Rosenheck, R. A. (2002). Population attributable fractions of psychiatric disorders and behavioral outcomes associated with combat exposure among U.S. men. *American Journal of Public Health, 92,* 59–63.

Rosenheck, R., & Fontana, A. (1994). Utilization of mental health services by minority veterans of the Vietnam era. *Journal of Nervous and Mental Disease, 182,* 685–691.

Rosenheck, R., & Fontana, A. (1995). Do Vietnam-era veterans who suffer from posttraumatic stress disorder avoid mental health services? *Military Medicine, 160,* 136–142.

Rosenheck, R., & Fontana, A. (1996). Race and outcome of treatment for veterans suffering from PTSD. *Journal of Traumatic Stress, 9,* 343–351.

Ruskin, P. E., Reed, S., Kumar, R., Kling, M., Siegel, E., Rosen, M., et al. (1998). Reliability and acceptability of psychiatric diagnosis via telecommunication and audiovisual technology. *Psychiatric Services, 49,* 1086–1088.

Ruskin, P. E., Silver-Aylaian, M., Kling, M. A., Reed, S. A., Bradham, D. D., Hebel, J. R., et al. (2004). Treatment outcomes in depression: Comparison of remote treatment through telepsychiatry to in-person treatment. *American Journal of Psychiatry, 161,* 1471–1476.

Rybarczyk, B., Lopez, M., Benson, R., Alsten, C., & Stepanski, E. (2002). Efficacy of two behavioral treatment programs for comorbid geriatric insomnia. *Psychology and Aging, 17,* 288–298.

Schnurr, P. P., Friedman, M. J., Sengupta, A., Jankowski, M. K., & Holmes, T. (2000). PTSD and utilization of medical treatment services among male Vietnam veterans. *Journal of Nervous and Mental Disease, 188,* 496–504.

Schnurr, P. P., & Spiro, A. (1999). Combat exposure, PTSD symptoms, and health behaviors as predictors of self-reported physical health in older veterans. *Journal of Nervous and Mental Disease, 187,* 353–359.

Scholle, S. H., Weismean, C. S., Anderson, R., Weitz, T., Freund, K. M., & Binko, J. (2000). Women's satisfaction with primary care: A new measurement effort from the PHS national centers of excellence in women's health. *Women's Health Issues, 10,* 1–9.

Seal, K. H., Berenthal, D., Miner, C. R., Sen, S., & Marmar, C. (2007). Bringing the war back home: Mental health disorders among 103,788 U.S. veterans returning from Iraq and Afghanistan seen at department of veterans affairs facilities. *Archives of Internal Medicine, 167,* 476–482.

Seal, K. H., Maguen, S., Cohen, B., Gima, K. S., Metzler, T. J., Ren, L., et al. (2010). VA mental health services utilization in Iraq and Afghanistan veterans in the first year of receiving new mental health diagnoses. *Journal of Traumatic Stress, 23,* 5–16.

Shore, J. H., & Manson, S. M. (2005). A developmental model for rural telepsychiatry. *Psychiatric Services*, *56*, 976—980.

Simpson, J., Doze, S., Urness, D., Hailey, D., & Jacobs, P. (2001). Evaluation of a routine telepsychiatry service. *Journal of Telemedicine and Telecare*, *7*, 90—98.

Solomon, S. D., & Davidson, J. R. (1997). Trauma: Prevalence, impairment, service use, and cost. *Journal of Clinical Psychiatry*, *58*, 5—11.

Stecker, T., Fortney, J. C., Hamilton, F., & Ajzen, I. (2007). An assessment of beliefs about mental health care among veterans who served in Iraq. *Psychiatric Services*, *58*, 1358—1361.

Tanielian, T., & Jaycox, L. H. (2008). *Invisible woundsofwar: Psychological and cognitive injuries, their consequences, and services to assist recovery*. Santa Monica, CA: RAND Center for Military Health Policy Research.

Thomas, J. L., Wilk, J. E., Riviere, L. A., McGurk, D., Castro, C. A., & Hoge, C. W. (2010). Prevalence of mental health problems and functional impairment among active component and National Guard soldiers 3 and 12 months following combat in Iraq. *Archives of General Psychiatry*, *67*, 614—623.

Thorp, S. R., & Stein, M. B. (2005). Posttraumatic stress disorder and functioning. *PTSD Research Quarterly*, *16*, 1—7.

Thorp, S. R., & Stein, M. B. (2008). Occupational disability. In G. Reyes, J. Elhai, & J. Ford (Eds.): *Encyclopedia of psychological trauma* (p.453). Hoboken, NJ: John Wiley & Sons.

Trott, P., & Blignault, I. (1998). Cost evaluation of a telepsychiatry service in northern Queensland. *Journal of Telemedicine and Telecare*, *4*, 66—68.

Tuerk, P. W., Grubaugh, A. L., Hamner, M. B., & Foa, E. B. (2009). Diagnosis and treatment of PTSD-related compulsive checking behaviors in veterans of the Iraq war: The influence of military context on the expression of PTSD symptoms. *American Journal of Psychiatry*, *166*, 762—767.

Tuerk, P. W., Yoder, M., Grubaugh, A., Myrick, H., Hamner, M., & Acierno, R. (2011). Prolonged exposure therapy for combat-related posttraumatic stress disorder: An examination of treatment effectiveness for veterans of the wars in Afghanistan and Iraq. *Journal of Anxiety Disorders*, *25*, 397—403.

U.S. Department of Veterans Affairs. (2008). VHA Handbook 1160.01: Uniformed mental health services in VA medical centers and clinics. Washington, DC: Author.

U.S. Department of Veterans Affairs. (2012). About the Office of Rural Health. Retrieved from U.S. Department of Veterans Affairs, Office of Rural Health. <http://www.ruralhealth.va.gov/about/index.asp>.

Vogt, D., Bergeron, A., Salgado, D., Daley, J., Ouimette, P., & Wolfe, J. (2006). Barriers to veteran health administration care in a nationally representative sample of women veterans. *Journal of General Internal Medicine*, *21*, S19—S25.

Wagner, T. H., Harris, K. M., Federman, B., Dai, L., Luna, Y., & Humphreys, K. (2007). Prevalence of substance use disorders among veterans and comparable nonveterans from the national survey on drug use and health. *Psychological Services*, *4*, 149—157.

Wallace, A. E., Weeks, W. B., Wang, S., Lee, A. F., & Kazis, L. E. (2006). Rural and urban disparities in health-related quality of life among veterans with psychiatric disorders. *Psychiatric Services*, *57*, 851—856.

Wang, P. S., Lane, M., Olfson, M., Pincus, H. A., Wells, K. B., & Kessler, R. C. (2005). Twelve-month use of mental health services in the United States: Results from the national comorbidity survey replication. *Archives of General Psychiatry*, *62*, 629—640.

Washington, D. L., Yano, E. M., Simon, B., & Sun, S. (2006). To use or not to use: What influences why women veterans choose VA health care. *Journal of General Internal Medicine, 21*, S11–S18.

Weeks, W. B., Kazis, L. E., Shen, Y., Cong, Z., Ren, X. S., Miller, D., et al. (2004). Differences in health-related quality of life in rural and urban veterans. *American Journal of Public Health, 94*, 1762–1767.

Weeks, W. B., Mahar, P. J., & Wright, S. M. (2005). Utilization of VA and Medicare services by Medicare-eligible veterans: The impact of additional access points in a rural setting. *Journal of Healthcare Management, 50*, 95–106.

Weeks, W. B., Wallace, A. E., Wang, S., Lee, A., & Kazis, L. E. (2006). Rural–urban disparities in health-related quality of life within disease categories of veterans. *Journal of Rural Health, 22*, 204–211.

Werner, A. (2001). Unanswered questions about telepsychiatry. *Psychiatric Services, 52*, 689–690.

Westermeyer, J., Canive, J., Thuras, P., Chesness, D., & Thompson, J. (2002). Perceived barriers to VA mental health care among upper Midwest American Indian Veterans: Description and associations. *Medical Care, 40*, 62–70.

Yoder, M., Tuerk, P. W., Price, M., Grubaugh, A. L., Strachan, M., Myrick, H., et al. (2012). Prolonged exposure therapy for combat-related posttraumatic stress disorder: Comparing outcomes for veterans of different wars. *Psychological Services, 9*, 16–25.

Zarate, C. A., Weinstock, L., Cukor, P., Morabito, C., Leahy, L., Burns, C., et al. (1997). Applicability of telemedicine for assessing patients with schizophrenia: Acceptance and reliability. *Journal of Clinical Psychiatry, 58*, 22–25.

Zaylor, C., Whitten, P., & Kingsley, C. (2000). Telemedicine services to a county jail. *Journal of Telemedicine and Telecare, 6*, S93–S95.

13 Videoteleconferencing in Forensic and Correctional Practice

Ashley B. Batastini, Brendan R. McDonald and Robert D. Morgan

Department of Psychology, Texas Tech University

Videoteleconferencing Health in Forensic and Correctional Practices

The Development of Videoteleconferencing in Forensic and Correctional Settings

Over recent decades, videoteleconferencing (VTC) has gained increasing attention (Manfredi, Shupe, & Batki, 2005). VTC is a data transmission system used by providers to deliver services over a distance. In health care contexts, VTC is often interchangeable with other terms depending on the application (e.g., telehealth, telemental health, telepsychiatry, telelaw). In the current state of technology, this form of communication is typically conducted using "real-time" audiovisual monitors to connect agencies in need of services (i.e., the originating or remote site) to agencies that render such services (i.e., the distant or hub site (Ax, Fagan, Magaletta et al., 2007)). The specific terminology used in this chapter to describe these sites was adopted from The American Telemedicine Association [ATA], 2012). Other terms may be encountered elsewhere. VTC appears to be a promising method for extending health care services to a variety of underserved populations, including inmates with mental illness (Larsen, Stamm, Davis, & Magaletta, 2004).

Elements of VTC have been used across the United States in medical settings for diagnosis, patient care, and professional education for over 30 years. In 1991, there were four telemedicine networks nationally; merely 5 years later, there were approximately 160. Between 1993 and 1996, video consultations increased from 1750 to 18,766 across both correctional and noncorrectional populations (T. W. Miller, Clark, Veltkamp, Burton, & Swope, 2008).The first use of telehealth in a prison system began at the University of Miami in 1974, where physicians treated inmates at three facilities using microwave transmission. However, this method of service delivery did

Telemental Health. DOI: http://dx.doi.org/10.1016/B978-0-12-416048-4.00013-0

not last long due to operation and maintenance costs. With advancements in technology, telehealth reappeared in corrections around the 1990s (Doarn, Justis, Chaudhri, & Merrel, 2005). Common modes of transmission include both analog and digital. Analog modes use wavelengths to transmit high-resolution video images through bandwidth capacities that may include satellite, microwave, or T1 links. However, this mode is often associated with higher costs, complex hardware in higher bandwidths, and jerky or delayed audiovisuals in lower bandwidths. Digital modes transmit data in the form of a digital byte-stream consisting of zeros and ones. This mode is generally more advantageous given the lower transmission costs, reduced equipment size, ease of operation, and higher quality images (T. W. Miller et al., 2008).

Currently 26 states operate telehealth programs that reach over 400 correctional facilities in the country (Larsen et al., 2004). About 20% of all telemedicine applications involve correctional health care (Lowes, 2001), and interventions that target the needs of inmates with mental illness are one of the most frequently cited uses in correctional settings (Ax, Fagan, Magaletta et al., 2007). At time of this publication, there were over 80 organizational members of the ATA, who provide health care services to correctional and noncorrectional populations across the country. Common uses of telehealth in corrections include legal consultation and court testimony, forensic mental health assessment (e.g., competency determinations, sexually violent predator evaluations), juvenile rehabilitation, psychiatric medication management, group treatment for inmates in segregation, and training and continuing education (Larsen et al., 2004).

A closer look at legal applications. Although not directly related to mental health care, understanding the use of VTC in legal proceedings, labeled telelaw (TL), is important for providing justice-involved persons with a full range of quality services. The first signs of TL in the courts began in 1995 with the Prison Litigation Reform Act. This legislation encouraged federal courts to conduct pretrial hearings through telecommunications whenever possible, so as to prevent the removal of prisoners from correctional facilities (Johnson & Wiggins, 2006). In 2001, amendments to the Federal Rules of Criminal Procedure were passed that authorize the use of VTC during criminal proceedings (Wiggins, Dunn, & Cort, 2003). Currently, TL methods are permissible in court for a variety of trial-related purposes, including initial appearances, arraignments, testimony, and sentencing (Johnson & Wiggins, 2006; Wiggins et al., 2003). For example, VTC may be used to obtain testimony from witnesses who are incarcerated, medically handicapped, or located in remote regions (Wiggins, 2006). This modality may also be a viable alternative for witnesses who are uncomfortable confronting criminal defendants (e.g., sexual assault cases (Yiming & Fung, 2003)). VTC may also be used to obtain testimony from expert witnesses (including those who offer opinions regarding a defendant's mental functioning (Brett & Blumburg, 2006; T. W. Miller et al., 2008). Other uses of TL include pretrial consultations, conferences, depositions, probable cause hearings, competency hearings, and pretrial motion hearings (Johnson & Wiggins, 2006; T. W. Miller et al., 2008; Wiggins, 2006). Today, approximately 85% of federal courts have access to VTC technology (Wiggins et al., 2003) and 60% of state courts report using this modality in some capacity during criminal proceedings (National Center for State Courts, 2010). The widespread use of VTC in courtroom settings calls for further investigation of its effectiveness.

Barriers to Health Care

Incarcerating the mentally ill. Of the nearly 2.5 million adult inmates detained in jails or prisons, more than half report experiencing at least some symptoms associated with mental illness (James & Glaze, 2006). According to a survey by the Bureau of Justice Statistics (James & Glaze, 2006), the most commonly reported mental health problems among this subgroup of inmates were related to major depressive disorder and mania, with symptom prevalence rates falling anywhere between 6% for suicidal ideation and 50% for persistent anger or irritability. Symptoms of psychotic disorders (i.e., hallucinations and delusions) were reported by about 5−18% of inmates with mental illness. In a more recent prevalence study (Steadman, Osher, Robbins, Case, & Samuels, 2009), the rate of serious mental illness (SMI) was 14.5% for male inmates and 31% for female inmates in a sample of five Northeastern jails. Currently, there are about three times as many persons with serious and persistent mental illnesses in jails and prisons than in all state psychiatric hospitals across the country (Abramsky & Fellner, 2003; Torrey, Kennard, Eslinger, Lamb, & Pavle, 2010). Although nearly all correctional institutions screen inmates for mental health concerns or provide at least some level of psychological services (Beck & Maruschak, 2001), programming for inmates is generally underfunded and inadequate for addressing the unique treatment needs of inmates (Manfredi et al., 2005). A 2001 report estimated that only 33% of state prisoners, 25% of federal prisoners, and 16% of jailed inmates with mental health problems receive treatment (e.g., psychotropic medication, short-term counseling) after admission (Beck & Maruschak, 2001).

Persons with mental illness have particular difficulty coping with the stressors encountered behind prison walls (e.g., conforming to highly restricted and regimented routines, long hours of confinement and isolation (Metzer & Fellner, 2010)). Bizarre, annoying, or dangerous behaviors are often tolerated without considering their association with mental health functioning, because many facilities and their staff (e.g., correctional officers, prison officials) lack the resources to appropriately handle disordered individuals (Metzer & Fellner, 2010). In the absence of adequate treatment services and specialty providers, responses to inmates with SMI are often no different from responses to other inmates who break institutional rules (Metzer & Fellner, 2010). Untreated psychological problems manifested as overt symptoms can lead to continued disciplinary consequences, which in turn exacerbate distress (H. A. Miller & Young, 1997). Mental health concerns in corrections are not only debilitating for the inmates experiencing psychological distress and the staff involved in managing symptoms, but they are also problematic from a public safety perspective. One study (Cloyes, Wong, Latimer, & Abarca, 2010), for example, found that inmates with SMI were reincarcerated after a median of 385 days as compared to 743 days for inmates without SMI. However, it should be noted that alleviating mental health symptoms alone is not enough to reduce recidivism (Peterson, Skeem, Hart, Vidal, & Keith, 2010). Offenders with mental illness have been shown to endorse similar patterns of criminal thinking when compared to nonmentally disordered offenders (Morgan, Fisher, Duan, Mandracchia, & Murray, 2010; Wolff, Morgan, Shi, Fisher & Huening, in press), and the link between mental illness and criminal justice involvement may be moderated by an individual's social context, including poverty, homelessness, and unemployment (Draine, Salzer, Culhane, & Hadley, 2002).

The growth of rural prisons. Drastic increases in the incarceration rate created a demand for prison expansion. This problem, coupled with the economic hardships faced by rural communities, led to the construction of correctional facilities as an attractive approach to addressing the fiscal issues of these areas (Hooks, Mosher, Rotolo, & Lobao, 2004). Prisons and jails are often viewed as a strategy for reviving employment rates and increasing local government revenue, despite research that fails to support such economic benefits (Glasmeier & Farrigan, 2007; King, Mauer, & Hurling, 2004). Consequently, rural prison expansion has become big business (Hooks et al., 2004). Unfortunately, these remote facilities experience a deficit in quality health care that is common to rural areas (Ax, Fagan, & Holton, 2002). In fact, many problems encountered by inmates in rural correctional facilities appear to be driven by placement in a rural facility. For example, distance often leads to the separation of urban offenders from their social support systems, including family members, significant others, peers, and attorneys. Additionally, inmates may feel alienated from the local culture, further complicating their ability to adjust to life behind bars (Ax, Fagan, & Holton, 2002). Notably, poor adjustment can create or aggravate psychological distress (Metzer & Fellner, 2010). Another dilemma faced by rural prisons and jails is limited access to appropriate health care professionals. There seems to be an overwhelming difficulty in securing full-time providers who are willing to offer their services in these settings because of the resources (e.g., time and money) necessary to work on-site (Manfredi et al., 2005).

Current trends in correctional health care. The rising costs of health care preclude access to services for many who are in need. The costs for an off-site service provider are estimated to be as high as $1000 per inmate visit (Zollo, Kienzle, Loeffelholz, & Sebille, 1999). If federal air transport is required, this number can reach up to $10,000 (Magaletta, Fagan, & Ax, 1998). These costs include the actual services rendered (e.g., medical, dental, psychiatric), travel expenses, and salaries for personnel (e.g., drivers, security, physician assistants) who need to accompany inmates on visits. Additionally, the absence of competition among "specialty" providers (e.g., orthopedics, urology, forensic psychiatrists, counseling for inmates positive for human immunodeficiency virus (HIV), sex offender treatment, early parole assessments), particularly in rural areas, can increase the price of services to well above average (Magaletta, Fagan, & Ax, 1998).

The delivery of health care is further compromised by the general lack of qualified professionals willing to work with inmates. The high potential for burnout and low pay deters many service providers from seeking full-time employment in correctional settings (Daniel, 2007; Magaletta, Fagan, & Ax, 1998). The scarcity of trained professionals is again exacerbated in rural areas where facilities are sparsely located and commute times for providers are long (Manfredi et al., 2005). Even within the Federal Bureau of Prisons, where resources for health care services are typically more plentiful than many other correctional organizations, securing specialty providers who are familiar with inmate populations remains a challenge. When services are eventually obtained, they are often not delivered in a timely or consistent manner (Magaletta, Fagan, & Ax, 1998).

Another trend that has introduced new challenges in correctional health care is privatization. Traditionally, corrections departments hired their own staff and clinics to directly administer medical care (including mental health care) to inmates (Daniel, 2007); however, the growing costs of health care and the shortage of service providers has led many states to privatize services for inmates. In 2000, 34 states had privatized health care contracts and 24 state corrections systems were run completely by private contractors (Montague, 2003). This number has likely increased over the past decade. A popular approach for many correctional facilities is to contract with medical schools or university medical centers. In these types of contracts, there is an equitable exchange of benefits: correctional institutions gain access to quality treatment services and can form working alliances with newly trained professionals, while the medical schools expand revenues by providing a needed public service and gain the opportunity to conduct correctional research (Daniel, 2007). Although this seems like a viable remedy to the health care problem, profit motives can sometimes outweigh incentives for quality care, thereby compromising ethical standards of practice (Daniel, 2007). In addition, community-based contract providers who are not sensitive to the correctional environment may recommend treatment options that conflict with security and management needs; this lack of understanding often translates to ineffective care and rehabilitation for inmates (Magaletta, Fagan, & Ax, 1998).

How Can VTC Improve Services in Criminal Justice Settings?

The most apparent benefit of VTC is heightened security and safety for the inmates, staff, and the public. When criminal defendants or inmates are transported off-site (e.g., court hearings, medical facilities, mental health agencies), there is an increased risk of escape and harm to staff or civilians (Zaylor, Nelson, & Cook, 2001). VTC allows inmates to receive services (legal or health) within the confinements of secure perimeters (Larsen et al., 2004). Services delivered through VTC also offer the advantage of reduced wait-times because many of the steps involved in connecting inmates to necessary services are eliminated (e.g., transportation and security procedures, travel time (National Institute of Justice, 1999)). Furthermore, motivation to provide services to this population may increase if the mechanism of delivery is more convenient. Inmates whose needs are addressed promptly may be less likely to become agitated or volatile. Responding more proactively to requests for services may increase inmates' trust in the justice system, and—in doing so—may enhance compliance with treatment or legal procedures. Less aggression from inmates will also impact the emotional and behavioral milieu within the jail or prison setting (Magaletta, Fagan, & Ax, 1998). A safer and more controlled environment alleviates stress and anxiety among correctional employees, who will be able to focus on running a safe facility, rather than attending to custody and disciplinary problems (Magaletta, Fagan, & Ax, 1998; Zaylor, Whitten, & Kingsley, 2000). Lastly, psychiatric emergency care situations (e.g., suicide prevention) can be handled more quickly through the use of VTC when on-site providers are not readily available (Magaletta, Fagan, & Peyrot, 2000).

Using VTC to specifically address mental health problems, often referred to as telemental health (TMH), has become a common application. Understanding the effectiveness of TMH in identifying and targeting the treatment needs of inmates could have significant implications for correctional programming and subsequent community safety. TMH has the potential to provide easier access to services for underserved populations, including inmates. In particular, mental health services via TMH can easily connect correctional institutions with forensic specialists who are familiar with inmate needs. This linkage will ultimately improve the quality of care for inmates (Khalifa, Saleem, & Stankard, 2008; Magaletta, Fagan, & Ax, 1998). TMH may also create more seamless systems of treatment (Magaletta, Fagan, & Ax, 1998; Magaletta, Fagan, & Peyrot, 2000). For example, inmates who are being discharged from a forensic mental health hospital to a secure correctional facility could have their first few sessions with continuing care providers while still at the medical center. Similarly, TMH can assist correctional psychologists in coordinating community resources (e.g., parole officers, health care providers, job supervisors) for inmates preparing for release. Special needs cases requiring highly scheduled care that combines psychological and medical services (e.g., substance abuse treatment and infectious disease specialists for HIV-positive inmates) can also be accommodated through TMH. These advantages of TMH services may increase compliance and reduce psychological or behavioral relapse (Magaletta, Fagan, & Ax, 1998).

Moreover, TMH has the ability to involve persons outside the institution walls in the inmate's treatment (Magaletta, Fagan, & Peyrot, 2000). Family therapy, including parenting counseling, is more likely to be effective if significant others can participate alongside the incarcerated person from a remote site. This capacity may be particularly beneficial for incarcerated youth (Kaliebe, Heneghan, & Kim, 2011), who often require comprehensive treatments that involve persons from multiple domains. For example, multisystemic therapy—a well-established intervention shown to reduce delinquency among violent juvenile offenders (Schaeffer & Borduin, 2005)—includes a network of caregivers, school officials, peers, and neighbors to promote positive behavioral changes. TMH could assist in building better connections among these individuals by offering a faster, more convenient mode of communication.

Demonstrating the Effectiveness of VTC

Cost-effectiveness. At present, cost-effectiveness evaluations are the most robust (Ax, Fagan, Magaletta et al., 2007) of studies examining VTC. It is estimated that a conventional, face-to-face consultation for an inmate carries an average cost of $173 compared to $71 per telemedicine consultation (National Institute of Justice, 2002). Texas and Ohio—two states that have substantial TMH networks—report saving approximately $200–1000 every time consults are conducted electronically (Kinsella, 2004); however, some service providers and policy-makers are reluctant to develop TMH programs because of high initial start-up costs (Ax, Fagan, Magaletta et al., 2007). Such resistance may be unwarranted as software, hardware, and signal transmission costs have decreased dramatically over the years (T. W. Miller et al., 2008). For example, in 1992, interactive multimedia equipment could have cost agencies over $100,000. Just 8 years later, the same equipment was available for less than $20,000 (Baker, 2000). Today, high-definition videoconferencing systems can be purchased for as low as about $8000 (Technology Marketing Corporation, 2009). However, it should be noted that the costs associated with videoconferencing equipment can vary depending on the quality of the system and its applications. Furthermore, funding for initial equipment costs could be awarded through government subsidies, and most operating jurisdictions are projected to experience monthly savings of about $14,200 (National Institute of Justice, 1999). For agencies looking to develop TMH programs, the National Institute of Justice (2002) has proposed a cost-estimation model to help determine the costs and benefits of applying this method of service delivery specifically to prison environments. The suggested model takes into account the cost of facility modifications and installation of equipment, training costs, long-term costs of maintaining system operations, costs of employing off-site personnel to provide services, cost savings that accrue by replacing conventional health care with TMH, transportation cost savings, and the estimated savings that continue to accrue after payback of the initial TMH acquisition costs.

Demonstrating the cost-effectiveness of this modality bolsters its marketability and may increase its acceptability among policy-makers as an alternative option for health care providers. As some researchers have argued, "the issue of cost and cost-effectiveness is at the heart of the debate of whether or not telepsychiatry has a future" (Monnier, Knapp, & Frueh, 2003, p. 1607). However, Zollo et al. (1999) caution against assuming instantaneous savings; rather, a properly planned and implemented TMH program is likely to be "cost acceptable." Cost-effectiveness can only be achieved as the demand for TMH contacts increases (Zollo et al., 1999).

Acceptability of services. Another major area of research in correctional TMH has addressed the acceptability of service modality from the patient perspective. In a survey (Magaletta, Fagan, & Peyrot, 2000) of 75 adult male inmates who received psychiatry consultations via TMH, 81% of respondents rated treatment positively, 83% reported that they would seek help again, 71% said they would recommend it to other inmates, and 35% preferred it over face-to-face interactions. Similarly, Morgan, Patrick, and Magaletta (2008) examined the impact of treatment modality on the therapeutic relationship and found no significant between-group differences regarding inmates' post-session mood, perceptions of the working alliance, and overall satisfaction with the provider and treatment modality. Brodey, Claypoole, Motto, Arias, and Goss (2000) also found moderately high satisfaction with psychiatric interviews via VTC with no significant differences in satisfaction from inmates interviewed in-person. In a sample of male and female jailed patients receiving a total of 264 mental health consultations (70 initial visits, 194 follow-up or continuing care visits) through VTC, Zaylor, Whitten, and Kingsley (2000) reported high satisfaction as demonstrated by compliance and cooperation with treatment. Additionally, jail staff perceived TMH services as easily integrated into routine care (Zaylor, Whitten, & Kingsley, 2000). Results from this line of research suggest that the method of service delivery is not a primary factor influencing the therapeutic relationship from the perspective of the inmate being treated. In fact, some inmates may actually prefer TMH to in-person consultations for discussing difficult issues like sexual abuse (Khalifa et al., 2008). Likewise, on-site TMH visits eliminate the embarrassment of being treated in the community wearing prison clothing and shackles (Zollo et al., 1999).

The acceptability of TMH has been further demonstrated in juvenile populations. In one study (Myers, Valentine, Morganthaler, & Melzer, 2006), a remote psychiatrist provided diagnostic evaluations, needs assessments, initial medication treatment, and brief follow-up consultations to juveniles incarcerated in a rural, minimum-security correctional facility. A global rating of client satisfaction, rated by the adolescents themselves, suggested that participants were satisfied with the services they received ($M = 3.97$ on a five-point scale). Furthermore, the participating psychiatrist denied any problems establishing interpersonal rapport and expressed comfort in treating seriously impaired youth via this modality. In another study (Fox, Connor, McCullers, & Waters, 2008) of delinquent youths (ages 12–19) receiving behavioral health counseling via TMH, participants actually reported that they perceived the provider to be more focused on them as compared to their previous experiences with in-person interactions. Likewise, providers perceived that participants were more open to sharing their thoughts and feelings through interactive video than through face-to-face contact. Despite the anecdotal nature of this evidence, it nonetheless implies that TMH can be an appropriate and beneficial tool for treating incarcerated youth—perhaps even more so than traditional approaches. With the changing technological climate (so embraced by this nation's youth), it is likely that future research will continue to demonstrate adequate acceptability of TMH services among this group.

Forensic mental health assessment. The literature on TMH in forensic populations has also focused on the reliability of assessment outcomes. One study evaluated the use of TMH for determining competency to stand trial (Manguno-Mire et al., 2007). Inmates were randomly assigned to either an in-person or VTC interview. Results showed strong inter-rater reliability ($r = 0.92$ for in-person; $r = 0.93$ for telemedicine) among forensic evaluators in both conditions. Participants also expressed high levels of satisfaction with the VTC interview process. Additionally, Lexcen, Hawk, Herrick, and Blank (2006) reported good to excellent inter-rater reliability ($r = 0.69–0.82$) between TMH and in-person forensic mental health assessments using the Brief Psychiatric Rating Scale-Anchored Version (Overall & Gorham, 1962) and the MacArthur Competence Assessment Tool—Criminal Adjudication (Poythress et al., 1999). In another study of jailed inmates receiving TMH services, Nelson, Zaylor, and

Cook (2004) found significant positive correlations between patient and provider symptom impressions, particularly with regard to suicidal ideation. However, this study did not include a face-to-face comparison group. Despite the emergence of promising evidence, more research is needed to determine the reliability and validity of clinical diagnoses and treatment recommendations derived from VTC assessments, particularly when persons with severe cognitive or behavioral disturbances are being evaluated.

Treatment outcome. Some preliminary studies on treatment outcomes have shown support for the use of TMH. Zaylor, Nelson, and Cook (2001) examined whether TMH services are longitudinally effective in improving psychological functioning. Results indicated a significant time effect, such that patients reported experiencing less distress over time and psychiatrists rated patients as less "ill" over time. In their review of TMH programs, Antonacci, Bloch, Saeed, Yildirim, and Talley (2008) also suggested that interventions delivered through TMH and face-to-face modalities appear to yield the same treatment effects. However, the majority of studies included in this review examined medication management consultations or short-form cognitive–behavioral therapy, and only five specifically targeted forensic populations.

The ability of TMH to produce positive treatment outcomes among juvenile offenders has also been explored. Fox et al. (2008) evaluated the efficacy of a behavioral health program conducted through TMH at four adolescent detention facilities. Results showed that the number of goals identified and the proportion of participants who were able to successfully achieve those goals significantly increased following the implementation of TMH. Given the lack of a controlled comparison group, it cannot be concluded that these outcomes were caused by the intervention. Overall, the available literature supporting TMH as a viable method for implementing interventions that bring about long-term, clinically significant changes, particularly to justice-involved individuals, is weak (Antonacci et al., 2008). Implications for future research will be discussed later in this chapter.

Legal proceedings. The results of existing studies suggest several advantages of TL in court-related matters. Goodman et al. (1998) evaluated the credibility of children's eyewitness testimony delivered over TL using a sample of mock jurors. Despite rating video witnesses as less credible than in-person witnesses, jurors were able to discriminate between accurate and inaccurate testimony regardless of modality. Additionally, jurors' perceptions regarding the culpability of the defendant did not differ across modalities. This study further demonstrated that witnesses who provided testimony via TL were significantly less anxious, and in general, were more accurate than those testifying in open court. Another study (Price & Sapci, 2007) reported that psychiatric involuntary commitment hearings conducted via TL increased staff productivity, improved staff and patient safety, and preserved patients' dignity by eliminating the discomfort of appearing in court. Additionally, studies surveying perceived acceptability among judges, attorneys, law enforcement officers, and court clerks generally indicate favorable views of court testimony provided through TL (Khalifa et al., 2008; Williams, 1998). Based on these limited research findings, it seems that the potential problems resulting from the use of TL in legal proceedings are likely a small price to pay for the abundance of potential benefits.

Challenges Facing VTC in Corrections

Despite the anticipated benefits of VTC in justice settings, there are a number of potential consequences that challenge widespread acceptability of this service delivery modality. For example, the most cited barrier to advancing TMH services in correctional and forensic practice is provider resistance (Antonacci et al., 2008; Khalifa et al., 2008; Magaletta, Fagan, & Ax, 1998; Magaletta, Fagan, & Peyrot, 2000; Manguno-Mire et al., 2007; Merideth, 1999). Manguno-Mire et al. (2007) found a significant difference in provider satisfaction between telemedicine and in-person competency evaluations, such that providers reported less overall satisfaction with the former modality despite nonsignificant differences in patient satisfaction and inter-rater test agreement. Furthermore, Zollo et al. (1999) revealed that perceived effectiveness of TMH in determining appropriate mental health diagnoses was rated the lowest by service providers. Many professionals hesitate to embrace TMH due to the "distance" between provider and patient. Psychologists are typically trained in models of therapy that assume clients will receive face-to-face services in the same-room. Magaletta, Fagan, and Peyrot (2000) suggest that repeated exposure to the pairing of interpersonal and physical space has come to define the therapeutic relationship as a tangible attachment. The remoteness of TMH leads psychologists to fear losing emotional connectedness with patients (Magaletta, Fagan, & Peyrot, 2000). Given the extant research on patient satisfaction (Antonacci et al., 2008; Leonard, 2004; Magaletta, Fagan, & Ax, 1998; Magaletta, Fagan, & Peyrot, 2000; Morgan, Patrick, & Magaletta, 2008) with mental health treatments rendered via TMH, this belief appears to be more salient for the provider. Regarding legal applications, anecdotal evidence seems to suggest that judges, attorneys, law enforcement, and courtroom personnel may be more accepting of VTC as a method of service delivery than mental health providers (Khalifa et al., 2008). Most of the reported resistance among legal professionals relates to the constitutionality or admissibility of VTC in court proceedings (Johnson & Wiggins, 2006; Poulin, 2004).

Limits to confidentiality and concerns over privacy constitute another concern of professionals with the use of TMH specifically (Antonacci et al., 2008; Manguno-Mire et al., 2007). Because patients in correctional facilities cannot be left unsupervised, particularly with technological equipment, it will most likely be standard procedure to require at least one staff member present during the TMH consultation. This reduces the level of privacy typically afforded in the patient/ therapist relationship. In face-to-face sessions, security officers are available for emergency assistance but are generally not admitted into the treatment room. In addition, transmitting inmate files and medical reports electronically or via facsimile may increase the opportunity for breeches of confidentiality. Aside from providers, inmates have also expressed some hesitation regarding privacy (Antonacci et al., 2008). Although there is no known research indicating that confidentiality is a reported concern in legal matters, it is likely that similar apprehensions exist in this context, as well.

Equipment failure and maintenance problems also cause concern (Darkins, 2001; Khalifa et al., 2008). Magaletta, Fagan, and Peyrot (2000) described an incident in which the transmission of quick verbal exchanges was delayed, thereby interrupting the "turn-taking" aspect of communication between patient or defendant and provider (the authors termed this as "walking" on the other person's transmitted speech). In this scenario, neither party hears the other properly. Such problems can frustrate and overwhelm the inmate, which may often lead to increased hostility and volatility. Advances in computer science may help reduce the occurrence of audiovisual difficulties (T. W. Miller et al., 2008). Another argued consequence of VTC is its potential inability to accurately capture relevant physical and emotional data. For example, TMH treatment for mental illness may lead to inaccuracies in diagnosis due to factors such as physical, emotional, and cognitive disturbances that may not be observed optimally through video monitoring (Magaletta, Fagan, & Ax, 1998; Magaletta, Fagan, & Peyrot, 2000), resistance among inmates with Axis II and thought disorders (Magaletta, Fagan, & Peyrot, 2000), and delayed team-based treatment decisions due to the need to coordinate multiple providers, such as on-site prison physicians, medical assistants, and remote specialists (Zollo et al., 1999). Likewise, in legal proceedings, judges and juries may misperceive certain characteristics of defendants, such as their remorse or competency (Johnson & Wiggins, 2006).

The Need for Specialty Best Practice Guidelines

The establishment of universal guidelines describing legal and ethical standards of TMH practice may alleviate concerns regarding privacy and the possibility of technology transmission failure (Leonard, 2004; T. W. Miller et al., 2008). The American Psychological Association (APA) recently formed a task force on telepsychology with the goal of creating a standard set of practice guidelines (Novotney, 2011). Other organizations, such as the TeleMental Health Institute, have also endeavored to provide resources and training opportunities for the professional use of this technology in delivering clinical interventions. Several recommendations for general uses include technological awareness (e.g., adjusting the camera to eye level, explaining to clients what it means if the provider looks away, maintaining appropriate tone of voice), exerting caution when transmitting electronic data, creating a safety plan in case of disconnection, and ensuring a complete understanding of procedures (Novotney, 2011).

However, the unique culture of a correctional setting highlights the importance of specific guidelines that are tailored to fit the needs of those who live and work within it. Beyond the suggestions listed above, correctional staff and mental health providers must be prepared to deal with a number of additional issues. Some considerations include factors such as: (a) the need to balance security with privacy, (b) specialized training for off-site providers regarding the treatment needs of correctional populations and the limitations of their environment, (c) the ability of correctional staff to implement treatment recommendations in the absence of the provider, and (d) the use of a safety plan in the event that patient problems arise when the provider is not available, either during connection failures or outside the appointment (Khalifa et al., 2008; Magaletta, Fagan, & Peyrot, 2000). In addition, the ability to establish a working alliance on-screen may be especially important for this group given the high prevalence of distrust of authority, particularly health care providers (Howerton et al., 2007). TMH may create extra weariness for defensive offenders. This apprehension could be mitigated through open and honest communication, which may require different interpersonal skills than those afforded in face-to-face interactions (Leonard, 2004).

Future Directions

The variety of ways in which VTC is currently being applied to the delivery of forensic and correctional services far exceed the magnitude of empirical investigations that support such applications. Given the increasing volume of mental health contacts conducted via TMH, research efforts must continue to focus on uncovering the factors that foster successful utilization, such as factors related to the patient, the provider, and the infrastructure, as well as those that hinder utilization. Some suggested areas for future study are provided next.

Acceptability of services. Future research is necessary to identify which concerns encourage or discourage patients and providers to seek and use VTC. Magaletta, Fagan, and Peyrot (2000) offered some initial clues on the part of patients. Of the 20 (5%) inmates who refused to attend their telepsychiatry session, 11 reported that they did not want any form of consultation, 6 indicated suspicion about the medium being used, 2 expressed anger with the telepsychiatry provider, and 1 did not provide a clear reason. Interestingly, of those inmates who refused services due to the medium itself, all were given prior Axis II diagnoses, such as antisocial, paranoid, and narcissistic personality disorders. Perhaps reluctance or willingness to engage in TMH-based services is a function of individual factors such as the patient's perceived level of distress, prior experiences with the health care and criminal justice systems, exposure to similar forms of technology (e.g., the Internet), or the nature and severity of symptoms. Furthermore, because privacy limitations have been cited as a primary issue for patients (Antonacci et al., 2008), it will be particularly important to understand specific fears are most commonly involved in receiving services through TMH, including discomfort with the presence of security, distrust of the provider, or mishandling of confidential materials (T. W. Miller et al., 2008).

As mentioned previously, provider resistance is one of the major barriers to implementing TMH services (Antonacci et al., 2008; Magaletta, Fagan, & Ax, 1998). Aside from a general aversion to treatments delivered over a distance that seem to contradict the traditional structure of psychotherapy, some mental health professionals may also be cognizant of the increased job competition that TMH will likely bring. This is, with greater accessibility, the market for off-site specialty providers (e.g., those who offer forensic mental health assessments, sex offender treatment, early release assessments) is expected to expand (Magaletta, Fagan, & Peyrot, 2000). Instead of rejecting the integration of VTC into forensic and correctional practice, continued attention will hopefully increase familiarity and comfort with this technology, such that providers will begin to acknowledge its benefits for a growing, yet underserved population. However, future research is necessary to identify more precisely the concerns held by both patients and providers that restrict the demand for VTC services. Efforts can then be made to alleviate these concerns through proper education and training.

Forensic mental health assessment. The use of VTC in assessing the mental health needs of justice-involved persons is a burgeoning area of empirical investigation. Yet, the literature is still quite sparse considering the wide variety of psychological assessments that are conducted for forensic purposes. For example, a forensic mental health assessment (FMHA) may be aimed at identifying a person's mental capacity to waive Miranda Rights; competency to stand trial, plead, waive counsel, testify, be sentenced, or be executed; criminal culpability at the time an offense was committed; and risk for future offending (e.g., aggression, sexual offending, general recidivism). FMHAs are also used to provide opinions regarding civil justice issues, such as involuntary civil commitment due to dangerousness and family court decisions involving parental rights or child custody (Heilbrun, Grisso, & Goldstein, 2009). Providing recommendations for mental health treatment is often a component of FMHA, as well.

Despite these applications, only two known studies (Lexcen et al., 2006; Manguno-Mire et al., 2007) have scrutinized a particular type of FMHA. Both studies looked at the inter-rater reliability of specialized forensic assessment instruments used to draw clinical inferences about an evaluee's competency to stand trial. Other investigations (Nelson et al., 2004) of assessment feasibility focus primarily on the reliability of nonforensic clinical tools in determining the mental health functioning of defendants and inmates. Several additional research initiatives within this domain are presented next.

First, it may be the case that some legal issues can be addressed with greater ease and accuracy via VTC than other issues. Likewise, individual characteristics of the evaluee such as cognitive degeneration, psychotic features, or malingering may affect the quality of observable information obtained through video interactions. Research that employs high methodological standards is needed to parse apart those instances in which VTC can effectively assist in the collection and integration of relevant data. Second, future studies should consider comparing clinical decisions that are based on an entire battery of assessments, rather than one specific instrument, across TMH and face-to-face modalities. This procedure more closely approximates the comprehensiveness of a typical FMHA. Third, because FMHA often requires the inclusion of collateral informants, research might address the utility of TMH as a convenient way to access and interview these individuals. Lastly, longitudinal studies examining the link between treatment recommendations made through FMHAs, treatment decisions based on those recommendations, and subsequent treatment outcomes are also important to the field's understanding of TMH and its capacities.

Treatment outcome. Although research on the use of TMH in corrections is flourishing, one domain that remains vastly unknown is the efficacy of interventions implemented through TMH in reducing psychological and behavioral symptoms for inmates with mental illness. Despite preliminary evaluations (Zaylor, Whitten, & Kingsley, 2000) that provide initial evidence for the positive treatment outcomes associated with TMH service delivery, existing research is severely limited by the lack of sound methodology. Treatment outcome research that includes baseline and follow-up data on relevant clinical markers (e.g., disciplinary infractions, crisis interventions), comparison groups (e.g., treatment as usual), larger sample sizes, multiple outcome measures, and statistical analyses is necessary to draw firmer conclusions regarding the effective use of TMH in addressing the mental health and behavioral symptoms of justice-involved persons (Antonacci et al., 2008; Ax, Fagan, Magaletta et al., 2007; Morgan, Patrick, & Magaletta, 2008; Novotney, 2011). Additional research should further investigate potential clinical applications of TMH including psychotherapy, cognitive—behavioral therapy, psychosocial interventions, and family counseling, as well as the possibility that TMH may require different therapeutic skills, such as alternative approaches to communicating and delivering information (Leonard, 2004). There is also a need to explore the strengths and limitations of TMH in serving various forensic subpopulations, including individuals who are thought disordered, personality disordered, neurologically or cognitively impaired, suicidal, high security (e.g., segregated, violent), female, and juveniles (Antonacci et al., 2008; Magaletta, Fagan, & Peyrot, 2000).

Legal proceedings. Because courthouses and correctional facilities are steadily gaining access to interactive video technology (National Center for State Courts, 2010; Wiggins et al., 2003), it is becoming more imperative to expand the research base in this domain. One area of study might focus on factors that affect the attorney—client relationship in pretrial consultations. Interpersonal communication skills and concern for defendants' well-being are associated with inmates' perceptions of attorney competence and expertise (Boccaccini & Brodsky, 2001; Feldman & Wilson, 1981; O'Brien, Pheterson, Wright, & Hostica, 1977). Future research should investigate the ability of VTC to facilitate a working alliance between attorneys and their clients. A study currently being conducted by two of the authors (McDonald and Morgan) is attempting to determine whether or not key elements of the attorney—client relationship, including the clients' perceptions of working alliance, trust, procedural fairness, and satisfaction, are affected during consultations provided through VTC. Other suggested areas of investigation include: (a) the impact of video testimony on judicial decision-making (e.g., do certain behaviors of witnesses such as remorse, honesty, and deceit become more salient or diluted?), (b) the utility of VTC when applied to psychologically or cognitively impaired defendants (e.g., are these defendants able to cooperate and work as effectively with counsel when communication is digital and remote?), (c) the possibility of changes in defendants' composure when appearing in court through VTC (Johnson & Wiggins, 2006), and (d) the consistency of imposed legal sanctions (e.g., sentence severity, conditions of release) for defendants who appear in-person and those who appear via VTC.

Spotlight on TMH and TL Programs

Telemental health. The Center for Telemedicine at Texas Tech University Health Sciences Center (TTU HSC), located in Lubbock, Texas, began in 1989 as a grant-funded research project. Although uses within correctional facilities were not part of the initial aims of the program, by 1994, it had extended its services to this population. TTU HSC currently services 30% of inmates detained in the Texas Department of Criminal Justice—consisting of approximately 32,000 inmates housed in 23 prison units. A variety of specialty services are offered to state inmates, including orthopedics, general surgery, internal medicine, urology, gastro-enterology, pediatrics, and psychology and psychiatry (Texas Tech University Center for Telemedicine, 2012a). More than 4500 prison consultations are conducted via telehealth each year (Texas Tech University Center for Telemedicine, 2012b). In servicing correctional populations, TTU HSC relies on the use of T1 secure phone lines (supported by the Polycom® corporation) to transmit audiovisual data between sites. At this time, TTU HSC only operates within male populated prisons.

In keeping with the focus of this chapter, the procedures for providing inmates with mental health services via telehealth will be described in an attempt to illustrate how a university-based program may operate. When an inmate requests medical or mental health services by submitting a "sick call" form describing his complaint to the medical unit, an on-site nurse schedules the inmate for an initial consultation. For mental health issues, the first contact the inmate typically receives is with a master's-level clinician, who conducts a thorough psychological screening assessment of emotional and behavioral functioning for the purpose of determining treatment needs. This clinician is located at a secure psychiatric prison in Lubbock. For 1-day, twice per month, the clinician travels to 12 remote facilities across western Texas for face-to-face consultations. Once these available sessions are filled, inmates are then assigned to TMH services. Texas state law requires that medical contact be initiated with inmates no later than 2 weeks following their written request for services. In most cases, appointments are made on a first-come-first-serve basis, such that inmates are assigned to the treatment modality that is most readily available. However, under circumstances in which emergency care may be required or symptoms are considered especially severe, inmates can be evaluated at an earlier time. Again, modality choice depends on which one is available first. However, due to the limited number of inmates who can be seen during the remote visits, most assessments are rendered through TMH. In this case, the clinician is seated in an office at the psychiatric prison that is equipped with a television monitor and camera, while the inmate is seated in a similar room at his respective housing facility. Inmates are closely monitored by on-site security and medical staff.

These screening assessments frequently result in a referral for other relevant services, such as psychiatric medication consultations, inpatient psychiatric care, and medical care. When the psychological interview results in a referral for psychiatric consultation or inpatient psychiatric care, the inmate is scheduled to follow up with a licensed psychiatrist who is an employee of TTU HSC. He or she derives a formal diagnosis and determines what type of intervention is warranted based on the screening information, the inmate's self-report, behavioral indicators, and his or her own clinical judgment. Follow-up consultations are most often conducted remotely via VTC, but inmates may occasionally be evaluated on-site. When follow-up consultations are provided through TMH, the technological set-up is largely the same as that described above, although providers may also use a viewing room located on the TTU HSC campus, rather than traveling to the psychiatric prison facility. For more severe cases of mental illness, or when a psychiatric consultation is not readily available, the initial mental health clinician may recommend that the inmate be transferred directly to the psychiatric prison for inpatient supervision. Under these circumstances, the distressed inmate will bypass the follow-up consultation until he arrives on-site at the psychiatric unit. An evaluation of these services is currently being developed by the first and third authors in collaboration with prison staff.

The Kansas University Center for Telemedicine and TMH (KUCTT), part of the Kansas University Medical Center, is another major telehealth program in the country. In addition to psychiatric assessment and consultations, KUCTT offers some psychotherapy services to inmates. For example, one unique and promising use that is now under empirical investigation by two of the authors (Batastini & Morgan) in collaboration with the Kansas Department of Corrections (KDOC) Mental Health Department is the delivery of a group formatted cognitive−behavioral-based intervention to inmates in long-term segregation (LTS). This program uses high-definition (HDX) digital multimedia equipment and software available through Polycom Teleprescence Solutions®. Inmates confined in LTS units typically spend 23−24 h a day in isolation. Aside from creating physical limitations on behavior, segregated placement is associated with a number of psychological consequences. When compared to inmates in the general population, inmates in segregation report significantly more feelings and thoughts related to interpersonal inferiority, hostility, and impulsivity (H. A. Miller & Young, 1997). Additionally, isolation can lead to adjustment disorders, increased risk of suicide, and aggravation of existing mental health problems (Chaiken & Shull, 2007). Mental health services in segregation are even more limited due to security restrictions and typically consist of psychotropic medication management, brief check-ins at the inmate's cell front, and occasional meetings in private with a clinician (Metzer & Fellner, 2010). TMH group treatments, like that offered through KUCTT and KDOC, may improve access to quality mental health care for inmates in segregation by offering a safer alternative to service delivery. For example, providers can participate without entering a highly dangerous unit and inmates can engage each other interpersonally without the threat of physical aggression. This may allow for the inclusion of more intensive psychotherapy that covers a larger number of inmates in need. Ultimately, the use of TMH for this purpose may not only keep inmates out of segregation but also out of the criminal justice system once released.

Telelaw. One example of TL applications is also taking place in Lubbock, Texas. Through an organization of criminal defense attorneys, the Caprock

Regional Public Defender Clinic (CRPDC), VTC modalities are being used to facilitate pretrial consultations with clients. Pretrial consultations may include an explanation of the charges and subsequent legal proceedings, a discussion of relevant documents, requests for additional information or evidence to assist in case development, and preparation for cross-examination. The CRPDC's caseload consists of indigent criminal defendants who reside in 16 rural counties in northeast Texas. The attorneys at the CRPDC communicate with their clients via a digital audiovisual communications platform, Microsoft® Lync® 2010, that is fully integrated with desktop software. This equipment allows attorneys to initiate audio, video, and web conferences, or make a phone call to clients. Their clients, on the other hand, are located in nearby courthouses and detention centers that house similar technologies. The second and third authors, in conjunction with the CRPDC, are in the process of evaluating this program—in comparison to in-person contact—from the client and attorney perspective (see above).

Summary

VTC presents a practical and cost-effective modality for delivering quality care, legal and health related, to justice-involved clients by trained professionals. Additionally, it has the added benefit over in-person contacts of improved safety and security for off-site providers, on-site staff, the patient, and the public, as well as more efficient access to care, and the inclusion of multiple parties in the assessment and treatment process. Existing research shows that patients and consumers are generally more accepting of VTC than providers, and there is some preliminary evidence to support the use of TMH and TL in addressing psychiatric and legal issues. However, the current knowledge base does not fully support the frequency and breadth of TMH uses among this population. More progress needs to be made in the way of understanding the conditions in which VTC will be most effective as a method of service delivery and establishing uniform best practice guidelines that safeguard against misuse, intentional or unintentional. If this chapter leaves readers with a single, resonating message, let it be this: the advancement of VTC in criminal justice settings is contingent upon the availability of rigorous, empirical investigations and the establishment of high-quality, professional training opportunities—both of which are noticeably absent from the available literature summarized here.

References

Abramsky, S., & Fellner, J. (2003). *Ill-equipped prisons and offenders with mental illness.* New York, NY: Human Rights Watch.

Antonacci, D. J., Bloch, R. M., Saeed, S. A., Yildirim, Y., & Talley, J. (2008). Empirical evidence on the use and effectiveness of telepsychiatry via videoteleconferencing:

Implications for forensic and correctional psychiatry. *Behavioral Sciences and the Law*, *26*, 253–269. doi:10.1002/bsl.812.

Ax, R. K., Fagan, T. J., & Holton, S. M. B. (2002). Individuals with serious mental illnesses in prison: Rural perspectives and issues. In S. B. Hudnall (Ed.), *Rural behavioral health care: An interdisciplinary guide* (pp. 203–215). Washington, DC: American Psychological Association.

Ax, R. K., Fagan, T. J., Magaletta, P. R., Morgan, R. D., Nussbaum, D., & White, T. W. (2007). Innovations in correctional assessment and treatment. *Criminal Justice and Behavior*, *34*, 893–905. doi:10.1177/0093854807301555.

Baker, D. B. (2000). PCASSO: A model for the safe use of the Internet in health care. *Journal of the American Health Information Management Association*, *71*, 33–36 Retrieved March 4, 2012, from <http://library.ahima.org/xpedio/groups/public/documents/ahima/bok2_000473.hcsp?dDocName = bok2_000473>

Beck, A. J., & Maruschak, L. M. (2001). *Mental health treatment in state prisons, 2000*. Retrieved April 5, 2012, from <http://bjs.ojp.usdoj.gov/index.cfm?ty = pbdetail&iid = 788>.

Boccaccini, M. T., & Brodsky, S. L. (2001). Characteristics of the ideal criminal defense attorney from the client's perspective: Empirical findings and implications for legal practice. *Law and Psychology Review*, *25*, 81–117.

Brett, A., & Blumburg, L. (2006). Video-linked court liaison services: Forging new frontiers in psychiatry in Western Australia. *Australian Psychiatry*, *14*, 53–56. doi:10.1080/j.1440-1665.2006.02236.x.

Brodey, B. B., Claypoole, K. H., Motto, J., Arias, R. G., & Goss, R. (2000). Satisfaction of forensic psychiatric patients with remote telepsychiatric evaluation. *Psychiatric Services*, *51*, 1305–1307.

Chaiken, S., & Shull, J. (2007). Mental health treatment of inmates in segregated housing. In O. J. Thienhaus, & M. Piasecki (Eds.), *Correctional psychiatry: Practice guidelines and strategies* (pp. 7.2–7.21). Kingston, NJ: Civic Research Institute, Inc.

Cloyes, K. G., Wong, B., Latimer, S., & Abarca, J. (2010). Time to prison return for inmates with serious mental illness released from prison: A survival analysis. *Criminal Justice and Behavior*, *37*, 175–187. doi:10.1177/0093854809354370.

Daniel, A. E. (2007). Care of the mentally ill in prisons: Challenges and solutions. *The Journal of the American Academy of Psychiatry and the Law*, *35*, 406–410.

Darkins, A. (2001). Program management of telemental health care services. *Journal of Geriatric Psychiatry and Neurology*, *14*, 80–87.

Doarn, C. R., Justis, D., Chaudhri, M. S., & Merrel, R. C. (2005). Integration of telemedicine practice into correctional medicine: An evolving standard. *Journal of Correctional Health Care*, *11*, 253–270.

Draine, J., Salzer, M. S., Culhane, D. P., & Hadley, T. R. (2002). Role of social disadvantage in crime, joblessness, and homelessness among persons with serious mental illness. *Psychiatric Services*, *53*, 565–573.

Feldman, S., & Wilson, K. (1981). The value of interpersonal skills in lawyering. *Law and Human Behavior*, *5*, 311–324.

Fox, K. C., Connor, P., McCullers, E., & Waters, T. (2008). Effect of a behavioural health and specialty care telemedicine programme on goal attainment for youth in juvenile detention. *Journal of Telemedicine and Telecare*, *14*, 227–230. doi:10.1258/jtt.2008.071102.

Glasmeier, A. K., & Farrigan, T. (2007). The economic impacts of the prison development boom on persistently poor rural places. *International Regional Science Review*, *30*, 274–299. doi:10.1177/0160017607301608.

Goodman, G. S., Tobey, A. E., Batterman-Faunce, J. M., Orcutt, H. K., Shapiro, C. M., & Thomas, S. (1998). Face-to-face confrontation: Effects of closed circuit technology on children's eyewitness testimony. *Law and Human Behavior, 22*, 165−203.

Heilbrun, K., Grisso, T., & Goldstein, A. (2009). *Foundations of forensic mental health assessment*. New York, NY: Oxford University Press.

Hooks, G., Mosher, C., Rotolo, T., & Lobao, L. (2004). The prison industry: Carceral expansion and employment in U. S. counties, 1969−1994. *Social Science Quarterly, 85*, 37−56.

Howerton, A., Byng, R., Campbell, J., Hess, D., Owens, C., & Aitken, P. (2007). Understanding help seeking behavior among male offenders: Qualitative interview study. *British Medical Journal, 334*, 303−306 doi:110.1136/bmj.39059.594444.AE

James, D. J., & Glaze, L. E. (2006). *Mental health problems of prison and jail inmates*. Retrieved April 5, 2012, from <http://bjs.ojp.usdoj.gov/index.cfm?ty = pbdetail&iid = 789>.

Johnson, M. T., & Wiggins, E. C. (2006). Videoteleconferencing in criminal proceedings: Legal and empirical issues and directions for research. *Law and Policy, 28*, 211−227. doi:10.1111/j.1467-9930.2006.00224.x.

Kaliebe, K. E., Heneghan, J., & Kim, T. J. (2011). Telepsychiatry in juvenile justice settings. *Child and Adolescent Psychiatric Clinics of North America, 20*, 113−123. doi:10.1016/j.chc.2010.09.001.

Khalifa, N., Saleem, Y., & Stankard, P. (2008). The use of telepsychiatry within forensic practice: A literature review on the use of videolink. *The Journal of Forensic Psychiatry and Psychology, 19*, 2−13. doi:10.1080/14789940701560794.

King, R. S., Mauer, M., & Hurling, T. (2004). An analysis of the economics of prison sitting in rural communities. *Criminology and Public Policy, 3*, 453−480. doi:10.1111/j.1745-9133.2004.tb00054.x.

Kinsella, C. (2004). *Corrections health care costs*. Retrieved April 5, 2012, from <www.csg.org/knowledgecenter/docs/TA0401CorrHealth.pdf>.

Larsen, D., Stamm, B. H., Davis, K., & Magaletta, P. R. (2004). Prison telemedicine and TMH utilization in the United States: State and federal perceptions of benefits and barriers. *Telemedicine and e-Health, 10*, 81−89.

Leonard, S. (2004). The development and evaluation of a telepsychiatry service for prisoners. *Journal of Psychiatric and Mental Health Nursing, 11*, 461−468.

Lexcen, F. J., Hawk, G. L., Herrick, S., & Blank, M. B. (2006). Use of video conferencing for psychiatric and forensic evaluations. *Psychiatric Services, 57*, 713−715. doi:10.1176/appi.ps.57.5.713.

Lowes, R. (2001). Telemedicine. *Medical Economics, 78*, 24.

Magaletta, P. R., Fagan, T. J., & Ax, R. K. (1998). Advancing psychology services through TMH in the Federal Bureau of Prisons. *Professional Psychology: Research and Practice, 29*, 543−548.

Magaletta, P. R., Fagan, T. J., & Peyrot, M. F. (2000). TMH in the federal bureau of prisons: Inmates' perceptions. *Professional Psychology: Research and Practice, 31*, 497−502. doi:10.1037//0735-7028.31.5.497.

Manfredi, L., Shupe, J., & Batki, S. L. (2005). Rural jail telepsychiatry: A pilot feasibility study. *Telemedicine and e-Health, 11*, 574−577.

Manguno-Mire, G. M., Thompson, J. W., Shore, J. H., Croy, C. D., Artecona, J. F., & Pickering, J. W. (2007). The use of telemedicine to evaluate competency to stand trial: A preliminary randomized controlled study. *The Journal of the American Academy of Psychiatry and the Law, 35*, 481−489.

Merideth, P. (1999). Forensic applications of telepsychiatry. *Psychiatric Annals, 29,* 429−431.

Metzer, J. L., & Fellner, J. (2010). Solitary confinement and mental illness in U.S. prisons: A challenge for medical ethics. *The Journal of the American Academy of Psychiatry and the Law, 38,* 104−108.

Miller, H. A., & Young, G. R. (1997). Prison segregation: Administrative remedy or mental health problem? *Criminal Behavior and Mental Health, 7,* 85−94.

Miller, T. W., Clark, J., Veltkamp, L. J., Burton, D. C., & Swope, M. (2008). Teleconferencing model for forensic consultation, court testimony, and continuing education. *Behavioral Sciences and the Law, 26,* 301−313. doi:10.1002/bsl.809.

Monnier, J., Knapp, R. G., & Frueh, B. C. (2003). Recent advances in telepsychiatry: An updated review. *Psychiatric Services, 54,* 1604−1609.

Montague, E. (2003). *Prison health care: Healing a sick system through private competition.* Retrieved February 11, 2012, from <http://www.wips.org/ConOutPrivatization/PNPrisonHealthCare03-08.html>.

Morgan, R. D., Fisher, W., Duan, N., Mandracchia, J. T., & Murray, D. (2010). Prevalence of criminal thinking among state prison inmates with serious mental illness. *Law and Human Behavior, 34,* 324−336. doi:10.1007/s10979-009-9182-z.

Morgan, R. D., Patrick, A. R., & Magaletta, P. R. (2008). Does the use of telemental health alter the treatment experience? Inmates' perceptions of telemental health versus face-to-face treatment modalities. *Journal of Consulting and Clinical Psychology, 76,* 158−162. doi:10.1037/0022-006X.76.1.158.

Myers, K., Valentine, J., Morganthaler, R., & Melzer, S. (2006). Telepsychiatry with incarcerated youth. *Journal of Adolescent Health, 38,* 643−648. doi:10.1016/j.jadohealth.2005.07.015.

National Center for State Courts. *NCSC Videoteleconferencing survey.* (2010). Retrieved January 19, 2012, from <http://www.ncsc.org/services-and-experts/areas-of-expertise/technology/ncsc-video-conferencing-survey.aspx>.

National Institute of Justice. *Telemedicine can reduce correctional health care costs: An evaluation of a prison telemedicine network.* (1999). Retrieved February 10, 2012, from <www.ncjrs.gov/pdffiles1/175040.pdf>.

National Institute of Justice. *Implementing telemedicine in correctional facilities.* (2002). Retrieved April 5, 2012, from <www.ncjrs.gov/pdffiles1/nij/190310.pdf>.

Nelson, E., Zaylor, C., & Cook, D. (2004). A comparison of psychiatrist evaluation and patient symptom report in a jail telepsychiatry clinic. *Telemedicine Journal and e-Health, 10,* 54−59.

Novotney, A. (2011). A new emphasis on Telemental Health: How can psychologists stay ahead of the curve—and keeping patients safe? *Monitor on Psychology, 42,* 40−44.

O'Brien, S., Pheterson, S., Wright, M., & Hostica, C. (1977). The criminal lawyer: The defendant's perspective. *American Journal of Criminal Law, 5,* 283−312.

Overall, J., & Gorham, D. (1962). The brief psychiatric rating scale. *Psychological Reports, 10,* 799−812.

Peterson, J., Skeem, J. L., Hart, E., Vidal, S., & Keith, F. (2010). Analyzing offense patterns as a function of mental illness to test the criminalization hypothesis. *Psychiatric Services, 61,* 1217−1222. doi:10.1176/appi.ps.61.12.1217.

Poulin, A. B. (2004). Criminal justice and videoteleconferencing technology: The remote defendant. *Tulane Law Review, 78,* 1089−1167.

Poythress, N. G., Nicholson, R. A., Otto, R. K., Edens, J. F., Bonnie, R. J., Monahan, J., et al. *The MacArthur competence assessment tool—Criminal adjudication (MacCAT−CA) professional manual.* Odessa, FL: PAR.

Price, J., & Sapci, H. (2007). Telecourt: The use of videoteleconferencing for involuntary commitment hearings in academic health centers. *Psychiatric Services, 54*, 17−18.

Schaeffer, C. M., & Borduin, C. M. (2005). Long-term follow-up to a randomized clinical trial of multisystemic therapy with serious and violent juvenile offenders. *Journal of Consulting Psychology, 73*, 445−453. doi:10.1037/0022-006X.73.3.445.

Steadman, H. J., Osher, F. C., Robbins, P. C., Case, B., & Samuels, S. (2009). Prevalence of serious mental illness among jail inmates. *Psychiatric Services, 60*, 761−765 doi:0.1176/appi.ps.60.6.761

Technology Marketing Corporation. *Can you afford telepresence systems?* (2009). Retrieved April 7, 2012, from <http://www.tmcnet.com/usubmit/2009/05/20/4190361.htm>.

Texas Tech University Center for Telemedicine. *Correctional telemedicine.* (2012a). Retrieved March 11, 2012 from <http://www.ttuhsc.edu/telemedicine/tdcj.aspx>.

Texas Tech University Center for Telemedicine. *The history of telemedicine at Texas Tech.* (2012b). Retrieved March 11, 2012, from <http://www.ttuhsc.edu/telemedicine/history. aspx>.

The American Telemedicine Association. *Telemedicine/telehealth terminology.* (n.d.) Retrieved April 5, 2012, from <http://www.americantelemed.org/files/public/abouttele-medicine/Terminology.pdf>.

Torrey, E. F., Kennard, A. D., Eslinger, D., Lamb, R., & Pavle, J. (2010). *More mentally ill persons are in jails and prisons than hospitals: A survey of the states.* Arlington, VA: Treatment Advocacy Center.

Wiggins, E. C. (2006). The courtroom of the future is here: Introduction to emerging technologies in the legal system. *Law and Policy, 28*, 182−191.

Wiggins, E. C., Dunn, M. A., & Cort, G. (2003). Survey on courtroom technology. Washington, DC: Federal Judicial Center.

Williams, G. A. (1998). Video technology and children's evidence: International perspectives and recent research. *Medicine and Law, 17*, 263−281.

Wolff, N., Morgan, R. D., Shi, J., Fisher, W., & Huening, J. (2012). Comparative analysis of thinking styles and emotional states of male and female inmates with and without mental disorders. (Manuscript submitted for publication.)

Yiming, C., & Fung, D. (2003). Child sexual abuse in Singapore with special reference to medico-legal implications: A review of 38 cases. *Medicine Science and Law, 43*, 260−266.

Zaylor, C., Nelson, E., & Cook, D. J. (2001). Clinical outcomes in a prison telepsychiatry clinic. *Journal of Telemedicine and Telecare, 7*, 47−49.

Zaylor, C., Whitten, P., & Kingsley, C. (2000). Telemedicine services to a county jail. *Journal of Telemedicine and Telecare, 6*, 93−95.

Zollo, S., Kienzle, M., Loeffelholz, P., & Sebille, S. (1999). Telemedicine in Iowa's correctional facilities: Initial clinical experience and assessment of program costs. *Telemedicine Journal, 5*, 291−301.

Section Five

Assessment and Intervention

14 Special Considerations in Conducting Neuropsychology Assessment over Videoteleconferencing

C. Munro Cullum and Maria C. Grosch

University of Texas Southwestern Medical Center at Dallas, Dallas, TX

Background and Scope

There has been an explosive growth in telemedicine technology applications over the past decade. Modern telecommunications and videoteleconferencing (VTC) provide greatly enhanced audiovisual transmission and real-time interactions as compared with earlier technology, and increasingly reduced costs of VTC provide for more ready access in a variety of settings. Significant advances have been made in the field of telemedicine applications since the term "telemedicine" was introduced by Dwyer in 1973, and there are now at least four journals that focus on telemedicine and telehealth. One of the largest growth areas in telehealth applications has been in telepsychiatry (Wootton & Craig, 1999; Wootton, Yellowlees, & McLaren, 2003), which is used widely in mental health programs across the world, including major telemental health initiatives in the VA Hospital system (Darkins, 2006). A recent literature search of Medline, PsychInfo, and PubMed using the terms "telepsychiatry" and "telemental" resulted in a total of 233 citations since 1973, reflecting a three- to fourfold increase over the past 10 years. Telestroke programs are also growing rapidly (156 citations over the past 5 years), allowing specialists to see and examine patients in remote settings that might not have access to specialty care. In comparison, the terms "teleneuropsychology," "telecognitive assessment," and "neuropsychology" combined with "telemedicine," "telehealth," or "videoconference" resulted in only three references. Nevertheless, application of neuropsychological assessment procedures in the VTC context is growing, although only a handful of tests have undergone psychometric investigation when administered in traditional face-to-face versus VTC fashion, as reviewed below.

Telemental Health. DOI: http://dx.doi.org/10.1016/B978-0-12-416048-4.00014-2

Why Teleneuropsychology?

One of the major advantages of telemedicine is its potential to reach patients in rural areas and provide access to specialists and specialized services that may otherwise be unavailable or difficult to obtain (Darkins, 2006; Hilty, Yellowlees, & Nesbitt, 2006). In reviewing 200 consecutive first-time Telepsychiatry consultations, Hilty, Nesbitt, Kuenneth, Cruz, and Hales (2007) concluded that, "Telepsychiatry programs may enhance access, satisfaction, and quality of rural care." Similar conclusions have been reached by others reviewing the literature, including Norman's (2006) overview of the use of telepsychiatry in the United Kingdom. Many other countries have developed telemedicine programs in psychiatry, dermatology, and radiology, and the future appears bright for increased utilization of VTC in the clinical neurosciences. This includes growing opportunities in the diagnosis and management of dementia (Shores et al., 2004; Vilalta-Franch, Garre-Olmo, López-Pousa, Coll-De Tuero, & Monserrat-Vila, 2007), stroke, and sports concussion. Although telehealth research with pediatric populations is limited, child and adolescent telepsychiatry programs have shown promise (Pesämaa et al., 2004).

Extrapolating the benefits of telehealth-based care to neuropsychological services, both in terms of teleassessment (Cullum, Weiner, Gehrmann, & Hynan, 2006) as well as telerehabilitation efforts (e.g., Brennan et al., 2010; McCue, Fairman, & Pramuka, 2010) is a natural extension of the movement in health care to expand the availability of specialty services. Because neuropsychological assessment represents an approved and recognized neurodiagnostic procedure (American Academy of Neurology, 1996) that is useful in many conditions across the life span, this will continue to be an area of growth across the globe as the population expands as telehealth, e-health, and mobile health technologies evolve. At present, there are only a few thousand clinical neuropsychologists in North America (almost 800 with board certification from the American Board of Professional Psychology as of 2011), and these tend to be in more populated areas, often leaving rural patients and health care facilities with limited options for obtaining neuropsychological services. The additional opportunities for bringing cutting-edge research into such settings are also promising.

Limiting Factors

Availability of Equipment

Despite the growth and promise of telemental health and telepsychology applications, limitations to VTC-based evaluations and care also exist (McGinty, Saeed, Simmons, & Yildirim, 2006). These include technological issues such as equipment availability and data transmission speeds to allow adequate audiovisual communication, in addition to the start-up and maintenance costs of VTC systems at both ends. However, Darkins (2006) noted that at least several years ago, the major barrier to more widespread telemental health utilization has been acceptance by patients and practitioners. As more and more vendors develop VTC equipment and hospitals and clinics embrace the technology, availability will become widespread.

Data Transmission Speeds

The speed at which audiovisual data can be transmitted, or *bandwidth* (commonly reflected by the number of kilobits per second, or kbs), is an important factor for clinical and research applications of VTC. Bandwidth must be sufficient to eliminate jerkiness of movement, which can be visually distracting or hamper behavioral observations. Early studies with low bandwidth (<384 kbs) sometimes reported poor image quality due to tiling and pixelation with movement (Jones, Johnston, Reboussin, & McCall, 2001), although some telemedicine programs have been effective with lower bandwidth (e.g., Zaylor, Whitten, & Kingsley, 2000), depending upon what services are being provided and how important real-time interactions are to the process. At slower connection speeds (i.e., 128 kbs), there can be a slight delay (0.5−1.0 s) in transmission, but at 512 kbs or faster, the interaction virtually replicates live interactions. With ongoing technological advances, speed is unlikely to represent a major barrier in most settings at this point.

Distance between home and remote sites can have an impact on the coordination of images and sound, with greater distance sometimes resulting in greater delay of sound. Fortunately, with a good, consistent link, such image/sound disconnects usually do not severely compromise interactions, but they can be distracting and can briefly disrupt smooth communication, which may be particularly important with regard to neuropsychological testing. Modern data transmissions speeds and equipment reliability have significantly reduced distance as a barrier to VTC-based interactions, however. In our own experience of over 200 telecognitive research assessment sessions at a distance of 200 miles, for example, we experienced audio or transmission disturbances in less than 5% of cases.

Cost has been posited as one of the most significant limiting factors to the adoption of VTC-based health care services, although decreasing costs of equipment and data transmission, in addition to more widespread equipment availability and advances in technology, have made a major impact on cost reduction. In the past, start-up costs were prohibitive, but VTC systems are becoming available in more and more settings across the globe. While the issue of cost is difficult to ascertain in an absolute sense due to the myriad of factors involved (e.g., see Kennedy, 2005), most authors have concluded that telemental health is ultimately cost-effective (Hilty, Luo, Morache, Marcelo, & Nesbitt, 2002; Monnier, Knapp, & Frueh, 2003; Schopp, Johnstone, & Merrell, 2000), particularly when improved access to care is considered as a counterbalancing factor (Kennedy, 2005). In practical terms, Ruskin et al. (2004) calculated that at 22 miles distance, costs of in-person versus VTC visits were equivalent, but at distances more than 22 miles, VTC was less expensive. Based upon data from a large ($N = 495$) randomized clinical trial (O'Reilly et al., 2007), VTC-based interventions were found to be at least 10% less costly on average than in-person sessions. Shore, Brooks, Savin,

Manson, and Libby (2007) compared the direct costs of conducting structured psychiatric interviews via VTC compared with in-person interviews and found that VTC-based contacts were more costly than in-person interviews in 2003, although significant cost *savings* were realized through the use of VTC-based interviews in 2005 as a result of decreased equipment and transmission costs. Thus, at this point, cost does not appear to be a major limiting factor.

VTC Environment

Clearly, the VTC environment poses limits in terms of the nature and types of neurocognitive tests that can be administered. Most traditional neuropsychological tests involve paper—pencil and question—answer types of tasks. Many standard neurocognitive tests are highly verbal, relying upon questions and instructions from the examiner and verbal responses from patients. Many such tests lend themselves very well to VTC-based interactions and should not require modification for valid response recording, scoring, and interpretation (e.g., WAIS-IV Vocabulary, etc.). Caution must be used, however, in the VTC setting, as this environment is more susceptible to factors that might influence test performance (see Table 14.1 for a list of some of the more obvious limitations).

Obviously, since there are limitations within the VTC context, portions of the neuropsychological examination may require modification, and certain tasks would need to be omitted because of the lack of direct patient contact and availability of test stimuli at the remote site, unless assistants are used. For example, remote administration of measures requiring psychomotor responses such as the Trail Making Test poses a challenge in terms of close patient monitoring and corrections during the test, not to mention the need for remote availability of test forms and stimuli. Administration of some standard measures, such as the Wechsler Scales,

Table 14.1 Potential Factors Influencing Test Results in the VTC Environment

Problem	Example
(a) Inadvertent interruption or presence of additional persons at the remote site	Others entering into remote site during test session
(b) Less control over the environment	Subject responding to a phone call in the middle of a test may be more likely without an examiner present in the room
(c) VTC connection instability/ interruption	Subject becomes unable to view the examiner or test stimuli fully, or sound is interrupted to one or both ends
(d) Limited ability to provide corrections during nonverbal tests	Client makes error on the Trail Making Test, and examiner is limited to verbal intervention without being able to point
(e) Reduced ability to observe patient behaviors	Field of view more limited with camera

includes various test stimuli or props pose additional challenges such as availability and need for manipulation of test materials at the remote site. One solution is to have an assistant at the remote end who can help with test materials and aspects of administration, although the extent to which such an individual becomes involved with the examination may increase costs or render moot the need for a VTC-based assessment (i.e., if a technician is available who administers the tests). Nevertheless, standard instructions might require modification in the VTC environment, and the potential effects of altered test instructions on test performance would need to be carefully evaluated and considered in interpretation of results. Tablet-based devices and computer-assisted testing may be ways of overcoming some of these limitations, however, particularly as computer-assisted interactive systems evolve. A related issue would be the applicability of existing test norms to VTC-based test administration to ensure that telecognitive test results could be interpreted in the same way as standard testing. Revised instructions/procedures might require different norms.

Setting Up Teleneuropsychology Services

Many of the considerations for developing a practice in teleneuropsychology are the same as for a traditional practice, although some factors have even greater importance for the VTC experience. Some practical VTC environmental considerations are outlined in Table 14.2.

Table 14.2 Practical Considerations for Telecognitive Assessment

Room and Equipment	Examiner	Procedures
• Quiet, private room for testing • Comfortable seating • Even and adequate lighting at both ends; avoid glare • Plain/nondistracting visual background • Appropriate distance from cameras/monitors to allow visibility of upper torso and mobility of camera(s) • Adequacy of video and sound, with local adjustability	• Wear contrasting solid colors and avoid busy patterns/lines that might be distracting over video • Enunciate clearly • Look at camera, as opposed to monitor, when addressing patient • Establish rapport and provide introduction to VTC experience • Reduce background noise (e.g., tapping of pen, rustling of papers) • Avoid excessive and rapid movements (e.g., hand gestures, chair movement)	• Consideration of whether special assistance at the remote end will be needed for each patient • Assess patient's hearing or visual limitations that might require adaptation • Identify everyone in the room at both sites • Consideration of stimuli and materials required at remote site to complete desired testing • Ensure that all necessary materials are within patient's reach

Evidence for VTC-Based Diagnosis and VTC-Based Cognitive Assessment

Despite technological and practical limitations, good agreement between in-person and VTC-based clinical diagnoses have generally been supported in the literature. For example, the diagnosis of dementia has been reported in US (Frueh et al., 2000) and non-US samples (Lee et al., 2000), suggesting both efficacy and cross-cultural applicability. Adaptation of some clinical assessment procedures may be required in the VTC environment given the constraints of the technology (e.g., camera location, field of view, and mobility; also see Table 14.1), but for many mental status examination procedures that are predominantly verbal in nature, this does not pose significant problems, and many mental status examinations can be carried out by VTC as if the patient and clinician were in the same-room. As an example, Clement, Brooks, Dean, and Galaz (2001) provided an overview of their neuropsychology telemedicine clinic at Brooke Army Medical Center. Whereas their use of VTC was limited to follow up feedback sessions, the authors concluded that VTC was an effective means for extending neuropsychological services beyond the clinic. Similar positive results have been found in administering a modified neurologic examination (Larner, 2011), including the evaluation and follow-up of patients with Parkinson's disease (Samii et al., 2006). Shores et al. (2004) reported 100% diagnostic agreement in their elderly subjects, and Loh, Donaldson, Flicker, Maher, and Goldswain (2007) and Loh, Ramesh et al. (2004) reported a kappa of 0.8 for the diagnosis of dementia. Such findings support the use of VTC-based diagnostic evaluations and follow-up care for patients with cognitive disorders such as dementia, particularly in rural and underserved areas (Vilalta-Franch et al., 2007).

In contrast to the widespread applications of telepsychiatry, very little has been done to explore the utility of VTC in the assessment of neuropsychological functioning. Neuropsychological testing is widely used to detect, characterize, and quantify cognitive impairment in children and adults, and forms an integral component of the comprehensive neurodiagnostic evaluation (Cullum, Paulman, Koss, Chapman, & Lacritz, 2003). Neuropsychological testing is an accepted neurodiagnostic procedure, strongly indicated in some disorders and useful in a wide range of neurobehavioral disturbances across the life span (American Academy of Neurology, 1996). However, the clinical utility of neuropsychological testing has, with few exceptions, been limited by the need for face-to-face contact with subjects, making it largely unavailable to persons who live in remote or underserved areas lacking in clinical neuropsychologists.

As advances have been made in telemedicine over the past decade, a growing number of studies suggest feasibility, validity, and resounding patient acceptance in psychiatry (Yellowlees, Shore, & Roberts, 2010). Thus, there are significant implications for the use of neuropsychological assessment as an adjunct to telepsychiatry and geropsychiatry applications, not to mention the many opportunities for pediatric applications (even though there is no research regarding feasibility, reliability, or validity in this area). As noted above, modern telecommunications and VTC provide for greatly enhanced audiovisual transmission and near real-time interactions compared with early studies, and reduced costs and greater availability of this technology provide for more ready access in a variety of settings all over the world. Along these lines, the potential for teleneuropsychological applications is equally promising, but available evidence-based support for many neuropsychological tools administered via VTC remains limited.

A review of neuropsychological tests that have been utilized in studies pertaining to VTC-based testing is summarized in Table 14.3. We present a list of tests by cognitive domain, including the source of information and whether modifications to instructions were reported. This review includes 14 data-based publications that utilized quantitative neurocognitive tests, generally focusing on healthy subjects and older patients. Most samples have been small, and diagnostic procedures were sometimes poorly described, thus limiting our knowledge regarding the potential applications and sensitivity of tests across disorders. It is also rather striking to note that we were unable to identify any teleneuropsychology studies as of 2011 that included children, and very few have included rural or ethnically diverse groups with cognitive disorders.

Most studies have compared VTC-based testing with traditional in-person or face-to-face testing either using the same instrument(s) administered twice or utilizing alternate forms of tests. There are methodological limitations to either approach that need to be considered, as test—retest correlations are naturally higher when the same test is administered twice to the same subjects (also increasing the likelihood of higher scores upon readministration due to practice effects). This is especially a concern for tests with no alternate versions, for then the results of the test—retest comparison speaks more to the reliability of the test itself rather than addressing the potential role of the VTC versus face-to-face test condition. Thus, it is important to consider the known test—retest reliabilities of the measures under investigation to see how VTC versus face-to-face retest results actually might differ. When alternate test forms are used in VTC investigations, the comparability of the test forms outside the VTC environment also represents an important piece of information to consider in the interpretation of results. Some alternate forms show strong correlations with original test versions, while others are lower and may depend upon the samples studied. In addition to counterbalancing the order of test forms, counterbalancing test *condition* is an additional important factor in VTC-based test validation research, though most studies have utilized such a design. Another issue is the time between examinations, which have varied widely, from back-to-back examinations to months in between test sessions. Whereas most studies have addressed these issues to some extent, only a handful of investigations have examined the psychometric properties of more than a few instruments at a time. Nevertheless, the evidence in support of the use and validity of teleneuropsychological assessment is growing (Cullum, Weiner et al., 2006) and although questions remain regarding the applicability of existing test norms, based on the available evidence, it appears that separate normative data may not be necessary for some tests, particularly those that require only verbal instructions and responses.

Table 14.3 Neuropsychological Tests Empirically Studied Using VTC-Based
Administration and Modifications Incorporated

Neuropsychological Measure	Administration Modifications
Global Cognitive Functioning and Intelligence	
Ammons Quick Test (Kirkwood, Peck, & Bennie, 2000)	None reported
CAMCOG (Ball & Puffett, 1998)	None reported
MMSE (Ball, Scott, McLaren, & Watson, 1993; Barton, Morris, Rothlind, & Yaffe, 2011; Ciemins, Holloway, Coon, McClosky-Armstrong, & Min, 2009; Cullum, Weiner et al., 2006; Loh, Donaldson et al., 2007; Loh, Ramesh et al., 2004; McEachern, Kirk, Morgan, Crossley, & Henry, 2008; Montani et al., 1997)	None reported (Loh, Donaldson et al., 2007; Loh, Ramesh et al., 2004; Montani et al., 1997); visual stimuli enlarged (Ball et al., 1993); staff at remote site presented materials to participants (McEachern et al., 2008); administered at remote site (Barton et al., 2011)
National Adult Reading Test (NART) (Kirkwood, Peck, & Bennie, 2000)	None reported
Short Portable Mental Status Questionnaire (Menon et al., 2001)	None reported
WASI (Temple, Drummond, Valiquette, & Jozsvai, 2010) *Vocabulary* (Hildebrand, Chow, Williams, Nelson, & Wass, 2004), *Block Design, Similarities, Matrix Reasoning* (Hildebrand et al., 2004)	Staff at remote site presented materials to participants
Attention and Processing Speed	
Adult Memory and Information Processing Battery *Information Processing A* (Kirkwood, Peck, & Bennie, 2000)	None reported
Brief Test of Attention (Hildebrand et al., 2004; McCue, Fairman, & Pramuka, 2010)	None reported
Digit Span (Barton et al., 2011; Cullum, Weiner et al., 2006)	None reported
Seashore Rhythm Test (Jacobsen, Sprenger, Andersson, & Krogstad, 2003)	None reported
Symbol Digit Modalities Test (Jacobsen et al., 2003)	Record form located at remote site; test demonstrated via document camera to ensure participant used correct recording sheet
Trail Making Test (Barton et al., 2011)	Limited information provided, but staff available at remote site; instructions and scoring via VTC, but tests sent to local site
Memory	
Adult Memory and Information Processing Battery *Story Recall, List Learning, Figure Recall* (Kirkwood, Peck, & Bennie, 2000)	None reported

(*Continued*)

Table 14.3 (Continued)

Neuropsychological Measure	Administration Modifications
Benton Visual Retention Test (Jacobsen et al., 2003)	Record booklet at remote site; results transmitted via document camera
CVLT-II *Short Form* (Barton et al., 2011)	None reported
Dementia Rating Scale *Memory* (Barton et al., 2011)	None reported
Hopkins Verbal Learning Test (Cullum, Weiner et al., 2006)	None reported
Modified Rey−Osterrieth Complex Figure Test (Barton et al., 2011)	Limited information provided, but staff available at remote site; responses scored via VTC and sent to local site
Rey Auditory Verbal Learning Test (Hildebrand et al., 2004)	None reported
WMS-R *Logical Memory* (Jacobsen et al., 2003)	None reported
Language	
WAIS-III *Vocabulary* (Hildebrand et al., 2004; Jacobsen et al., 2003)[a]	None reported
BDAE *Picture Description (auditory response version)* (Vestal, Smith-Olinde, Hicks, Hutton, & Hart, 2006)	None reported
Verbal Fluency (Barton et al., 2011; Cullum, Weiner et al., 2006; Hildebrand et al., 2004; Vestal et al., 2006)	None reported
Boston Naming Test *60-item* version (Barton et al., 2011), *15-item version* (Cullum, Weiner et al., 2006)	None reported
MAE *Aural Comprehension, Token Test* (Vestal et al., 2006)	Token Test stimuli located at remote site; clinician-generated template used to aid participants in correct reformation of tokens
Visuospatial	
Clock Drawing (Barton et al., 2011;Cullum, Weiner et al., 2006; Hildebrand et al., 2004; Montani et al., 1997)	None reported, though some administered remotely and scored locally; document camera used in some
WAIS-III *Matrix Reasoning* (Hildebrand et al., 2004; Jacobsen et al., 2003)[b]	None reported
Visual Object and Space Perception (Jacobsen et al., 2003) *Silhouettes*	All items and responses transmitted via document camera
Beery VMI (Temple et al., 2010)	Staff at remote site presented materials; all records sent to local site for scoring

(Continued)

Table 14.3 (Continued)

Neuropsychological Measure	Administration Modifications
Motor Function	
Grooved Pegboard (Ball & Puffett, 1998; Ball et al., 1993; Barton et al., 2011; Ciemins et al., 2009; Cullum, Weiner et al., 2006; Hildebrand et al., 2004; Jacobsen et al., 2003; Kirkwood et al., 2000; Loh, Donaldson et al., 2007; Loh, Ramesh et al., 2004; McEachern et al., 2008; Menon et al., 2001; Montani et al., 1997; Temple et al., 2010; Vestal et al., 2006)	Pegboard located at remote site; test demonstrated via document camera

BDAE, Boston Diagnostic Aphasia Examination; Beery VMI, Beery-Buktenica Developmental Test of Visual−Motor Integration; CAMCOG, Cambridge Examination for Mental Disorders, Cognitive Portion; CVLT-II, California Verbal Learning Test, Second Edition; MAE, Multilingual Aphasia Exam; MMSE, Mini Mental State Examination; NART, National Adult Reading Test; WAIS-III, Wechsler Adult Intelligence Scale-Third Edition; WASI, Wechsler Abbreviated Scale of Intelligence; WMS-R, Wechsler Memory Scale-Revised.
[a]WAIS Norwegian version.
[b]Digit Span not from the WAIS-III.

Prior to 2000, only a few investigations examined the use of neurocognitive testing in the VTC context, and all focused on brief cognitive screening tasks in small samples (Ball & Puffett, 1998; Ball et al., 1993; Montani et al., 1997). In some of the early studies, it was noted that VTC picture quality was limited, and subjects' written responses sometimes could not be scored. Nevertheless, it was noted that despite variability in correlational results on some items, overall reliability for VTC-based cognitive screening appeared promising.

Since 2000, a variety of neurocognitive measures have been examined in VTC compared to face-to-face testing conditions, but research in this area remains relatively scarce, despite the widespread growth of telehealth services. Samples have ranged from 10 to 73 and have included healthy individuals (Hildebrand et al., 2004; Jacobsen et al., 2003) as well as groups of patients with medical disorders (Ciemins et al., 2009; Menon et al., 2001), alcohol abuse (Kirkwood, Peck, & Bennie, 2000), dementia (Barton et al., 2011; Cullum, Weiner et al., 2006; McEachern et al., 2008; Vestal et al., 2006), intellectual disability and autism spectrum disorders (Temple et al., 2010), or mixed diagnoses (Loh, Donaldson et al., 2007; Loh, Ramesh et al., 2004). Thus, a number of research questions remain, as discussed below. At this point, the most widely studied neurocognitive test administered via VTC is the Mini Mental Status Examination (MMSE), followed by Clock Drawing, verbal fluency, Boston Naming Test, and Digit Span, all used in at least two published investigations. Tests of verbal memory (i.e., word lists or paragraph recall) have also been included in a number of investigations as noted in Table 14.3, but few of these tests have been examined in more than one or two studies. The literature is even weaker for other popular neuropsychological tests, although some probably require little additional validation in the VTC environment. For example, questionnaire-based surveys and tests requiring exclusively verbal instructions as well as responses (e.g., word definitions and other typical question—answer tasks) should not be adversely affected much or at all by the VTC interface (assuming good visual and sound connections, adequate rapport, etc.). However, as noted earlier, some visuospatial tasks and tests requiring manipulable stimuli or special administration interactions with patients may require, at a minimum, altered instructions, and/or the need for test materials or an assistant at the remote end. Such altered administration procedures require special attention to validity issues to ensure that existing norms are appropriate for standard clinical interpretation.

In terms of availability of information based on VTC administration of a more comprehensive battery of tests, we published a summary of data from an initial pilot study that formed the basis for a larger investigation of telecognitive assessment that is under way. This was one of the first studies to examine VTC-based administration of a brief yet multidomain battery of common neuropsychological tests used in dementia evaluations (Cullum, Weiner et al., 2006). Participants included 33 individuals with a diagnosis of mild cognitive impairment or Alzheimer's disease, ranging in age from 51 to 84, with a mean education of 15 years (range = 8—20). Comparison of VTC-based with face-to-face assessment using alternate test forms in counterbalanced fashion (also counterbalanced for test condition) resulted in highly similar results on most test scores examined, with intraclass correlations (ICC) across primary test scores averaging 0.73 (Figure 14.1). Findings supported the feasibility and reliability of neurocognitive evaluations in this population but also demonstrated some limitations, as some subscores showed lower reliabilities as reflected by ICC. For example, whereas the ICC for the total learning score from the Hopkins Verbal Learning Test-Revised (HVLT-R) was 0.77, the ICC for delayed recognition was 0.68, and for delayed

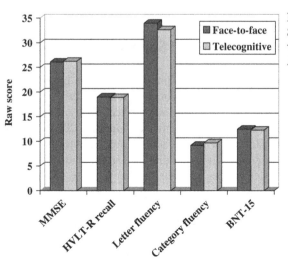

Figure 14.1 Comparability of Scores Obtained Face-to-Face versus via Telecognitive Assessment.

recall, 0.61, followed by 0.54 for delayed recall percent retention. Category fluency also showed a lower ICC of 0.58, whereas the ICC for letter fluency was 0.83. Such findings merit further investigation, as some scores were less reliable than others, although most were above 0.70 or 0.80. One possible reason for the lower reliability on certain scores may relate to inherent differences in the alternate test forms used, as no systematic advantage to VTC or face-to-face test condition was seen on most measures. However, a tendency for higher HVLT-R percent retention scores was seen in the face-to-face condition, which merits further exploration in larger samples.

We found that telecognitive testing was well tolerated by all subjects across a range of cognitive impairments. MMSE scores in our pilot study averaged 26, although we have since completed more than 100 teleneuropsychological evaluations in cognitively impaired adults with MMSE scores as low as 15. Subjects have adapted readily to the VTC environment, and contrary to our initial concerns, we did not have an assistant or relative present in the room with the subject during the VTC sessions (though we did have staff nearby). Only one subject with dementia wandered out of the testing room and needed to be redirected; all others were successfully tested and managed remotely via VTC.

Whereas most studies have reported good agreement between VTC and face-to-face test results overall in the measures studied to date, some individual tests have shown lower correlations, with greater variability in results. Tests that have tended to show more variability and lower correlations between test conditions have primarily been measures of delayed paragraph recall and visuospatial tasks (e.g., see Hildebrand et al., 2004; Jacobsen et al., 2003; Kirkwood et al., 2000). Reasons for this may include the inherent test–retest variability of some measures and of some alternate forms, as well as differences in samples, and/or different means of obtaining and scoring data (i.e., remote vs. local scoring, scoring done via VTC vs. in-person).

Consumer Satisfaction with VTC-Based Services

In terms of VTC-based psychiatric evaluations and interventions, it is important to note that patients as well as clinicians report levels of satisfaction with VTC-based services at least as high as with traditional face-to-face services (Hilty, Luo et al., 2002; Hilty, Nesbitt et al., 2007; Kobak, 2004; Shore & Manson, 2005; Shores et al., 2004; O'Reilly et al., 2007). In reviewing the initial 5 years of the University of Arizona Teleconsultations Program, Cruz, Krupinski, Lopez, and Weinstein (2005) reported a total of 1086 telemedicine consults on 206 patients. High satisfaction was reported with the services, although 17% of patients and 18% of providers found equipment problems distracting at times. Shores et al. (2004) reported that while many subjects indicated that they would have preferred to see a physician in person, 94% felt they could communicate with the physician via VTC as well as in person, and 76% of Kobak's (2004) subjects said they preferred telepsychiatry services to traveling long distances to a doctor's office. Menon et al. (2001) found that ratings of subject satisfaction with the interview and testing procedures across conditions were similar, and Vestal et al. (2006) reported acceptance of VTC-based aphasia testing procedures was high in 9/10 participants. Many subjects in the Hildebrand et al. (2004) study expressed a preference for face-to-face testing (44%), but 39% indicated no preference, reflecting good acceptance of VTC-based assessment.

In our own ongoing research of the feasibility and reliability of telecognitive assessment in older adults with and without dementia, we found a 98% satisfaction rating for VTC-based assessment among 40 participants who were tested in person and via VTC, and a majority (59%) found either approach acceptable (Parikh et al., 2012). It is also worth noting that in completing over 200 VTC-based evaluations, no participants have expressed significant problems with VTC interactions with examiners or visual/audio quality, and while some have noted a preference to be in the room with the examiner, most have indicated that VTC would be an acceptable alternative, particularly if they were to have to drive a long distance to obtain such an examination.

Practical and Ethical Issues in Teleneuropsychology

The American Psychological Association has issued preliminary statements regarding telemedicine-based psychological applications (American Psychological Association Practice Organization, 2010), as has the American Telemedicine Association (Yellowlees et al., 2010). However, there has been very little written with regard to practice and ethical issues in teleneuropsychology specifically. Recently, Grosch, Gottlieb, and Cullum (2011) outlined a number of practical and ethical considerations relevant to telecognitive assessment, including issues involving: (1) informed consent, (2) privacy and confidentiality, (3) competence, (4) licensure, (5) assessment, and (6) technology. For example, telecognitive practice should include modification of informed consent procedures to reflect the unique nature of the assessment (e.g., providing increased information regarding security and storage of private health information transmitted over the Internet or videoconferencing connection). Because the practice of teleneuropsychology necessitates an increased concern for privacy and confidentiality, the authors recommend taking precautions such as establishing security protocols as well as making patients aware of all individuals involved in the VTC interactions. With regard to assessment measures themselves, it is recommended that neuropsychologists use tests that have been empirically demonstrated to be appropriate for use in telemedicine whenever possible. Clinical or research reports should describe any administrative modifications or other unique situations factors and how they may have affected outcome. Finally, Grosch et al. (2011) provide discussion and recommendations regarding issues such as practitioner competence, licensure and billing, as well as technology and equipment.

Mobile Teleneuropsychology Applications

The concept of "brain health" has become a popular topic in our culture, and many Internet sites and downloadable smart phone applications are available that include some sort of "cognitive testing," "memory assessment," "IQ test," and/or games/ activities purportedly designed to enhance memory or other cognitive skills. Whereas most of these offerings are of a commercial nature for the general public and have limited or no data behind their validity, a growing number of bona fide computerized neuropsychological assessment tools and systems have become available in recent years, with appropriate psychometric studies to support their use in some clinical settings. Most rely upon personal computer platforms, with some being Internet-based or with Internet-connectivity capability. Advantages include accurate measurement of reaction times and standardization of administration, as well as the convenience of automatic test scoring and reporting of results. Such systems have particular appeal in specialized contexts such as settings that call for large numbers of brief evaluations (e.g., baseline and follow-up testing following concussion in sports). Most of the existing test systems constitute a relatively brief (i.e., 30 min) assessment of a limited range of cognitive abilities consistent with the concept of cognitive screening, and many can be administered via laptop, lending mobility to these examinations.

Computerized cognitive testing has grown most rapidly in the context of sports concussion assessment due to the need for brief evaluation of large numbers of individuals. In this context, "baseline," or preinjury test performance is often obtained for postconcussion evaluation comparisons. In this way, in addition to normative comparisons, individuals can be compared with their own premorbid performance levels. Issues such as test-taking attitude/effort on the part of examinees are sometimes a question, particularly in the absence of neuropsychologist-monitored proctoring, and the computer environment poses various limitations to cognitive assessment versus traditional neuropsychological evaluation tools. A review of the various strengths and weaknesses of computerized neurocognitive testing is beyond the scope of this chapter and is available in a variety of sources (Elsmore, Reeves, & Reeves, 2007; Naglieri et al., 2004; Schatz & Browndyke, 2002; Wild, Howieson, Webbe, Seelye, & Kaye, 2008). Laptop administration of tests provides for some mobility, but as an extension of the computerized testing movement, there have been several mobile or handheld/self-contained neuropsychological assessment tools developed in recent years.

A related, emerging area is the development of mobile/handheld and smartphone-based neurocognitive testing tools. Initial applications include sports concussion assessment (e.g., see Gioia & Mihalik, 2011; Inc., 2011) and remote cognitive testing in the military and aerospace (Design Interactive, 2011; Elsmore et al., 2007; Reeves et al., 2007). Cognitive screening batteries such as the Cognistat Assessment System (Cognistat, 2011) and CANTAB (Ltd., 2011) have recently been adapted to mobile formats as well. Benefits of this type of platform include portability, brief administration, automated scoring, immediate comparison to normative data, and electronic data storage. Initial findings suggest good correlations between traditional and handheld testing formats (Elsmore et al., 2007), although it should be noted that this technology remains in its infancy, and these platforms await systematic validation. Furthermore, there are inherent limitations of such platforms, including limited screen size (hence limiting the size and legibility of stimuli and response options), restricted audio options, battery life, and potential for data loss. Clearly many traditional neuropsychological tests would not be suitable for this type of administration and response recording, although some challenges can be overcome, and the technology holds promise for new test development and standardization.

Future Directions

Few investigations to date have systematically examined VTC-based neurocognitive assessment in patients at various levels of cognitive impairment and with different disorders across the life span, with no studies in children. Furthermore, questions still exist regarding the utility and validity of telecognitive assessment in underserved, rural, and ethnic minority populations, although the opportunities for telehealth service provision to such groups is tremendous. For example, with the rapid growth of the elderly segment of our population, particularly among ethnic minorities, in conjunction with the growing awareness of the prevalence of dementia among the aging population, there will be an increasing need for widespread availability of specialty evaluations for both diagnosis and monitoring of progression, treatment, and need for placement. Another area ripe for investigation of VTC-based neuropsychological assessment is in sports concussion, where neurocognitive assessment is an important component but may not be readily available given the scope of the problem. Opportunities also exist for the development of new tests amenable to VTC administration, and there will no doubt be an expansion of integrated computer-interface/VTC assessment systems as well as increased adaptation of neurocognitive assessment/monitoring to mobile e-health applications.

Summary

These preliminary results add to the emerging literature suggesting that VTC-based neuropsychological assessment is feasible in persons with known or suspected cognitive impairment, and that VTC-based testing produces valid and reliable results similar to face-to-face testing. Several limitations of this line of research have been the limited sample sizes and limited number and types of neuropsychological assessment tools studied to date, however. Nevertheless, in most of the tests studied to date, it appears that results will generally be similar to those obtained via conventional face-to-face interactions as long as standard instructions are not varied too much. However, there is sparse information available regarding more detailed neuropsychological tests and test batteries administered in this fashion, and modifications to some measures would need to be more extensive such that demonstration of equivalence would be required. Thus, at this early stage in research, it appears that separate normative data for the neuropsychological tests studied thus far administered via VTC are probably not necessary for some tests, although additional reliability/validity data are needed, and additional measures merit examination in the VTC context. Fortunately, as with other telehealth applications, teleneuropsychology appears to be well accepted by patients, particularly when remote travel would be an issue to obtain services.

References

American Academy of Neurology (1996). Assessment: Neuropsychological testing of adults. *Neurology, 47*, 592−599.

American Psychological Association Practice Organization (2010). Telehealth: Legal basics for psychologists. *Good Practice, 41*, 2−7.

Ball, C., & Puffett, A. (1998). The assessment of cognitive function in the elderly using videoconferencing. *Journal of Telemedicine and Telecare, 4*, 36−38.

Ball, C., Scott, N., McLaren, P., & Watson, J. (1993). Preliminary evaluation of a low-cost videoconferencing (LCVC) system for remote cognitive testing of adult psychiatric patients. *British Journal of Clinical Psychology, 32*, 303−307.

Barton, C., Morris, R., Rothlind, J., & Yaffe, K. (2011). Video-telemedicine in a memory disorders clinic: Evaluation and management of rural elders with cognitive impairment. *Telemedicine and e-Health, 17*, 789−793.

Brennan, D. M., Tindall, L., Theodoros, D., Brown, J., Campbell, M., Christiana, D., et al. (2010). A blueprint for telerehabilitation guidelines. *Telemedicine and e-Health, 17*, 662−665.

Ciemins, E. L., Holloway, B., Coon, P. J., McClosky-Armstrong, T., & Min, S. J. (2009). Telemedicine and the mini-mental state examination: Assessment from a distance. *Telemedicine and e-Health, 15*, 476−478.

Clement, P., Brooks, F., Dean, B., & Galaz, A. (2001). A neuropsychology telemedicine clinic. *Military Medicine, 166*, 382−384.

Cognistat, I. (2011). CAS: Cognistat assessment system.

Cruz, M., Krupinski, E., Lopez, A., & Weinstein, R. (2005). A review of the first five years of the University of Arizona telepsychiatry programme. *Journal of Telemedicine and Telecare, 11*, 234−239.

Cullum, C. M., Paulman, R., Koss, E., Chapman, S., & Lacritz, L. (2003). Evaluation of cognitive functions. In M. Weiner & A. Lipton (Eds.), *The dementias: Diagnosis, treatment, and research* (3rd ed., pp. 285−320). Washington, DC: American Psychiatric Publishing.

Cullum, C. M., Weiner, M. F., Gehrmann, H. R., & Hynan, L. S. (2006). Feasibility of telecognitive assessment in dementia. *Assessment, 13*, 385−390.

Darkins, A. (2006). Changing the location of care: Management of patients with chronic conditions in Veterans Health administration using care coordination/home telehealth. *Journal of Rehabilitation Research and Development*, *43*. vii-xii

Design Interactive, I. (2011). CogGauge: A cognitive assessment tool.

Dwyer, T. F. (1973). Telepsychiatry: Psychiatric consultation by interactive television. *American Journal of Psychiatry*, *130*, 865−869.

Elsmore, T. F., Reeves, D. L., & Reeves, A. N. (2007). The ARES test system for palm OS handheld computers. *Archives of Clinical Neuropsychology*, *22*, 135−144.

Frueh, B. C., Deitsch, S. E., Santos, a. B., Gold, P. B., Johnson, M. R., Meisler, N., et al. (2000). Procedural and methodological issues in telepsychiatry research and program development. *Psychiatric Services*, *51*, 1522−1527.

Gioia, G., & Mihalik, J. (2011). *Concussion Recognition and Response (CRR) [app]*. Psychological Assessment Resources (PAR). Retrieved from <http://www4.parmc.com/Products/Product,aspx?ProductID = CRR-APP/>.

Grosch, M. C., Gottlieb, M. C., & Cullum, C. M. (2011). Initial practice recommendations for teleneuropsychology. *The Clinical Neuropsychologist*, *25*, 1119−1133.

Hildebrand, R., Chow, H., Williams, C., Nelson, M., & Wass, P. (2004). Feasibility of neuropsychological testing of older adults via videoconference: Implications for assessing the capacity for independent living. *Journal of Telemedicine and Telecare*, *10*, 130−134.

Hilty, D. M., Luo, J. S., Morache, C., Marcelo, D. A., & Nesbitt, T. S. (2002). Telepsychiatry: An overview for psychiatrists. *CNS Drugs*, *16*, 527−548.

Hilty, D. M., Nesbitt, T. S., Kuenneth, C. a, Cruz, G. M., & Hales, R. E. (2007). Rural versus suburban primary care needs, utilization, and satisfaction with telepsychiatric consultation. *Journal of Rural Health*, *23*, 163−165.

Hilty, D. M., Yellowlees, P. M., & Nesbitt, T. S. (2006). Evolution of telepsychiatry to rural sites: changes over time in types of referral and in primary care providers' knowledge, skills and satisfaction. *General Hospital Psychiatry*, *28*, 367−373.

Inc., I. (2011). SCAT2 Sport Concussion Assessment Tool.

Jacobsen, S. E., Sprenger, T., Andersson, S., & Krogstad, J.-M. (2003). Neuropsychological assessment and telemedicine: A preliminary study examining the reliability of neuropsychology services performed via telecommunication. *Journal of the International Neuropsychological Society*, *9*, 472−478.

Jones, B. N., Johnston, D., Reboussin, B., & McCall, W. V. (2001). Reliability of telepsychiatry assessments: subjective versus observational ratings. *Journal of Geriatric Psychiatry and Neurology*, *14*, 66−71.

Kennedy, C. A. (2005). The challenges of economic evaluations of remote technical health interventions. *Clinical and Investigative Medicine*, *28*, 71−74.

Kirkwood, K. T., Peck, D. F., & Bennie, L. (2000). The consistency of neuropsychological assessments performed via telecommunication and face to face. *Journal of Telemedicine and Telecare*, *6*, 147−151.

Kobak, K. A. (2004). A comparison of face-to-face and videoconference administration of the Hamilton depression rating scale. *Journal of Telemedicine and Telecare*, *10*, 231−235.

Larner, A. (2011). Teleneurology: An overview of current status. *Practical Neurology*, *11*, 283−288.

Lee, J. H., Kim, J. H., Jhoo, J. H., Lee, K. U., Kim, K. W., Lee, D. Y., et al. (2000). A telemedicine system as a care modality for dementia patients in Korea. *Alzheimer Disease and Associated Disorders*, *14*, 94−101.

Loh, P.-K., Donaldson, M., Flicker, L., Maher, S., & Goldswain, P. (2007). Development of a telemedicine protocol for the diagnosis of Alzheimer's disease. *Journal of Telemedicine and Telecare, 13*, 90−94.

Loh, P. -K., Ramesh, P., Maher, S., Saligari, J., Flicker, L., & Goldswain, P. (2004). Can patients with dementia be assessed at a distance? The use of telehealth and standardized assessments. *Internal Medicine Journal, 34*, 239−242.

Ltd., C. C. (2011). CANTAB Mobile.

McCue, M., Fairman, A., & Pramuka, M. (2010). Enhancing quality of life through telerehabilitation. *Physical Medicine and Rehabilitation Clinics of North America, 21*, 195−205.

McEachern, W., Kirk, A., Morgan, D. G., Crossley, M., & Henry, C. (2008). Reliability of the MMSE administered in-person and by telehealth. *Canadian Journal of Neurological Sciences, 35*, 643−646.

McGinty, K. L., Saeed, S. A., Simmons, S. C., & Yildirim, Y. (2006). Telepsychiatry and e-mental health services: Potential for improving access to mental health care. *Psychiatric Quarterly, 77*, 335−342.

Menon, A., Kondapavalru, P., Krishna, P., Chrismer, J., Raskin, A., Hebel, J., et al. (2001). Evaluation of a low cost videophone system in the assessment of depressive symptoms and cognitive function in elderly medically ill veterans. *Journal of Nervous and Mental Disease, 189*, 399−401.

Monnier, J., Knapp, R. G., & Frueh, B. C. (2003). Recent advances in telepsychiatry: An updated review. *Psychiatric Services, 54*, 1604−1609.

Montani, C., Billaud, N., Tyrrell, J., Fluchaire, I., Malterre, C., & Lauvernay, N., et al. (1997). Psychological impact of a remote psychometric consultation with hospitalized elderly people. *Journal of Telemedicine and Telecare, 3*, 140−145.

Naglieri, J. A, Drasgow, F., Schmit, M., Handler, L., Prifitera, A., Margolis, A., et al. (2004). Psychological testing on the Internet: New problems, old issues. *The American Psychologist, 59*, 150−162.

Norman, S. (2006). The use of telemedicine in psychiatry. *Journal of Psychiatric and Mental Health Nursing, 13*, 771−777.

O'Reilly, R., Bishop, J., Maddox, K., Hutchinson, L., Fisman, M., & Takhar, J. (2007). Is telepsychiatry equivalent to face-to-face psychiatry? Results from a randomized controlled equivalence trial. *Psychiatric Services, 58*, 836−843.

Parikh, M., Grosch, M., Graham, L., Weiner, M., Hynan, L., Shore, J., et al. (2012). Consumer acceptability of teleneuropsychology, In *Paper session presented at the meeting of the international neuropsychological society*. Montreal, Quebec, Canada.

Pesämaa, L., Ebeling, H., Kuusimäki, M. -L., Winblad, I., Isohanni, M., & Moilanen, I. (2004). Videoconferencing in child and adolescent telepsychiatry: A systematic review of the literature. *Journal of Telemedicine and Telecare, 10*, 187−192.

Reeves, D., Elsmore, T., Wiederhold, M. D., Wood, D., Murphy, J., Center, C., et al. (2007). Handheld computerized neuropsychological assessment in a virtual reality treatment protocol for combat PTSD. *Annual Review of Cybertherapy and Telemedicine, 5*, 1−12.

Ruskin, P. E., Silver-Aylaian, M., Kling, M. A., Reed, S. A, Bradham, D. D., Hebel, J. R., et al. (2004). Treatment outcomes in depression: comparison of remote treatment through telepsychiatry to in-person treatment. *American Journal of Psychiatry, 161*, 1471−1476.

Samii, A., Ryan-Dykes, P., Tsukuda, R. A., Zink, C., Franks, R., & Nichol, W. P. (2006). Telemedicine for delivery of health care in Parkinson's disease. *Journal of Telemedicine and Telecare, 12*, 16−18.

Schatz, P., & Browndyke, J. (2002). Applications of computer-based neuropsychological assessment. *Journal of Head Trauma Rehabilitation, 17*, 395−410.

Schopp, L., Johnstone, B., & Merrell, D. (2000). Telehealth and neuropsychological assessment: New opportunities for psychologists. *Professional Psychology: Research and Practice, 31*, 179−183.

Shore, J. H., & Manson, S. M. (2005). A developmental model for rural telepsychiatry. *Psychiatric Services, 56*, 976−980.

Shore, J. H., Brooks, E., Savin, D. M., Manson, S. M., & Libby, A. M. (2007). An economic evaluation of telehealth data collection with rural populations. *Psychiatric Services, 58*, 830−835.

Shores, M. M., Ryan-Dykes, P., Williams, R. M., Mamerto, B., Sadak, T., Pascualy, M., et al. (2004). Identifying undiagnosed dementia in residential care veterans: Comparing telemedicine to in-person clinical examination. *International Journal of Geriatric Psychiatry, 19*, 101−108.

Temple, V., Drummond, C., Valiquette, S., & Jozsvai, E. (2010). A comparison of intellectual assessments over video conferencing and in-person for individuals with ID: Preliminary data. *Journal of Intellectual Disability Research, 54*, 573−577.

Vestal, L., Smith-Olinde, L., Hicks, G., Hutton, T., & Hart, J. J. (2006). Efficacy of language assessment in Alzheimer's disease: Comparing in-person examination and telemedicine. *Clinical Interventions in Aging, 1*, 467−471.

Vilalta-Franch, J., Garre-Olmo, J., López-Pousa, S., Coll-De Tuero, G., & Monserrat-Vila, S. (2007). Telemedicine and dementia: A need for the 21st century. *Revista de Neurologia, 44*, 556−561.

Wild, K., Howieson, D., Webbe, F., Seelye, A., & Kaye, J. (2008). Status of computerized cognitive testing in aging: A systematic review. *Alzheimer's and Dementia, 4*, 428−437 (The Alzheimer's Association)

Wootton, R., & Craig, J. (1999). *Introduction to telemedicine.* London: Royal Society of Medicine Press. p. 220.

Wootton, R., Yellowlees, P., & McLaren, P. (2003). *Telepsychiatry and e-Mental Health.* London: Royal Society of Medicine Press. p. 368.

Yellowlees, P., Shore, J., & Roberts, L. (2010). Practice guidelines for videoconferencing-based telemental health—October 2009. *Telemedicine and e-Health, 16*, 1074−1089.

Zaylor, C., Whitten, P., & Kingsley, C. (2000). Telemedicine services to a county jail. *Journal of Telemedicine and Telecare, 6*, S93−S95.

15 Special Considerations for Conducting Psychotherapy over Videoteleconferencing

Eve-Lynn Nelson[a,b,]*, Angela Banitt Duncan[b] and Teresa Lillis[b]

[a]Pediatrics Department, University of Kansas Medical Center, Kansas City, KS, [b]KU Center for Telemedicine and Telehealth, University of Kansas Medical Center, Kansas City, KS

Considerations for Conducting Psychotherapy over VTC

Videoteleconferencing (VTC) continues to be an innovative approach to address the striking access gaps to mental health services, particularly in rural communities. From the beginning, mental health disciplines (e.g., psychology, psychiatry, counseling, social work, developmental medicine, and related disciplines) have been among the most active users of real-time VTC, to provide services usually delivered in-person. This chapter focuses on reimbursable telehealth services using room-based equipment or personal, computer-based systems to connect the mental health provider within an outreach setting. The authors illustrate VTC basics around the *why, where, who,* and *what* of psychotherapy. The authors generalize lessons presented for academic psychology (Nelson & Velasquez, 2011) to broader psychotherapy providers. Due to space considerations, the authors focus on direct clinical services with clients presenting with primary mental health concerns. While very important, health psychology interventions over VTC (Davis, Boulger, Hovland, & Hoven, 2007; Van Allen, Davis, & Lassen, 2011), neuropsychological testing (Jacobsen, Sprenger, Andersson, & Krogstad, 2003), prevention services over VTC (Grady et al., 2011), and related behavioral health topics are beyond the chapter's scope. The use of VTC for neuropsychological and primary health-care services is addressed in other chapters of this text. The conclusion addresses how ongoing telemental health practice to date informs how to best use emerging VTC technologies, including home telehealth and mobile devices.

* Corresponding Author: Eve-Lynn Nelson, 2012 Wahl Annex, MS 1048, 3901 Rainbow Blvd., Kansas City, KS 66160. Tel.: 913-588-2413, Fax: 913-588-2227, E-mail: enelson2@kumc.edu.

Telemental Health. DOI: http://dx.doi.org/10.1016/B978-0-12-416048-4.00015-4

Why Deliver Psychotherapy over VTC?

The overall rationale for VTC has remained constant over the last two decades, with a focus on using the technology to bridge the gap between the high need for psychotherapy and limited or no access to the growing number of empirically supported interventions. Despite advanced treatments, the vast majority of individuals with behavioral health concerns do not receive any therapy, let alone evidence-based treatments delivered by mental health specialists (Substance Abuse and Mental Health Services Administration, SAMHSA, 2007). For instance, there are approximately 39 psychologists per 100,000 residents in urban/suburban areas (Metropolitan Statistical Areas) but only 16 psychologists per 100,000 residents in non-Metropolitan Statistical Areas according to a survey conducted by The Center for Health Policy, Planning & Research for the American Psychological Association (2007). Similar statistics are seen across mental health professionals. These access gaps have remained or worsened in the last two decades (Mohatt, Bradley, Adams, & Morris, 2006) as many rural communities have experienced shrinking populations, declining economies, and increasing poverty as well as delays to treatment, less access to mental health insurance, and limited transportation options. The burdens of traveling for mental health care are often magnified with psychotherapy, with the frequent standard of care for regular sessions sustained over a period of time. VTC provides an avenue to increase regular attendance by diminishing the financial and temporal barriers of extensive travel as well as the possibility of increased collaboration with community systems of care (e.g., primary care personnel, school personnel, and case managers).

The purpose of the psychotherapy clinic drives technology selection. It is sometimes difficult to avoid the marketing buzz for the newest technologies which may or may not be a fit for the psychotherapy purpose. For example, newer communicative technologies like smart phones and tablet computers would seem an ideal medium for the delivery of VTC services given the mobile nature of the devices and the ability of those services to be delivered "in-home." However, given the absence of research conducted with such technologies, exploration of their costs and benefits would need to be established before recommending their widespread use. Psychotherapy services require VTC equipment but not the more expensive peripherals needed for telemedicine applications (e.g., digital otoscope and stethoscope). Similar to other equipment purchases, therapists should talk not only with technology vendors but also with colleagues who have used the technology as well as national telehealth centers. In addition to the overarching purpose, therapists must outline the specific purpose of the VTC clinic, both for themselves and for the community. In most VTC clinics, the therapist collaborates with other professionals and parties (e.g., schools and primary care) and is independent from these other systems of care rather than a consultant working on their behalf.

The therapist must also bear in mind the individual setting when considering advantages/disadvantages related to technology and technology security. Many larger institutions select point-to-point encrypted technology rather than publically available VTC technologies (e.g., Skype). This is due to broader security concerns with the overall institutional network and with HIPAA (Health Insurance Portability Accountability Act, or Public Law 104−191)-compliance concerns related to data access through third-party servers. Therapists are also encouraged to consider their own individual and institutional requirements in consultation with practicing therapists and the federal telehealth resource centers (http://www.tele-healthresourcecenter.org/).

Where is Psychotherapy over VTC Delivered?

Technology makes it possible for therapists to provide psychotherapy to clients across the city, the state, the country, or even the world in real time. A community-focused approach is encouraged in considering where to pursue psychotherapy services using VTC. Shore and Manson's (2005) developmental model for rural telepsychiatry also enlightens psychotherapy over VTC and complements findings across telehealth readiness studies (Jennett, Gagnon, & Brandstadt, 2005).

Shore and Manson's (2005) first step is conducting a *needs assessment* that advises which communities are likely to be a better fit for psychotherapy over VTC and includes an ongoing series of written and verbal dialogues across constituents, including community leaders, community organizations, consumer groups, local mental health providers, local primary care providers, and other key partners. This step not only activates the therapist's relationships with the community but also allows the therapist to identify the target population and what specific mental health presentations, age groups, and interventions are of highest interest and will be more likely to support active clinics. Shore and Manson's (2005) second step is *completion of an infrastructure survey.* The survey includes a detailed assessment of the existing technological, organizational, and programmatic infrastructure at the client site as well as within the therapist's own organization. With VTC services, one must assess the equipment, clinical space, and connectivity available and/or needed, as well as the initial and ongoing expectations concerning who will pay for equipment/connectivity. In addition to the technology itself, the infrastructure survey addresses the organization's personnel related to VTC delivery, including a VTC coordinator. The VTC coordinator at the client site facilitates VTC encounters and is most often the site's "champion." The coordinator serves as the bridge between the therapist and the client/family at the client site. Of particular importance for therapists is discussing the target population and characteristics that will affect implementation of services (e.g., insurance status and transportation availability). The therapist and client site discuss the site's commitment to allow personnel time and space to complete psychotherapy encounters both at start-up and as client volumes increase. It is helpful to discuss up front the organization's policy toward opening up the site across community members or for use only within the organization. For example, a telemental health consultant may provide therapy services to a rural nursing home and then expand to provide services to elders in the larger community who may also need services.

Shore and Manson's (2005) third step is *exploring the involvement of local organizations with the proposed VTC clinics*. Reaching out early in the process will assist in building a collegial environment, with an emphasis on filling gaps in service rather than competing with existing services. It is helpful to engage the community's crisis services to assist clients if there are safety concerns during a psychotherapy session.

Shore and Manson's (2005) fourth step is *structure configuration*. This step defines the roles and responsibilities of the therapist and the community partners. This is accomplished through written protocols developed jointly in order to clarify expectations. Such protocols are a "work in progress" and are revised throughout the life of the VTC clinic. For example, protocols should be developed covering whom the patient should call if a problem arises between sessions, as the distant provider may prefer these questions be handled locally as much as possible. A key area to include in protocols is the client's right to choose to be seen via VTC or to utilize traditional psychotherapy services, such as traveling to non-VTC clinics. The *structure configuration* step outlines expectations concerning coverage of start-up costs at both the therapist and the client sites, including equipment and software costs, connectivity/line charges, installation costs, costs of remodeling or adding space, personnel costs associated with VTC training, and costs with adding staff or with changing workflow to meet VTC responsibilities.

Shore and Manson's (2005) fifth step focuses on a *pilot implementation*. This step stipulates a small-scale trial to make sure the procedures and processes outlines in the protocol will meet the community needs as anticipated. The final step, *solidification*, means implementation of the psychotherapy clinic with a wider client population.

Who Participates in Psychotherapy over VTC?

This section addresses the different people involved in VTC encounters, including the client and family, the therapist and trainees, the VTC coordinator, and the multiple informants. The authors describe a VTC model in which a VTC coordinator presents the patient and family at the client site. The authors are unaware of any telemental health programs at academic health centers or elsewhere using the client-only model without a trained assistant at the client site. This is due to the need to provide the client assistance related to presenting information, following recommendations, and addressing safety or other emergent concerns.

Clients and Family

Across telemental health clinics, clients tend to present with the same concerns as seen in traditional clinic settings (Grady et al., 2011). No presentation or diagnostic category has been excluded from mental health services over VTC. However, the same careful consideration used in traditional clinics is taken related to competence with the presenting concern as well as access to requisite resources, particularly with severely impaired clients. Of note, Sharp, Kobak, and Osman (2011) found that, in general, VTC is equivalent to face-to-face assessment and treatment of psychosis and that VTC is well tolerated and accepted by this population.

It has been noted that therapists have been slow to implement psychotherapy across the wide variety of clients who seek care through VTC. Such reluctance may contribute to increased comorbidity and severity of presentations for clients seen over VTC. The choice of who will be provided such services depends on developmental and diagnostic considerations, personnel, other resources at the client site, parents' or other caregivers' preferences if the client is under the age of 18 or living with a family member, and the therapist's comfort with the technology (Myers, Cain, Work Group on Quality Issues, & American Academy of Child and Adolescent Psychiatry Staff, 2008). Psychotherapy over VTC may be especially suited for youth who are often already comfortable with, and accepting of, the technology medium. Some studies suggest VTC offers unique advantages, including less self-consciousness and decreased confidentiality concerns as the therapist is outside of the local community (Himle et al., 2006; Simpson, Doze, Urness, Hailey, & Jacobs, 2001). Anecdotally, adolescent clients may respond particularly well to the distance and perceived control allowed by the VTC system.

Therapists and Trainees

There is no profile distinguishing between therapists who choose to engage in VTC or not. A major advantage of VTC is expanding services to high-need rural populations without having to be away from competing clinical, research, and teaching responsibilities. Disadvantages include already overbooked schedules, concerns about gaining proficiency with the technology, and limited availability of referral sources in the local setting.

National guidelines, as well as guidance from established telemental health programs, indicate the need for commitment at all organizational levels in order to build and sustain telemental health services. VTC services are outside of traditional workflow and require a strong commitment from upper administration. This upper level support is crucial in early VTC development due to the significant commitment to needs assessment and relationship building that is needed. Some departments embrace VTC as a way to "get the word out" and develop relationships that can grow referrals across the state.

Due to the newness of the field, there are no established performance competencies specific to technology, but telehealth guidelines provide direction (Grady et al., 2011; Myers, Cain et al., 2008; Yellowlees, Shore, & Roberts, 2009). Therapists need practice with the technology as well as cultural competence with the population served by the psychotherapy clinic. Ideally, therapists observe other telemental health providers and complete "test" runs in order to build confidence with the technology. Federally funded telehealth resource centers offer training related to these competencies (e.g., www.heartlandtrc.org, www.ctel.org, and www.cteconline.org). The telemental health guide developed by the University of Colorado in collaboration with the Substance Abuse and Mental Health Services Administration (SAMHSA) also provides excellent guidance about VTC practice for mental health professionals (see www.tmhguide.org). VTC offers unique training advantages as several trainees can be unobtrusive in the VTC room without crowding the client (Nelson, Bui, & Sharp, 2011; Szeftel et al., 2011). It is particularly valuable for student trainees who may otherwise have no opportunity to work with diverse rural patients.

VTC Coordinator

The VTC coordinator at the client site facilitates VTC encounters and is most often the site's "champion." Due to the needs of clients, most telepsychology programs utilize a coordinator to deliver clinical services. The coordinator serves as the bridge between the therapist and the client/family at the client site. The coordinator assists by promoting the psychotherapy service, scheduling the consult, compiling intake packets, socializing the client/family to VTC, utilizing the technology, assisting during the consultation, and helping the client/family follow-up on recommendations. Thus, the coordinator requires the support of upper level administrators in completing these many tasks as they are often outside of typical responsibilities.

Multiple Informants

VTC links together the systems of care by connecting the therapist with schools, rural clinics, primary care offices, and other systems of care. Increased communication across technology systems represented by these multiple informants is a chief advantage of VTC. If the client is under the age of 18, the parent/guardian dictates who participates in psychotherapy visits, but generally welcomes these additional support personnel in developing and implementing the treatment plan. The VTC visit allows all involved individuals to contribute their unique perspective to the diagnostic and treatment puzzle. Communication occurs not only with the therapist but also with each other. For example, it is a frequent situation in school-based clinics that parents and teachers have had very little or no direct communication about the child's behavior in different settings or about family stressors that may be impacting the child's functioning. Machalicek et al. (2009) provide an innovative VTC application across multiple informants in the classroom setting. They compared a VTC-based intervention of functional analysis of behavior (FAB) to typical classroom instruction in a sample of two elementary school-aged children with autism. The authors reported that the FAB intervention delivered over VTC resulted in significant reductions in challenging behavior. The authors concluded that their results provide preliminary support for the use of VTC-based implementation of FAB for students with autism.

In addition, having multiple informants present in the assessment of an adult client presenting with dementia is advantageous. Staff caring for the client can report on successes and challenges regarding activities of daily living, and children of the client can discuss their observations of the parent from visit to visit, noting any changes in cognition or behavior. The therapist can then synthesize the information from the interview with testing outcomes in order to develop an appropriate treatment plan.

There are also challenges with the involvement of multiple informants, including integrating the volume of clinical input and making sure that the participants are socialized to the high standards of confidentiality associated with psychology services. Additionally, client sites must consider rooms large enough to accommodate many participants as well as strategies to manage the participants in and out of the VTC room. Overall, VTC promotes a shared perspective around the diagnosis and a collective responsibility for implementing a treatment plan to support the client.

What Constitutes Psychotherapy over VTC?

In describing the "what," or the content of psychotherapy services delivered over VTC, the authors will summarize the research literature. Therapists' use of VTC for psychotherapy, while still limited, is increasing. For instance, psychologists' use of this technology increased from 2% to 10% from 2000 to 2008 (American Psychological Association Center for Workforce Studies, APACWS, 2010). Comprehensive literature reviews inform the content of psychotherapy services over VTC (Grady et al., 2011; Richardson, Frueh, Grubaugh, Egede, & Elhai, 2009). VTC allows the client and the therapist to talk with each other and observe nonverbal behavior in real time, approximating the relationship developed in face-to-face traditional therapy. Overall, diagnostic efficacy studies have shown good reliability between most diagnoses over VTC and face-to-face with both children and adults, particularly when well-validated assessment tools are utilized. In addition, a growing body of research suggests that VTC services are comparable to face-to-face services regarding quality of care and client/provider satisfaction with VTC for psychotherapy services. Furthermore, VTC is thought to create a social presence that promotes familiarity, connectedness, and comfort discussing complex topics (Myers, Palmer, & Geyer, 2011; Nelson & Bui, 2010). While it takes creativity and forethought to provide VTC service, the evidence to date does not preclude any diagnosis or any therapy strategy (Grady et al., 2011). The key component has been taking the best strategies available in the face-to-face setting and applying these evidence-supported approaches over VTC. The following sections describe therapy approaches across common presenting concerns (*depression, anger management, posttraumatic stress disorder (PTSD) and anxiety disorders, eating disorders, and substance abuse*), but many of the lessons in therapy over VTC apply across diagnoses.

Depression

There is increasing evidence from randomized trials that VTC interventions yield similar results as face-to-face encounters. For instance, one study comparing face-to-face delivery of cognitive–behavioral therapy (CBT) to VTC delivery of CBT for childhood depression found no differences between groups' response to treatment (Nelson, Barnard, & Cain, 2003). Additionally, a recent literature review found that telemedicine-based interventions for depression appear to be as effective as face-to-face interventions (Garcia-Lizana & Munoz-Mayorga, 2010). Emerging literature suggests that it is feasible to utilize VTC for suicide assessment with veterans (Godleski, Nieves, Darkins, & Lehmann, 2008). In terms of the assessment of depression across modalities, Kobak, Williams, Jeglic, Salvucci, and Sharp (2008) compared the remote administration of the Montgomery–Asberg Depression Rating Scale via televideo, telephone, and face to-face administration. Participants with depression were interviewed twice. The first interview occurred via face-to face and the second was conducted by either videoconference or teleconference. The authors found no significant assessment differences.

Anger Management

A recent study by Morland et al. (2010) compared therapist adherence to a manualized, cognitive–behavioral treatment for anger management therapy delivered via VTC and face-to-face. The authors found that the delivery of the intervention was similar across groups and that the VTC modality did not compromise the therapist's ability to structure sessions or manage care. The most challenging area was developing therapeutic alliance across group members. Greene et al. (2010) suggest that consistent monitoring is crucial to ensure that alliance is developed across group members. Greene et al.'s study is unique because clinically meaningful results were observed among veterans with anger problems (and often co-occurring PTSD and/or depression), a population in which it is challenging to establish trust with providers. Moreover, it demonstrates the feasibility of using VTC to conduct group therapy which is highly novel.

Posttraumatic Stress Disorder

Similarly, CBT interventions delivered face-to-face and over VTC were equally effective in improving overall functioning for clients with PTSD (Frueh, Monnier et al., 2007; Germain, Marchand, Bouchard, Drouin, & Guay, 2009). All interventions aimed to adapt the same elements that are the standard of care in face-to-face settings. Tuerk, Yoder, Ruggiero, Gros, and Acierno (2010) implemented prolonged exposure (PE) treatment over VTC to a group of veterans with combat-related PTSD and found a large reduction in their symptoms of PTSD and depression. The authors concluded that their results support the feasibility and safety of the VTC modality for the treatment of PTSD. Additionally, Freuh's research team (Frueh, Monnier et al., 2007) compared therapist adherence to and competence with the Social and Emotional Rehabilitation, a group therapy-based intervention designed for veterans with PTSD, delivered via either VTC or face-to-face. The authors found no statistically significant differences in adherence between modalities. The only difference found was in regard to how the therapist introduced and explained a new "flexibility" exercise, resulting in more favorable ratings on this item for the VTC delivery.

Another study assessing VTC-based delivery of an anger management intervention for PTSD reported that participants in both the VTC and the face-to-face groups showed clinically meaningful reduction in their anger symptoms (Morland et al., 2010). Additionally, the authors found no significant differences between groups on process variables, such as attrition, adherence, satisfaction, and treatment expectancy. In a follow-up study assessing group process variables, Greene et al. (2010) reported a stronger therapeutic alliance with the therapist in the face-to-face group versus the VTC group. However, they noted that this reduction in alliance was not strong enough to result in inferior outcomes among the VTC participants.

Similarly, Germain et al. (2009) evaluated the quality of the therapeutic relationship between VTC and face-to-face implementation of CBT for PTSD across different traumas. Twenty-nine participants with PTSD received CBT treatment for PTSD via face-to-face and 17 participants received the same treatment via VTC. The CBT treatment occurred over a period of 16−25 weeks, depending upon the severity of the trauma, and consisted of psychoeducational information about PTSD, training on anxiety management, imaginary and in vivo exposure to avoided situations, and strategies to prevent a relapse. The authors found that the therapeutic alliance was well developed in both groups and that there were no significant differences between the two. The authors concluded that the therapeutic alliance is not harmed by VTC delivery of therapy for individuals with PTSD.

As with assessment of depression over VTC, assessment of PTSD over VTC has been found comparable efficacy to face-to-face assessment of PTSD. Using the Clinician-Administered PTSD Scale, Porcari et al. (2009) compared the mental health evaluation of 20 men with PTSD over VTC and traditional face-to-face. The authors found no significant differences in administration across modalities and a moderate working alliance for both conditions. The authors noted that although participants reported general satisfaction with the VTC condition, most reported a preference for face-to-face delivery. However, the authors also noted that the participants reported feeling comfortable utilizing video-based delivery if there were barriers to direct care.

Other Anxiety Disorders

For clients with panic disorder and agoraphobia, those who received psychotherapy via VTC were just as likely to improve as those who received face-to-face therapy (Bouchard et al., 2004). CBT was delivered once per week for 12 weeks and included case conceptualization, education about the cognitive model for panic, cognitive restructuring techniques to assist with interpretation of bodily sensations, interoceptive exposure, and exposure to agoraphobic situations. The last component was relapse prevention. O'Reilly et al. (2007) randomized a group of 496 psychiatric patients with mixed psychiatric diagnoses, including depression, bipolar disorder, adjustment disorder, general anxiety disorders, and psychosis to receive their consultation sessions over a 4-month period with psychiatrists via either VTC or face-to-face. The authors found no differences in Brief Symptom Inventory scores between randomized face-to-face or televideo consultations for clients. The authors also noted that the cost of providing psychiatric services via VTC was 10% less expensive than the traditional face-to-face modality.

Himle et al. (2006) implemented Exposure and Response Prevention (ERP) therapy via VTC for three patients with obsessive compulsive disorder (OCD) over 12 weeks. Traditionally, an ERP intervention involves exposing a client to a given stimulus that normally elicit a strong desire to implement a ritualistic response pattern and having the client inhibit that response pattern. The ERP intervention implemented in this study also included analysis of OCD symptoms, review of causes of OCD, cognitive approaches to handling OCD symptoms, strategies for making the intervention more effective, and lifestyle issues associated with CBT. Additionally, family members were encouraged to attend the first and last session as well as the sixth session which centered on OCD and family issues. The authors reported decreases in symptoms over time, based on Yale-Brown Obsessive Compulsive Inventory, that were equivalent to face-to-face intervention-related symptom decline. The authors also reported that the patients reported satisfaction with the VTC modality and noted high levels of "telepresence" which made them feel as though they were in the room with the therapist.

Griffiths, Blignault, and Yellowlees (2006) implemented a 6- to 8-week course of CBT over VTC for 15 patients with mixed psychiatric diagnoses, including generalized anxiety disorder, major depressive disorder, and panic disorder with agoraphobia. Elements of CBT covered over VTC differed by diagnosis but often included relaxation training, managing avoidance, structured problem-solving and coping with setbacks, controlling hyperventilation, graded exposure, improving sleep, increasing activity, and encouraging eating behaviors. The study also utilized case managers who observed the VTC delivery of the CBT intervention and reinforced the intervention in subsequent face-to-face sessions with their clients after the VTC sessions. Though the authors did not include a control group in which the intervention(s) was delivered via face-to-face, they reported that the intervention(s) delivered over VTC resulted in significant reduction in symptoms. Additionally, the authors reported that participants, therapists, and case managers reported average or above-average satisfaction with the VTC modality. The authors noted that their study demonstrated the efficacy of a 6- to 8-week course of CBT versus the traditional 12-week course; however, they acknowledged that this effect could be due to the role of the case manager reinforcing the intervention with the client in person after each VTC session. Additionally, a case study by Cowain (2001) reported that CBT for agoraphobia delivered via VTC resulted in reduction in anxiety and depressive symptoms over time.

Eating Disorders

Mitchell et al. (2008) conducted a randomized controlled trial to assess the efficacy and acceptability of a manualized CBT course for bulimia nervosa (BN) delivered via VTC. Participants received 20 sessions of CBT over 16 weeks. The authors reported that posttreatment abstinence rates (no binging or purging behaviors having occurred in the past 28 days) were somewhat higher for the face-to-face group as compared to the VTC group; however, the authors noted the differences were not statistically significant. The authors also reported that patients in the face-to-face group experienced significantly greater reductions in eating disordered cognitions and interview-assessed depression than the VTC group. Despite these group differences, the authors concluded that VTC delivery of CBT for BN was roughly equivalent to face-to-face delivery in efficacy and acceptance. In a follow-up study using the same data, Ertelt et al. (2011) examined whether treatment delivery method differentially affected therapist and client ratings of the therapeutic alliance. The authors found that patients did not indicate a preference for either delivery method in terms of their ratings of factors associated with the therapeutic alliance. However, the authors noted that therapists tended to favor the face-to-face delivery over the VTC delivery. Importantly, the authors noted patients reported feeling equally comfortable with both delivery methods and indicated that they could be successful with both methods of delivery.

Crow et al. (2009) assessed the cost-effectiveness of delivery CBT treatment for BN over VTC as compared to face-to-face delivery. The authors found that VTC delivery of CBT was more cost effective per abstinent participant than face-to-face delivery; however, the cost differential was mostly related to travel time. As such, the authors noted that this method of treatment delivery may be especially cost effective in rural versus urban areas. The authors concluded overall, however, that VTC approaches for eating disorder may be particularly well suited, given the limited number of specialized treatment centers even within urban areas.

Substance Abuse

Frueh, Henderson, and Myrick (2005) and Ikelheimer (2008) both demonstrated positive results with VTC-based psychotherapy interventions for substance abuse. Additionally, VTC-based cognitive assessments of persons with a history of alcohol use disorders were found to be similar to face-to-face assessments, and participants were satisfied with the VTC examination (Kirkwood, Peck, & Bennie, 2006). Similarly, with respect to participant satisfaction, Baca and Manuel (2007) compared the delivery of motivational interviewing over VTC, telephone, and face-to-face in a sample of 29 self-identified problem drinkers. The authors found that participants were overall satisfied with all three methods of delivery of intervention. However, when asked to name their preferred method of delivery, the majority of participants (64.3%) chose VTC over audio (telephone) delivery of the intervention. Similarly, the study by King et al. (2009) comparing VTC-based delivery of intensified substance abuse counseling (*Getgoing*) versus traditional face-to-face reported that patients expressed a preference for the VTC-based service, noting the convenience and increased confidentiality as major reasons. A case study of an exposure-based intervention for pathological gambling delivered over VTC also reflected these reports of participant satisfaction with the mode of delivery (Oakes,

Battersby, Pols, & Cromarty, 2008), with the participant in this study reporting the VTC to be of great benefit and not distressing or anxiety-provoking.

Another example involves the use of VTC to assist with substance abuse prevention and treatment on rural college campuses. The authors are currently working on a VTC project of this nature. We are fortunate to have an array of affordable technology options available for the generally technology-friendly population including room-based VTC to the student health centers, PC-based VTC to the student's dorm or living arrangement, and VTC available through the students mobile tablet devices. In addition, there are numerous other technologies available that have the potential to support mental health on campuses, including e-mail, text messaging, virtual worlds, and social media. It remains an empirical question which set of interventions are best delivered by which technology (or technologies) for the individual rural college student, depending on their substance abuse needs (e.g., prevention, early intervention, and intensive treatment), co-occurring chronic health concerns (e.g., depression, diabetes, and obesity), personal preferences, therapist guidance/comfort, and safety concerns. Despite the many technology options, there are daunting workforce issues in having enough health professionals trained in substance abuse treatment in order to meet student demand in a timely fashion.

Additional Therapy Strategies over VTC

In addition to psychotherapy, therapists can complete not only psychotherapy over VTC but also the full range of support. This ranges from assisting patients with adherence to psychotropics over VTC (Fortney et al., 2006; Frangou, Sachpazidis, Stassinakis, & Sakas, 2005) to supporting psychoeducational components over VTC (Klaus, 2011). An emerging use of VTC is support for caregivers. Demiris, Oliver, Wittenberg-Lyles, and Washington (2011) provided problem-solving therapy for informal hospice caregivers over videophones. In addition to high levels of satisfaction with the CBT intervention, caregivers reported a slightly higher quality of life postintervention as well as lower levels of anxiety. Another newer technology-assisted application involves using the Internet to deliver parent–child interaction therapy directly to the home. Parents use a web camera and Bluetooth earpiece device to receive live, unobtrusive coaching from a therapist at the provider site (Comer, McNeil, & Eyberg 2011).

How is Psychotherapy over VTC Implemented?

While emerging research and VTC consensus guidelines provide direction, therapists using VTC must also refer to overall guidelines for ethical practice (Reed, McLaughlin, & Millholland, 2000). For example, the American Psychological Association, APA (2010) advises that psychologists "…take reasonable steps to ensure the competence of their work and to protect clients, students, supervisees, research participants, organizational clients, and others from harm". Consensus guidelines encourage transparency about VTC practice in dialogue with clients as well as the informed consent. Risks/benefits of therapy overall and VTC in particular are discussed over time in the context of the therapeutic relationship. Other treatment options within the community as well as travel to a medical center are noted in an attempt to encourage client choice, although this is difficult when there are few local options.

In addition to following ethical guidelines, therapists must think creatively about how to adapt the session needs to the VTC setting in order to approximate best practices, such as faxing handouts or supplying books to the client site ahead of the session (Shepherd et al., 2006). For example, homework required during CBT such as thought logs could be faxed or e-mailed to the provider site on the day of the session. Furthermore, the same good communication skills used on-site are even more important with VTC clients. It is important that the therapist is confident with the technology ahead of seeing patients in order to build a strong therapeutic alliance just as in on-site clinics. VTC etiquette includes rapport-building strategies and simple adaptations. For example, an adult client with depression was encouraged to reengage in photography to increase positive activities. The client brought in photos from her class and was able to show over the VTC system. Some programs have utilized innovative solutions such as a joint whiteboard, but lower cost measures such as mailing common materials/books is often beneficial (Jerome & Zaylor, 2000). Creativity and flexibility before, during, and after the psychotherapy visit facilitate relationship building just as in the face-to-face setting.

The therapist has less control of the physical environment at the client sites and works with the coordinator to develop a client-friendly room. The VTC office supports therapists with strategies to maximize the quality of the VTC encounter. Current VTC speeds have decreased the pixilation/tiling associated with earlier VTC and technical difficulties have decreased over time. The VTC office or coordinator assists with camera angle, monitor selection, and positioning to facilitate communication. Lighting is also important to clearly see facial expressions and affective responses. Therapists are encouraged to check in with clients to make sure that clients can see and hear therapists as anticipated. Just as important as technology encryption, it is important to establish the VTC room as a confidential clinical space. It is important that therapists scan the room at the client site to note who is present but not immediately visible on screen. Simple strategies such as signage noting the need for quiet can assist with establishing this expectation. The technology has some benefits not seen in the face-to-face setting, such as the ability to unobtrusively zoom in and note physical presentations, such as tics, gait, or in one case, suspected presence of Huntington's symptoms. While the technology has the ability to tape sessions, the therapists discuss with clients that sessions are not videotaped or archived in any way without the client knowledge and consent.

At the first VTC visit, the therapist and the VTC coordinator may complete paperwork with the client and socialize the client to the VTC format. For example, clients with dementia are socialized to the VTC equipment while accompanied by family and friends because comfort is facilitated by familiarity in this population. For these clients, it is important to identify any preexisting tendency toward hallucinations as this would preclude a successful VTC encounter. The introduction also includes a backup plan in case of technology difficulties (usually the telephone), as well as a safety plan should any concerns arise during the evaluation. For non-English-speaking VTC participants, a medical interpreter assists with this introductory description and throughout the session as needed.

Protocols drive the "how" of the VTC clinic. The authors include here a brief sample protocol for psychotherapy over VTC, but elements must be tailored to each VTC clinic. An example of key protocol components includes the following:

- The client's doctor or the client requests a VTC consult with a therapist trained in providing psychotherapy for depression. The VTC coordinator socializes the client to the VTC process and to psychotherapy.
- The VTC coordinator schedules appointment with the VTC office.
- The VTC coordinator distributes paperwork to the client and faxes back completed paperwork at least 1 week before the appointment. The VTC clinic utilizes the same history/ intake form, consents, HIPAA forms, and questionnaires as the traditional clinic setting. The client is required to have an identified primary care provider or be in the process of seeing a primary care provider ahead of the appointment.
- Rating scales are scored before the appointment and distributed to the clinical team for review. A completed intake is placed in the client's medical record at the therapist's site.
- On the appointment day, the site coordinator establishes the VTC connection and assists throughout the appointment with the client.
- Diagnoses and recommendations are shared with the client and faxed to the site coordinator. Recommendations may include continuing treatment over VTC as well as referral to community resources.

While the protocol details change based on the individual community and particular client site, the core elements remain the same. The protocol highlights the goal to approximate face-to-face services by completing the same intake as on-site clients. Protocols are updated over time and include backup plans with the local VTC coordinator in the event the client reports suicidal, homicidal, abuse, or other safety concerns. As in traditional settings, expectations concerning therapist coverage should be outlined within the informed consent. In addition to the safety plans, the informed consent delineates who the client should contact with crisis needs. As in the traditional clinic setting, it is important to socialize clients and families to the mental health system and client rights as well as responsibilities. VTC technicians assist with installation of equipment, training personnel at both the provider site and the outreach sites, and supporting personnel when technical problems arise. The VTC coordinator assists with scheduling the rooms, monitoring completion of the intake packet, and testing the equipment with new sites or sites that have been inactive to ensure the equipment if functioning adequately. While electronic health records (EHRs) have been described as the "vision for the future of psychotherapy practice," very few outreach clinics have adopted EHR for mental health purposes (Bray, 2009; Substance Abuse and Mental Health Services Administration, SAMHSA, 2011). Across EHRs and paper files at the client sites and the provider sites, it is crucial to have clear protocols for how the many personnel involved in telemedicine encounters send, receive, and maintain confidential protected health information.

Reimbursement is another important "how" of sustaining psychotherapy services over VTC. Mental health professionals have used varied initial funding for VTC, including institutional seed money, community and foundational support, state grants, federal funding, billing reimbursement, and contractual agreements. The ability to approximate face-to-face care led the Centers for Medicare and Medicaid Services and other insurers to reimburse VTC services (Centers for Medicare and Medicaid Services, CMMS, 2010). Thus, at least a half dozen states have legislative requirements that VTC services be reimbursed comparably to a face-to-face visit. A growing number of third-party insurers reimburse VTC services, including Medicare, the majority of state Medicaid policies, and many private insurers. Most individual therapy, group therapy, and health and behavior current procedural terminology (CPT) codes are covered over VTC (Centers for Medicare and Medicaid Services, CMMS, 2011) with the addition of the GT modifier (services occuring via interactive audio and video telecommunications system) to the billing code to denote the VTC delivery, including newer coverage related to the health areas including behavioral interventions for smoking cessation and newer sites including nursing home facilities. In addition, services are covered in some venues but not others. Some client sites are eligible for Medicare/Medicaid's originating site fees related to the VTC coordinator assistance, currently about US$27/client (Centers for Medicare and Medicaid Services, CMMS, 2010); see also http://www.telehealthresourcecenter.org/). Billing reimbursement is an important step in VTC sustainability, but the same challenges seen in on-site billing for mental health services remain over VTC. Another option is contractual agreements between the client sites and the therapists in order to cover both therapist time and related costs (e.g., line charges and office management).

There is limited state and national guidance concerning licensing specific to VTC practice. Without guidance, this creates a circular situation in which the lack of guidance potentially limits psychotherapy practice and the lack of volume does not make practice guidance a priority. Only a handful of state regulations mention VTC practice and this is not specific to the mental health arena. For example, Ohio psychologists have taken a leadership role across technologies and encourage best practices with existing regulations when using VTC and other technologies in practice (see www.ohpsych.org). Psychologists should consult their own state regulations concerning licensing implications related to the state in which they practice and the state in which the client is located (Harris & Younggren, 2011). Malpractice options are often covered under existing policies as well as options for VTC-specific coverage.

Conclusion

The lessons learned in VTC implementation, especially the importance of communication across client/family, therapist, and support staff, remain vitally important in successfully delivering psychotherapy over VTC. It is key to put the "how" and "what" of VTC practice within the context of the need in the community and the population to be served. The next vista is to match empirically supported treatments with technology delivery systems and tailor these strategies to best fit the individual clients within their unique community. Overall, the literature to date supports the use of VTC for the delivery of evidence-supported therapies, and satisfaction and outcomes have been similar to the face-to-face setting, although continued research is needed to better understand the unique benefits and challenges of VTC practice (Grady et al., 2011). Importantly, client satisfaction appears to be high, especially among those who otherwise may not receive treatment due to distance, cost, or other barriers.

It is an exciting time for VTC, with both federal agencies (Substance Abuse and Mental Health Services Administration, SAMHSA, 2011) and mental health associations (Vasquez, 2011) including goals around telehealth. Many new health technologies are emerging for mental health purposes, ranging from store-and-forward technology (Yellowlees et al., 2010) to mobile technologies (Clough & Casey, 2011), including secure videoconferencing on tablets and other devices. The future may see VTC paired with other technologies to deliver a stronger intervention maximizing each technology's benefit (Mohr, 2009). With such integration comes the potential for new paradigms of care that leverage the unique strengths offered by telecommunication technologies, but the same questions of who, what, where, and why will remain important related to the purpose of approximating face-to-face billable services and insuring the continued safety of clients when using technology for psychotherapy (see Chapter 4).

References

American Psychological Association, APA. *The critical need for psychologists in rural America.* (2007). <http://www.apa.org/about/gr/education/rural-need.aspx/> Accessed 20.10.11.

American Psychological Association, APA. *American Psychological Association ethical principles of psychologists and code of conduct.* (2010). <http://www.apa.org/ethics/code/index.aspx/> Accessed 20.10.11.

American Psychological Association Center for Workforce Studies, APACWS (2010). Telepsychology is on the rise. *Monitor on Psychology, 41,* 11.

Baca, C., & Manuel, J. (2007). Satisfaction with long-distance motivational interviewing for problem drinking. *Addictive Disorders and Their Treatment, 6,* 39–41.

Bouchard, S., Paquin, B., Payeur, R., Allard, M., Rivard, V., Fournier, T., et al. (2004). Delivering cognitive–behavior therapy for panic disorder with agoraphobia in videoconference. *Telemedicine Journal and e-Health, 10,* 13–25.

Bray, J. H. (2009). The future of psychological science. *Monitor on Psychology, 40,* 5.

Centers for Medicare and Medicaid Services, CMMS. (2010). *CMS final rule.* <http://www.ofr.gov/OFRUpload/OFRData/2010-27969_PI.pdf/> Accessed 20.10.11.

Centers for Medicare and Medicaid Services, CMMS (2011). *Telehealth service: Rural health fact sheet series.* Department of Health and Human Services. Revised March 2011. <https://www.cms.gov/MLNProducts/downloads/TelehealthSrvcsfctsht.pdf/>.

Clough, B. A., & Casey, L. M. (2011). Technological adjuncts to enhance current psychotherapy practices: A review. *Clinical Psychology Review, 31*, 279−292.

Comer, J. S., McNeil, C. B., & Eyberg, S. M. (2011). Development of an Internet-delivered protocol for in-home parent−child interaction therapy. In *45th Annual meeting of the association for behavioral and cognitive therapies.* Toronto, ON, Canada.

Cowain, T. (2001). Cognitive−behavioural therapy via videoconferencing to a rural area. *Austrailian and New Zealand Journal of Psychiatry, 35*, 62−64.

Crow, S. J., Mitchell, J. E., Crosby, R. D., Swanson, S. A., Wonderlich, S., & Lancanster, K. (2009). The cost effectiveness of cognitive behavioral therapy for bulimia nervosa delivered via telemedicine versus face-to-face. *Behavior Research and Therapy, 47*, 451−453.

Davis, G. L., Boulger, J. G., Hovland, J. C., & Hoven, N. T. (2007). The integration of a telemental health service into rural primary medical care. *Journal of Agricultural Safety and Health, 13*, 237−246.

Demiris, G., Oliver, D. P., Wittenberg-Lyles, E., & Washington, K. (2011). Use of videophones to deliver a cognitive−behavioural therapy to hospice caregivers. *Journal of Telemedicine and Telecare, 17*, 142−145.

Ertelt, T. W., Crosby, R. D., Marino, J. M., Mitchell, J. E., Lancaster, K., & Crow, S. J. (2011). Therapeutic factors affecting the cognitive behavioral treatment of bulimia nervosa via telemedicine versus face-to-face delivery. *The International Journal of Eating Disorders, 44*, 687−691.

Fortney, J. C., Pyne, J. M., Edlund, M. J., Robinson, D. E., Mittal, D., & Henderson, K. L. (2006). Design and implementation of the telemedicine-enhanced antidepressant management study. *General Hospital Psychiatry, 28*, 18−26.

Frangou, S., Sachpazidis, I., Stassinakis, A., & Sakas, G. (2005). Telemonitoring of medication adherence in patients with schizophrenia. *Telemedicine Journal of e-Health, 11*, 675−683.

Frueh, B. C., Henderson, S., & Myrick, H. (2005). Telehealth service delivery for persons with alcoholism. *Journal of Telemedicine and Telecare, 11*, 372−375.

Frueh, B. C., Monnier, J., Grubaugh, A. L., Elhai, J. D., Yim, E., & Knapp, R. (2007). Therapist adherence and competence with manualized cognitive−behavioral therapy for PTSD delivered via videoconferencing technology. *Behavior Modification, 31*, 856−866.

Garcia-Lizana, F., & Munoz-Mayorga, I. (2010). Telemedicine for depression: A systematic review. *Perspectives in Psychiatric Care, 46*, 119−126.

Germain, V., Marchand, A., Bouchard, S., Drouin, M. S., & Guay, S. (2009). Effectiveness of cognitive behavioural therapy administered by videoconference for posttraumatic stress disorder. *Cognitive Behavioral Therapy, 38*, 42−53.

Godleski, L., Nieves, J. E., Darkins, A., & Lehmann, L. (2008). VA telemental health: Suicide assessment. *Behavior Science Law, 26*, 271−286.

Grady, B., Myers, K. M., Nelson, E. L., Belz, N., Bennett, L., Carnahan, L., et al. (2011). Evidence-based practice for telemental health. *Telemedicne Journal and e-Health, 17*, 131−148.

Greene, C. J., Morland, L. A., Macdonald, A., Frueh, B. C., Grubbs, K. M., & Rosen, C. S. (2010). How does tele-mental health affect group therapy process? Secondary analysis of a noninferiority trial. *Journal of Consulting and Clinical Psychology, 78*, 746−750.

Griffiths, L., Blignault, I., & Yellowlees, P. (2006). Telemedicine as a means of delivering cognitive−behavioural therapy to rural and remote mental health clients. *Journal of Telemedicine and Telecare, 12*, 136−140.

Harris, E., & Younggren, J. N. (2011). Risk management in the digital world. *Professional Psychology: Research and Practice, 42,* 412–418.

Himle, J. A., Fischer, D. J., Muroff, J. R., Van Etten, M. L., Lokers, L. M., Abelson, J. L., et al. (2006). Videoconferencing-based cognitive–behavioral therapy for obsessive-compulsive disorder. *Behavior Research and Therapy, 44,* 1821–1829.

Ikelheimer, D. M. (2008). Treatment of opioid dependence via home-based telepsychiatry. *Psychiatric Services, 59,* 1218–1219.

Jacobsen, S. E., Sprenger, T., Andersson, S., & Krogstad, J. M. (2003). Neuropsychological assessment and telemedicine: A preliminary study examining the reliability of neuropsychology services performed via telecommunication. *Journal of the International Neuropsychological Society, 9,* 472–478.

Jennett, P. A., Gagnon, M. P., & Brandstadt, H. K. (2005). Preparing for success: Readiness models for rural telehealth. *Journal of Postgraduate Medicine, 51,* 279–285.

Jerome, L. W., & Zaylor, C. (2000). Cyberspace: Creating a therapeutic environment for telehealth applications. *Professional Psychology Research and Practice, 31,* 478–483.

King, V. L., Stoller, K. B., Kidorf, M., Kindbom, K., Hursh, S., Brady, T., et al. (2009). Assessing the effectiveness of an Internet-based videoconferencing platform for delivering intensified substance abuse counseling. *Journal of Substance Abuse and Treatment, 36,* 331–338.

Kirkwood, K., Peck, D., & Bennie, L. (2006). The consistency of neuropsychological assessments performed via telecommunication and face to face. *Journal of Telemedicine and Telecare, 6,* 147–151.

Klaus, N. (2011). *Teletherapy for children with mood disorders: Feasibility of adapting an evidence based treatment for videoconference delivery.* Powerpoint session presented at the psychiatry grand rounds of University of Kansas Medical School in Wichita, Wichita, KS.

Kobak, K. A., Williams, J. B., Jeglic, E., Salvucci, D., & Sharp, I. R. (2008). Face-to-face versus remote administration of the Montgomery–Asberg Depression Rating Scale using videoconference and telephone. *Depression and Anxiety, 25,* 913–919.

Machalicek, W., O'Reilly, M., Chan, J., Lang, R., Rispoli, M., Davis, T., et al. (2009). Using videoconferencing to conduct functional analysis of challenging behavior and develop classroom behavioral support plans for students with autism. *Education and Training in Developmental Disabilities, 44,* 207–217.

Mitchell, J. E., Crosby, R. D., Wonderlich, S. A., Crow, S., Lancaster, K., Simonich, H., et al. (2008). A randomized trial comparing the efficacy of cognitive–behavioral therapy for bulimia nervosa delivered via telemedicine versus face-to-face. *Behavior Research and Therapy, 46,* 581–592.

Mohatt, D. F., Bradley, M. M., Adams, S. J., & Morris, C. D. (2006). *Mental health and rural America: 1994–2005.* US Department of Health and Human Services. <ftp://ftp.hrsa.gov/ruralhealth/RuralMentalHealth.pdf/>.

Mohr, D. C. (2009). Telemental health: Reflections on how to move the field forward. *Clinical Psychology Science and Practice, 16,* 343–347.

Morland, L. A., Greene, C. J., Rosen, C. S., Foy, D., Reilly, P., Shore, J., et al. (2010). Telemedicine for anger management therapy in a rural population of combat veterans with posttraumatic stress disorder: A randomized noninferiority trial. *Journal of Clinical Psychiatry, 71,* 855–863.

Myers, K. M., Cain, S., & Work Group on Quality Issues of the American Academy of Child and Adolescent Psychiatry (2008). Practice parameter for telepsychiatry with children and adolescents. *Journal of the American Academy of Child and Adolescent Psychiatry, 47,* 1468–1483.

Myers, K. M., Palmer, N. B., & Geyer, J. R. (2011). Research in child and adolescent telemental health. *Child and Adolescent Psychiatric Clinics of North America, 20,* 155–171.

Nelson, E. L., Barnard, M., & Cain, S. (2003). Treating childhood depression over videoconferencing. *Telemedicine Journal and e-Health, 9,* 49–55.

Nelson, E. L., & Bui, T. (2010). Rural telepsychology services for children and adolescents. *Journal of Clinical Psychology, 66,* 490–501.

Nelson, E. L., Bui, T., & Sharp, S. (2011). Telemental health competencies: Training examples from a youth depression VTC clinic. In M. Gregerson (Ed.), *Techniques and technologies for medical and graduate education* (pp. 41–48). New York, NY: Springer.

Nelson, E. L., & Velasquez, S. E. (2011). Implementing psychological services over telemedicine. *Professional Psychology Research and Practice, 42,* 535–542.

O'Reilly, R., Bishop, J., Maddox, K., Hutchinson, L., Fisman, M., & Takhar, J. (2007). Is telepsychiatry equivalent to face-to-face psychiatry? Results from a randomized controlled equivalence trial. *Psychiatric Services, 58,* 836–843.

Oakes, J., Battersby, M. W., Pols, R. G., & Cromarty, P. (2008). Exposure therapy for problem gambling via videoconferencing: A case report. *Journal of Gambling Studies, 24,* 107–118.

Porcari, C. E., Amdur, R. L., Koch, E. I., Richard, D. C., Favorite, T., Martis, B., et al. (2009). Assessment of post-traumatic stress disorder in veterans by videoconferencing and by face-to-face methods. *Journal of Telemedicine and Telecare, 15,* 89–94.

Reed, G. M., McLaughlin, C. J., & Millholland, K. (2000). Ten interdisciplinary principles for professional practice in telehealth. *Professional Psychology Research and Practice, 31,* 170–178.

Richardson, L. K., Frueh, B. C., Grubaugh, A. L., Egede, L., & Elhai, J. D. (2009). Current directions in videoconferencing tele-mental health research. *Clinical Psychology (New York), 16,* 323–338.

Sharp, I. R., Kobak, K. A., & Osman, D. A. (2011). The use of videoconferencing with patients with psychosis: A review of the literature. *Annals of General Psychiatry, 10,* 1–11.

Shepherd, L., Goldstein, D., Whitford, H., Thewes, B., Brummell, V., & Hicks, M. (2006). The utility of videoconferencing to provide innovative delivery of psychological treatment for rural cancer patients: Results of a pilot study. *Journal of Pain Symptom Management, 32,* 453–461.

Shore, J. H., & Manson, S. M. (2005). A developmental model for rural telepsychiatry. *Psychiatric Services, 56,* 976–980.

Simpson, J., Doze, S., Urness, D., Hailey, D., & Jacobs, P. (2001). Telepsychiatry as a routine service—the perspective of the patient. *Journal of Telemedicine and Telecare, 7,* 155–160.

Substance Abuse and Mental Health Services Administration, SAMHSA (2007). *An action plan on behavioral health workforce development.* Washington, DC: US Government Printing Office.

Substance Abuse and Mental Health Services Administration, SAMHSA.*Leading change: A plan for SAMHSA's roles and actions 2011–2014.* (2011). <http://store.samhsa.gov/product/SMA11-4629/> Accessed 10.11.11.

Szeftel, R., Mandelbaum, S., Sulman-Smith, H., Naqvi, S., Lawrence, L., Szeftel, Z., et al. (2011). Telepsychiatry for children with developmental disabilities: Applications for patient care and medical education. *Child and Adolescent Psychiatric Clinics of North America, 20,* 95–111.

Tuerk, P., Yoder, M., Ruggiero, K., Gros, D., & Acierno, R. (2010). A pilot study of prolonged exposure therapy for posttraumatic stress disorder delivered via telehealth technology. *Journal of Traumatic Stress, 23,* 116–123.

Van Allen, J., Davis, A. M., & Lassen, S. (2011). The use of telemedicine in pediatric psychology: Research review and current applications. *Child and Adolescent Psychiatric Clinics of North America, 20,* 55–66.

Vasquez, M. J. (2011). Monitor columns by Dr. Vasquez. <http://www.apa.org/about/governance/president/index.aspx/> Accessed 10.11.11.

Yellowlees, P. M., Odor, A., Parish, M. B., Iosif, A. M., Haught, K., & Hilty, D. (2010). A feasibility study of the use of asynchronous telepsychiatry for psychiatric consultations. *Psychiatric Services, 61,* 838–840.

Yellowlees, P., Shore, J., & Roberts, L. (2009). *Practice guidelines for videoconferencing-based telemental health.* < http://www.americantelemed.org/i4a/pages/index.cfm?pageid=3311 > .

16 Special Considerations for Conducting Psychopharmacologic Treatment over Videoteleconferencing

Carol M. Rockhill[a,b,]*

[a]Department of Psychiatry and Behavioral Sciences, University of Washington School of Medicine, Seattle, WA, [b]Outpatient Child and Adolescent Psychiatry, Seattle Children's Hospital, Seattle, WA

Introduction

Psychiatry is a medical specialty well suited for delivery of health-care services via videoteleconferencing (VTC). Psychiatric evaluation and treatment depends largely upon a combination of observation, patient report, and collateral information from family members and other close contacts. The elements of the clinical examination can be readily ascertained through the visual and auditory media provided by VTC. The shortage of psychiatrists means that only a fraction of patients who need psychiatric care can find providers (Gabel, 2009; K. C. Thomas, Ellis, Konrad, Holzer, & Morrissey, 2009), with those in urban areas more likely to obtain care. The Institute of Medicine and the National Research Council (IOM/NRC) (2004) report argued that maximizing child health is critical to assuring national well-being. The IOM/NCR report highlighted the critical issues of availability, use and quality of health-care services, especially for those with special health-care needs and advocated for a comprehensive national strategy to make better use of existing resources and to identify the need for new methods and indicators. More recent reports from this group include a call to address the lack of access to care for vulnerable populations (McCormick et al., 2011). In addition, the President's New Freedom Commission in 2003 called for transformation of the public mental health system to one focusing on person-centered, recovery-focused, evidence-based, and quality-driven care (United States Department of Health and Human Services,

*Corresponding author: Carol M. Rockhill, Department of Psychiatry and Behavioral Sciences, University of Washington School of Medicine, Seattle, WA. Tel.: +1-206-987-2164, Fax: +1-425-637-5945, E-mail: carol.rockhill@seattlechildrens.org

Telemental Health. DOI: http://dx.doi.org/10.1016/B978-0-12-416048-4.00016-6

2003). Subsequent reports from the committee focus on the need for a community approach to preventing and treating illness, promoting well-being, and the need for accessibility of services (Power, 2009). The use of VTC has the potential to answer these calls.

A core component of evidence-based mental health care is pharmacological treatment. This chapter focuses on the guidelines for providing pharmacotherapy via VTC, generally referred to as telepsychiatry. To avoid confusion and to be specific, the term telemental health is used to refer to broad issues of mental health care, including therapy, provided through VTC, and the term telemedicine is used to refer to medical issues addressed through VTC. The fields of telepsychiatry, telemental health, and telemedicine are expanding rapidly and the state-of-the-art material presented here will likely need updating in the near future.

Background: The Case for Telepsychiatry

The evidence-base establishing telemental health as an effective vehicle for service delivery is growing. Most investigations have focused on access to services, the ability of providers to establish a therapeutic relationship through telemental health, and factors related to acceptability of this approach to patients, referring providers, and telemental health clinicians. The evidence-base for telepsychiatric services is reviewed below.

Access to Care

Telepsychiatry is generally requested when a community experiences a shortage of psychiatrists and seeks to increase access to services close to home, especially for individuals with chronic mental illness (Blackmon, Kaak, & Ranseen, 1997; Elford et al., 2000; Hilty, Cobb, Neufeld, Bourgeois, & Yellowlees, 2008; Hilty, Sison, Nesbitt, & Hales, 2000; Lopez, Avery, Krupinski, Lazarus, & Weinstein, 2005; Myers, Sulzbacher, & Melzer, 2004; Nelson, Barnard, & Cain, 2003; Saeed, Diamond, & Bloch, 2011). Lack of access to care is particularly challenging for individuals who are of low-income status and reside in rural areas (Institute of Medicine (IOM), 2004; MacDowell, Glasser, Fitts, Nielsen, & Hunsaker, 2010; K. C. Thomas et al., 2009; United States Department of Health and Human Services (USDHHS), National Advisory Committee on Rural Health and Human Services, 2004) as they do not have the means to commute to distant medical centers to obtain needed care, particularly ongoing care. The local primary care physician (PCP) becomes their default psychiatric provider. Tele-consultation to PCPs has been shown to be effective to provide support and improving PCPs' knowledge base for providing evidenced-based care to underserved populations (Lopez et al., 2005; Saeed et al., 2011) but is typically not reimbursed by insurance companies, making it difficult to sustain. Telepsychiatry services, in which psychiatrists provide direct care to patients via VTC, is a more sustainable option.

Establishing a Therapeutic Relationship

The overall issues relating to the establishment of therapeutic rapport and working alliance in telemental health are discussed in Chapter 3. This section covers the most salient aspects of rapport as related to prescribing psychiatric medications. Prescribing in telepsychiatry is neither about the technology nor about the medications. It is about taking care of people and empowering them to participate in decisions about their care. A telepsychiatry appointment includes supportive therapy and problem-solving in addition to medication decision-making and may also include other forms of therapy such as cognitive behavioral therapy. Establishing a therapeutic relationship is particularly important to build patients' confidence in the diagnosis and medication plan made by a psychiatrist they may be meeting for the first time. Considerable evidence supports the ability to establish a therapeutic relationship via VTC (Appel, Bleiberg, & Noiseuz, 2002; Fortney et al., 2007; Frueh et al., 2007; Gros et al., 2011; Hilty, Nesbit, Marks, & Callahan, 2002; Mitchell et al., 2008; Morland et al., 2010; Neufeld, Yellowlees, Hilty, Cobb, & Bourgeois, 2004; Ruskin et al., 2004).

Given the intimacy of the contact that patients have with their psychiatrists, primary concerns about the delivery of evaluation and treatment services through telepsychiatry include the patients' need to feel comfortable with the interactions, the patients' need to feel confident about the confidentiality of the information gathered, and the need for the management of symptoms and treatment to be well coordinated despite the distance between the coordinating sites. Differences in the interactions between clinicians and patients evaluated via telepsychiatry versus in person have been summarized by Hilty, Nesbit et al. (2002). Their review of the literature found both advantages and disadvantages of telepsychiatry. The chief advantages were the increased access to care and opportunities for education. Disadvantages for telepsychiatrists compared to psychiatrists consulting in person included noticing fewer nonverbal cues and requiring increased time needed to convey the same information. There was also an increased requirement for collaboration and coordination among parties involved in treatment, including the patient, the referring PCP, and the psychiatrist. Some accommodations must be made for these potential disadvantages. However, it should also be noted that no clinical condition has been deemed contraindicated for treatment through telepsychiatry specifically or telemental health more generally. Patients with most psychiatric illnesses have been treated through telepsychiatry, including severe disorders such as psychosis and mood disorders (Ruskin et al., 2004; Zarate et al., 1997). In addition, patients with hearing impairments are readily treated using sign language (S. Gibson, personal communication, 2012; J. Petersen, personal communication, 2012).

Additional evidence supporting the ability to establish therapeutic rapport during telemental health sessions comes from the success of psychotherapy interventions delivered through VTC. Several important studies have shown comparability of outcomes in the comparison of care provided through telemental health and in-person service delivery (Hilty, Nesbit et al., 2002; Neufeld et al., 2004; Ruskin et al., 2004). There is also evidence of equivalency of outcomes when receiving teletherapy for specific conditions such as self-regulation of chronic pain (Appel et al., 2002), treatment of depression (Fortney et al., 2007; Nelson, Barnard, & Cain, 2003; Ruskin et al., 2004), exposure-based therapy for participants with or at risk for posttraumatic stress disorder (Frueh et al., 2007; Gros et al., 2011), anger management therapy for participants with posttraumatic stress disorder (Morland et al., 2010), and for the treatment of bulimia (Mitchell et al., 2008). For telepsychiatry specifically, including medication management, psychoeducation, and supportive therapy, outcomes have also been found to be equivalent to in-person care (O'Reilly et al., 2007; Zaylor, 1999). These positive outcomes support the ability to establish therapeutic rapport in telepsychiatry and telemental health practice.

Feasibility and Acceptability of Telepsychiatry

An emerging literature regarding the use of telepsychiatry services indicates that both adult and youth patients are satisfied with treatment that is delivered through telepsychiatry (Appel et al., 2002; Bishop, O'Reilly, Maddox, & Hutchinson, 2002; Myers, Valentine, & Melzer, 2007; Myers, Valentine, Morganthaler, & Melzer, 2006; Nelson, Bui, & Velasquez, 2011; Ruskin et al., 2004). In addition, referring providers of adults (Hilty, Yellowlees et al., 2006) and children (Myers, Valentine, & Melzer, 2007) report satisfaction with the services their patients have received through telepsychiatry. Delivery of psychoeducation to referring providers has been shown to improve the knowledge base and skills of the referring providers regarding mental health treatment over time (Hilty, Yellowlees et al., 2006), suggesting that a good professional working relationship can be established through VTC.

One concern about the acceptability of telepsychiatry is that selection bias may result in significant differences in the patient populations and diagnostic groups served in person versus via telepsychiatry. Evidence to date does not support such differences. In fact, there is a striking commonality in the range of diagnoses given when comparing telepsychiatry with in-person care (Hilty, Nesbit et al., 2002; Myers, Sulzbacher, & Melzer, 2004; Singh, Arya, & Peters, 2007) and compared to the rates of psychiatric disorders in national samples (Myers, Valentine, & Melzer, 2007). Furthermore, studies have shown that assessment measures can be administered reliably via VTC (Zarate et al., 1997). As noted above, clinical outcomes for patients have been found to be similar across in-person and telepsychiatry care for similar diagnoses and procedures (O'Reilly et al., 2007; Zaylor, 1999). In addition, unpublished data from the Northern Arizona Regional Behavioral Health Association, a national model for providing telepsychiatry care, supports the equivalence of in-person versus telepsychiatry care across different clinics and treatment providers in the areas of medical costs, hospitalization rates, use of multiple pharmacologic agents, medication utilization, and functional and symptom improvement (NARBHA web site, Northern Arizona Regional Medical Health Authority (NARBHA), 2012; S. Gibson, personal communication, 2012). Therefore, the available data provide evidence that individuals evaluated and treated through telepsychiatry are similar to those treated in person.

Another concern regarding the feasibility and acceptability of telepsychiatry is cultural competence. Often the telepsychiatrist differs racially or ethnically from the patients residing in areas that are most underserved. This raises questions as to whether racial or cultural differences may pose barriers to care. However, current work suggests that this barrier is surmountable, as telepsychiatry has been used successfully across many racial and ethnic patient populations, including with patients of African–American (Cain & Spaulding, 2006), Hispanic (Harper, 2009), Native American (Savin, Garry, Zuccaro, & Novins, 2006; Shore et al., 2008), Chinese American (Yeung, Hails, Chang, Trinh, & Fava, 2011), and Hawaiian (Alicata, Guerrero, & Else, 2009) racial and ethnic groups, as well as with patients with a variety of cultural backgrounds (Mucic, 2010). Furthermore, there is no guarantee that patients will receive a racial or cultural "match" if they travelled to a distant site for in-person care. In fact, telepsychiatry may provide racial and cultural advantages as patients may bring their community with them to sessions. Family members, caregivers, therapists, or teachers who would not travel to a distant site to accompany the patient may attend a telepsychiatry session to provide information, support, and cultural and contextual relevance. Also, staff at the hosting telepsychiatry site may help the telepsychiatrist to develop competence by acting as a cultural interpreter regarding their community and its residents. More information regarding cultural issues in telepsychiatry can be found in Chapter 5.

Clinical and Financial Models of Telepsychiatry Practice

The telepsychiatrist is not just a "prescriber" but the director of a model of care for the patient. Multiple models have been used for the delivery of care through telepsychiatry, and differences in these models have fundamental implications for how the telepsychiatrist practices, staff needed at the patient sites, how reimbursement occurs, and the rate of reimbursement. Several commonly used models of telepsychiatric practice are briefly reviewed to exemplify the attendant issues.

Psychiatrists who are in private practice or who work for a major medical center are accustomed to a fee-for-service financial model. When providing telepsychiatry services to a distant private clinic, the telepsychiatrist may work with the referring PCP to develop a consulting or collaborative model of clinical care or may directly assume ongoing patient care. In this model, the telepsychiatrist bills third-party payers for the professional fee. The amount of time, division of costs and reimbursement strategies, and arrangements for billing third-party payers all need to be clarified when the partnership is established, as these administrative costs have implications for relative costs and benefits to the telepsychiatrist and the referral site. An important limitation of this model is that not all payers currently cover telepsychiatry. Twelve states mandate that insurers include telemedicine in their covered services. In other states, coverage may vary by insurer. For Medicaid, individual states determine whether or not to cover telemedicine, what types of telemedicine to cover, and where in the state such care can take place, such that reimbursement for care varies both between and within individual states, which can be challenging for providers to understand (http://www.medicaid.gov/Medicaid-CHIP-Program-Information/By-Topics/Delivery-Systems/Telemedicine.html). The appeal of fee-for-service models varies by state depending on private insurers and the state's Medicaid's policy for reimbursing a private practitioner or the institution, the billing codes allowed, and the rate of reimbursement for a specific service, i.e., a new evaluation or medication management appointment. To avoid nonpayment, an insurer's policy regarding reimbursement for telepsychiatry should be determined before attempting to bill for services. The site where the patient uses the VTC equipment generally bills a facility fee, while the provider's site generally bills for the professional services. Billing codes for the telepsychiatrist's professional fee are the same as used in usual outpatient psychiatric practice with a "gt modifier" added to indicate that the care is provided through VTC. Payers require this designation that care is being provided through VTC, although further details regarding the specifics of VTC are not usually requested, e.g., whether VTC is connected through high bandwidth endpoints or through desktop or mobile devices. With advances in technology and more common practice of telepsychiatry, it is possible that payers will request more specific technological information in the future. Sample templates for documenting provided services consistent with frequently used billing codes have been developed by this author's institution and are included in the appendices. These templates were developed for in-person care but are relevant to telepsychiatry as well. Billing codes include 90801 for a typical mental health intake (see Appendix A for a documentation template for a 90801 code) and 90862 for a typical follow-up medication management session (see Appendix B for a documentation template). If psychotherapy is added to a medication follow-up appointment, billing codes 90805, 90807, 90809 can be used (see Appendix C for a documentation template). For telepsychiatry appointments that are predominantly medically focused, the evaluation and management codes may be used and typically reimburse at a higher rate than the aforementioned codes, but they also require more specific and extensive documentation. Appendix D provides documentation templates for initial evaluations using billing codes for 99904 and 99205, while Appendix E provides comparable templates for the follow-up 99214 and 99215 appointments. Note that these evaluation and management codes may be billed on the basis of the number of elements covered during the clinical examination or on the basis of time. If billing on the basis of time, the telepsychiatrist indicates the total time spent in counseling and coordination of care, as indicated in the statement at the top of the templates in Appendices E and F. Also provided in Appendices F and G, respectively, are templates to be used with the evaluation and management codes for documentation of the patient's review of systems and the patient's past psychiatric, family, and social history. These documentation templates contain the same data as required for an in-person visit using comparable billing codes.

In another model, often termed a contractual model, a mental health or other health-care center contracts with a telepsychiatrist for a specific amount of time and range of services. The telepsychiatrist usually commits to a block of time with a guaranteed income for that dedicated time, and the community mental health center then recoups payment by billing public or commercial payers for services delivered. Sometimes, the telepsychiatrist provides diagnostic evaluations and medication recommendations to a clinic at which there is a prescribing nurse practitioner, physician's assistant, or PCP who "partners" with the telepsychiatrist. The on-site provider then writes the prescriptions, fields calls between visits, and manages interim care. The telepsychiatrist may take primary responsibilities for between-visit patient care during a trial of medication, in which case the on-site provider typically assumes care after the trial of a new medication is completed and a decision is made as to whether that medication and dose should be continued. The goal in this model is to optimally use the telepsychiatrist's time to evaluate as many new patients as possible, while providing ongoing consultation about patients while they are trying a new medication strategy.

Having an on-site prescribing clinician to partner with the telepsychiatrist can be expensive. Therefore, variations of this model include having an on-site registered nurse or licensed practical nurse or other trained staff member work with the telepsychiatrist in managing patient care in tasks other than direct prescribing. They may coordinate prescriptions written by the telepsychiatrist, for example, by phoning or faxing refill orders to pharmacies. In some states, the staff's time may be billed to third-party payers, including Medicare and Medicaid, under a case management code that helps the mental health center to offset some of the costs of providing this staff assistance.

Other practice models may be developed to optimally coordinate and reimburse the telepsychiatrist's services while conserving the agency's resources. Potential telepsychiatrists may be interested in exploring options with Federally Qualified Health Centers (FQHC) which receive special federal funding to obtain specialty health-care services (https://www.cms.gov/Center/Provider-Type/Federally-Qualified-Health-Centers-FQHC-Center.html?redirect=/center/fqhc.asp). Important issues include quality of care such that the model adequately serves patients' needs and sustainability of the clinic by providing appropriate time and support to a telepsychiatry practice.

Best Practices for Conducting Psychopharmacology via Telepsychiatry

The requirements and recommendations for completing a psychiatric evaluation, deciding on psychiatric medication treatment, and monitoring of psychiatric medication therapeutic benefits and side effects are the same regardless of whether the patient is evaluated and treated in person or via telepsychiatry. Psychiatrists should refer to evidence-based and/or consensus-based best practices for evaluation and treatment guidelines regarding specific diagnoses (American Academy of Child and Adolescent Psychiatry, 2011; American Psychiatric Association, 2011; Grady et al., 2011) and the relevant supporting technology (Grady et al., 2011). This section highlights issues that are important across diagnoses when evaluation and treatment are provided through telepsychiatry.

Practice Standards and Guidelines

Standards of practice apply including the essential need for confidentiality and informed consent for the treatment provided. The telepsychiatrist's services must conform to professional clinical standards, documentation must be adequate and confidential, and clinical guidelines should be based on empirical evidence when available or professional consensus if not. The integrity of the relationship between client and provider must be maintained, and telepsychiatrists should be licensed for the care they provide (Reed, McLaughlin, & Millholland, 2000). Licensure is required in the state in which the patient is receiving the care, in addition to the state in which the telepsychiatrist is located. Over the past decade, there has been considerable discussion of national licensure, but there is no pending action on this issue. This requirement for licensure in the patient's state could provide some challenges to continuity of care in selected circumstances, such as when a student moves on to college in another state. Further information on legal and regulatory issues is provided in Chapter 6.

All psychiatric diagnoses include consideration of medical problems in making a differential diagnosis and treatment plan. It is helpful to partner with the patient's PCP such that evaluation of potential medical causes of psychiatric symptoms or medical complications of psychiatric treatment can be comanaged. If a physical examination is needed in order to evaluate the patient, such as examination of cogwheeling for a patient on antipsychotic medication, the psychiatrist will need to train on-site staff and rely on their report. One way to alert PCPs to this issue is to add a statement to the referral document stating that before a patient is referred to telepsychiatry, the referring provider must have recently evaluated the patient and ruled out medical causes for psychiatric symptoms. When medication monitoring requires evaluation of physical symptoms, such as the use of the Abnormal Involuntary Movement Scale (AIMS) for patients prescribed antipsychotics or the evaluation of ataxia and tremor during treatment with lithium, the telepsychiatrist will be able to perform some of the examination over the monitor (AIMS, evaluation of tremor). Otherwise, the telepsychiatrist can train local staff to observe and report on other examination features (evaluation of gait, assessment of cogwheeling) (National Institutes of Mental Health, 2011). Websites are available that provide instruction for completing and scoring an AIMS evaluation (www.dr-bob.org/tips/aims.html) and a demonstration of conducting the AIMS over VTC is available at www.narbha.org.

Gathering of collateral information may be more difficult to accomplish when the patient is evaluated via telepspychiatry. Ideally, the telepsychiatrist should arrange with the patient site that persons involved in the visit but who are not needed in the room may sit in a waiting room. However, this may not be possible, as there may not be an adequate waiting room or staff to supervise accompanying siblings or other family members. The telepsychiatry space needs to afford confidential communication between the telepsychiatrist and the patient without risk of being overheard by the other parties in the office at the time. However, the severity of the patient's psychiatric symptoms and the needs of other patients at the patient site influence the feasibility of providing separate interviews for involved parties. Although these same factors may influence the ability of a psychiatrist conducting an in-person evaluation, they may be heightened by the telepsychiatrist's lack of physical presence to assess other options at the clinic to accommodate individuals accompanying the patient. The telepsychiatrist can utilize the distant clinic's staff to help with logistical issues, but may have to supplement the session with a follow-up telephone call to obtain collateral information from the patient or family.

Copies of commonly used questionnaires for screening and monitoring can be kept at the patient site for ease of use, and mailed, faxed, or emailed between sites for scoring, but confidentiality of the data needs to be protected regardless of the method used. Similarly, telepsychiatrists will either need to mail laboratory requisition forms for monitoring of medication or partner with a medical provider at the patient site for ordering of laboratory testing. Sharing and exchanging questionnaires, laboratory results, and other such information is most efficiently accomplished through e-mail. However, e-mail is not considered confidential unless the telepsychiatrist and patient site share an e-portal, an electronic medical record, or a virtual private network. In the absence of such shared systems, documents should be faxed, mailed, or deidentified for e-mailing.

Decisions Specific to Prescribing: Consenting Patients

As recommended in the American Psychiatric Association Practice Guidelines (American Academy of Child and Adolescent Psychiatry, 2011), patients should be informed about the expected time frame for therapeutic benefits of a medication and the potential for side effects, including the potential for urgent crisis symptoms. Ideally, patients sign an informed consent for each medication. However, the logistics of obtaining signed consent through telepsychiatry will vary greatly depending on supports at the patient site and may preclude this formality. If signing of informed consent is not possible, the telepsychiatrist should note the discussion of potential side effects in the clinic visit documentation, as well as noting that the patient and/or family agreed on a trial of the medication. Hopefully, e-consenting will soon be available as shared electronic systems are developed.

Decisions Specific to Prescribing: Choice and Logistics of Medication Provision

Preliminary work suggests that diagnoses made through VTC are consistent with diagnoses made during in-person evaluation (Cain, Nelson, & Khanna, 2009; Elford et al., 2000). Diagnoses made through telepsychiatry, as through in-person evaluation, will provide the basis for treatment planning. However, the choice of psychopharmacologic agent may be influenced by the practice of telepsychiatry. Although the same recommendations for treatment apply regardless of evaluation and treatment venue, the cumbersomeness of laboratory monitoring and vicissitudes of scheduling at the patient site may influence the telepsychiatrist's weighing of the pros and cons of a specific medication choice. For example, if laboratory testing occurs off-site, is not timely, and the method for sharing the results requires multiple steps, the provider may choose a medication alternative that requires less monitoring in order to minimize safety risks and optimize timely treatment. One example of such a decision is the choice of a mood-stabilizing agent for the treatment of bipolar disorder, depressed phase. Rather than prescribing a medication such as lithium or valproate, which require significant laboratory monitoring during the titration of dose, lamotrigine or an atypical antipsychotic may be chosen. The logistics of laboratory monitoring should be only one of many factors considered in making the best treatment decision in the context of the individual's life and treatment circumstances. Partnering with referring providers and asking that they oversee the laboratory testing may help to facilitate decision-making that minimizes the impact of logistical factors. However, other logistical factors should be considered, such as the distance a patient must travel to access a laboratory,

Risk management regarding medication side effects requires special attention for telepsychiatrists, given their distance from their patient. Monitoring of medication side effects is a requirement of safe psychiatric practice (American Psychiatric Association, 2011; Grady et al., 2011; Myers & Cain, 2008). Thus, the telepsychiatrist must either collaborate with referring PCPs to ask that they provide monitoring or see the patient back for ongoing management. A potential problem with the former approach is the difference in practice styles between PCPs and psychiatrists, with PCPs typically seeing patients less often than psychiatrists. To facilitate optimal care, the telepsychiatrist should provide specific recommendations to the patient and PCP regarding the frequency of follow-up visits, the requirements for monitoring of medication including laboratory studies, blood pressure, weight, and physical signs (Myers & Cain, 2008). In practice, a hybrid of PCP and telepsychiatry visits may be used. For example, the telepsychiatrist may manage the patient's treatment during initial stabilization and monitoring of side effects followed by an ongoing treatment and monitoring by the PCP, with the option of additional visits to the telepsychiatrist to address changes in symptoms or side effects over time.

Telepsychiatrists and their primary care partners need to develop a plan for addressing unanticipated events such as worsening of symptoms, acute side effects such as dystonia, and crisis events such as suicidal ideation, and this plan should be in place prior to initiating treatment and should be clearly conveyed to patients. PCPs and patients often prefer that the telepsychiatrist be available to provide crisis services, but crisis telepsychiatry services are generally very difficult to arrange not only due to other demands on the telepsychiatrists' time but also due to the need to coordinate with the equipment and staff involved at both the telepsychiatrist's and patient's sites. As such, managements in an emergency room or with the community crisis team are preferred approaches. Crisis visits with the PCP may be available and may best provide continuity of care. Referring PCPs and telepsychiatrists will need to establish mutually acceptable means of communication with each other, with the hosting telepsychiatry site, and with patients. For example, telepsychiatrists may establish e-mail or phone contact with PCPs to help them address patient questions and concerns that do not warrant emergency care, such as notification regarding a new side-effect of medication and decision-making regarding whether or not to continue that medication. Alternatively, the telepsychiatrist may offer patients direct telephone contact, such as in the case of medication concerns, that does not go through the PCPs office. If the patient is being treated through a contractual relationship with a mental health center, other arrangements may apply but should be agreed upon by all parties prior to commencement of practice. In all of these scenarios, it is important that the emergency room, referring provider, crisis team, or mental health center have information regarding the best way to reach the telepsychiatrist to discuss crisis management.

e-Prescribing

A new technological option for psychiatrists, including those practicing telepsychiatry, is e-prescribing, in which a prescriber is able to send a prescription directly to a pharmacy via an electronic interface. Prior to e-prescribing, options for telepsychiatrists included mailing prescriptions, having a local collaborator provide prescriptions, or phoning prescriptions into a pharmacy (which is not possible for Schedule II prescriptions such as stimulant medications). Although the practice of e-prescribing is new, there is emerging evidence that it is already reducing errors, especially those due to illegible handwriting of the prescriber (Abramson, Barrón, Quaresimo, & Kaushal, 2011; Kannry, 2011). Some e-prescribing programs come with features that provide medication decision support that also help to reduce errors, such as alerting the prescriber if the dose being prescribed is outside of the recommended range, indicating potential interactions with other prescribed medications, providing a list of formularies allowed by specific insurance companies, reviewing information about past agents used for this patient, and checking on the patient's allergies (Abramson et al., 2011; Grossman, Boukus, Cross, & Cohen, 2011; Kannry, 2011). Although these decision-support technologies hold promise for helping providers in the future, initial evidence indicates that providers have been slow to embrace such features. Cited reasons have included that the features are cumbersome and that the information gained has not been worth the time or financial investment needed to obtain them (Grossman et al., 2011). Indeed, an informal survey of several pharmacies indicated that e-prescribing would cost the pharmacy approximately US$0.17–US$0.20 for each e-script attributable to the costs of using the e-prescribing program (K. Myers, personal communication, May 2012). Design improvements in the ease of use of these features have potential to increase their use. Advances in decision-support systems are under way and hold great promise to improve the ease and safety of prescribing via telepsychiatry (Coleman, Nwulu, & Ferner, 2011). Financial implications remain unclear.

To date, controlled substances are not available to be e-prescribed, as pharmacies require written prescriptions with signatures. However, changes are under way in legislation regarding the prescription of controlled substances, and it is likely that they will be e-prescribed in the near future. A survey of providers' attitudes indicates some concerns about the potential requirements of e-prescribing stimulants, such as providers not wanting to carry an authentication device such as a random number generator or a universal serial bus drive for a specific computer interface, especially when they work at more than one location (C. P. Thomas et al., 2011). However, overall, the expectation of providers is that e-prescribing of controlled substances will reduce error and diversion of prescriptions to illegal use.

Current Controversy Regarding Prescribing Through VTC

Health-care professionals and the US Congress have long expressed concern about illicit online pharmacies that sell medications to consumers without adequate oversight by a qualified health professional. This concern led to proposal of the Online Pharmacy Safety Act. However, recently the Act was redrafted to be an amendment to a larger bill in Congress dealing with the Food and Drug Administration (H.R. 5651 and S. 2516). The proposal would create a federal definition of a "valid prescription" covering all prescriptions and all pharmacies. In part, it would require that the patient has had an in-person medical evaluation within the previous 24 months. It would also require the valid prescription to either (1) meet a Controlled Substances Act definition requiring the patient to be at a hospital or clinic or (2) be issued by a newly defined "qualified off-site telehealth practitioner" and based on an "instantaneous" communication with the patient. Completion of a questionnaire and/or a phone call would not be a sufficient basis for a prescription. Current and potential telepsychiatrists should monitor this and future proposed legislation regarding prescribing in telemedicine practice.

Conclusions

Telepsychiatry has arrived and is an accepted and necessary component to the provision of psychiatric treatment nationally. The technology is rapidly improving while costs are decreasing. T1 lines, integrated service delivery networks based on telephone lines, and broadband are being extended to the most distant communities. National health-care reform will mandate increased coverage for all citizens. Current projections indicate that the nation is unlikely to ever have a sufficient number of psychiatrists to meet the needs of citizens across the country. PCPs and patients welcome the option of receiving consultation and care at a distance. Telepsychiatry can efficiently redistribute the existing workforce so as to rectify these disparities and increase access to evidence-based psychiatric care for populations that are underserved due to geography, ethnicity, or other barriers. Developing and expanding a telepsychiatry workforce offers the most equitable of all the options that have been proposed to address the dire need for psychiatric care without compromising the level of expertise available to underserved populations.

Telepsychiatry has significant advantages over other proposed solutions such as offering prescribing privileges to psychologists or credentialing a broader range of nurse specialists or increasing expectations on already overworked PCPs to become expert in psychiatric care. The success of telepsychiatry has, and still does, rest upon its being a medical specialty with the same standards and practices expected of other medical specialists and the established ability to render care that is comparable to traditional in-person care, including the same high standard of confidentiality, accuracy of diagnosis, and reliability and safety in treatment. While the benefits of telepsychiatry have been most emphasized for patients, benefits for practicing psychiatrists must also be emphasized. Telepsychiatry offers psychiatrists the opportunity to reach new populations of interest without long absences from home, to explore new markets, and to adopt lifestyles that provide a better balance of work and personal life. The next step is for training programs and major medical centers to help more psychiatrists to participate in this method of treatment delivery.

Appendix A.
Template for Documentation of New Outpatient Visit
(Billing Codes 90801 or 90802 --- add "gt modifier" to code)

Date: ____/____/____   Length of Session: _____

Patient Age: _____   Patient Gender: ☐ male   ☐ female

Chief Complaint: _____
_____

History of Presenting Illness (including medications): _____
_____
_____
_____
_____
_____
_____
_____

Past (Patient Psychiatric), Family, and Social History: _____
_____
_____
_____

Patient Past Medical History:
_____
_____
_____

Documentation of patient's lack of development of verbal communication or verbal impairment (for code 90802 only)   ☐ NA
_____

Outpatient Record	**Patient ID #:** **Name:** **DOB:**

Psychiatric/Mental Status Examination:

Physical Appearance:	Behavior/Activity level	Speech:	Affect:
□ unremarkable	□ cooperative/normal	□ unremarkable	□ normal
□ distressed	□ guarded	□ loud/rapid rate	□ blunted
□ bizarre	□ withdrawn/slowed	□ slurred/inarticulate	□ flat
□ poor hygiene	□ hostile/erratic	□ pressured	□ labile
□ well groomed	□ fidgety	□ quiet/slowed rate	□ congruent
□ other:_____	□ other:_____	□ other:_____	□ incongruent

Thought Form:	Mood:	Thought Content:
□ organized/intact	□ angry	□ no concerns observed or reported
□ blocking	□ anxious	□ obsessions: _____
□ flight of ideas	□ apathetic	□ compulsions: _____
□ evasive	□ depressed	□ delusions: _____
□ latency of response	□ euphoric	□ hallucinations: _____
□ perseveration	□ excitable	□ magical thinking: _____
□ poor memory	□ irritable	□ suicidal ideation: _____
□ tangential	□ sad	□ homicidal ideation: _____
□ other:_____	□ other:_____	□ loose associations:_____

Orientation:	Abstraction:	Long-Term Memory:	Short-Term Memory:
□ oriented	□ age appropriate	□ age appropriate	□ age appropriate
□ confused	□ impaired	□ impaired	□ impaired
□ distorted	□ unknown	□ unknown	□ unknown

Judgment/Insight:	Intellectual Functioning:	Attention/Concentration:	Fund of Knowledge:
□ age appropriate	□ above average	□ attentive/good concentration	□ age appropriate
□ impaired	□ average	□ inattentive/poor concentration	□ impaired
□ unknown	□ below average	□ unknown	□ unknown

Clinical Impression :_____

_____

_____

_____

Multi-Axis Diagnosis:

Axis I: _____

_____

Axis II: _____

Axis III: _____

Axis IV: _____

Axis V: GAF (18 + years old) _____ CGAS (0–17 years old) _____

Initial Assessment and Recommended Treatment Plan: _____

_____

_____

_____

Provider Signature: _____ Billing #:_____

Date:_____ Time:_____a.m./p.m.

Outpatient Record	**Patient ID #:**
	Name:
	DOB:

Appendix B.
Template for Documentation of Medical Management Visit
(Billing Codes 90862 --- add "gt modifier" to codes)

Date:____/____/____ Time:_____ a.m./p.m.

Total time spent with patient and/or family and caregivers:_____ minutes

Interval History/Progress since last visit: _____

_____

_____

_____

Vital Signs: Height: _____Weight: _____ Blood Pressure: _____ Pulse: _____

Current Medications (Strength, Dose, Frequency):_____

_____

_____

Patient Allergies: □ No changes since last appointment □ Changes:_____

Patient Compliance with treatment plan:_____

_____

_____

Physician orders for laboratory studies or other diagnostic measures: □ NA

_____

Interpretation of laboratory studies or other diagnostic measures: □ NA

_____

Patient education regarding potential risks, benefits, side effects of treatment:

_____

Pertinent Psychiatric/Mental Status Examination:_____

_____

_____

Impression and Plan, including medication changes and rationale: _____

_____

_____

_____

Provider Signature:_____ Billing #:_____

Date:_____   Time:_____am/pm

Outpatient Record	**Provider ID #:**
	Name:
	DOB:

Appendix C.
Template for Documentation of Psychotherapy with Evaluation and Management
(Billing Codes 90805 to 90813 --- add "gt modifier" to code)

Date: ____/____/_____   Length of Session: _____

Patient Age: _____   Patient Gender: □ male   □ female

Vital Signs: Height: _____ Weight: _____ Blood Pressure: _____ Pulse: _____

Current Medications (dosage, strength, frequency): _____
_____

Patient Allergies: □ No change since last appointment   □ Changes _____
_____

Type of clinical/therapy intervention::_____
_____
_____

Patient's response to intervention: _____
_____
_____

Target symptoms and progress towards treatment goals: _____
_____
_____

Plans for laboratory/other diagnostic studies and/or review of new data since last visit: _____
_____

Patient education of potential risks, side effects, and benefits: _____
_____

Pertinent mental status examination:_____
_____

Diagnoses/impressions:_____
_____

Treatment plan (include any change-sin medication or therapy and expected response):_____
_____
_____

Outpatient Record	**Patient ID #:**
	Name:
	DOB:

Appendix D.
Template for Documentation of New Outpatient Visit
Using Evaluation and Management Codes
(99201 to 99205 Codes --- add "gt modifier" to code)

Date:____/____/_____   Time:_____ a.m./p.m.

Total time spent with patient and/or family and caregivers:_____ minutes
Chief Complaint:
_____
_____
_____

History of Present Illness:
_____
_____
_____
_____

Review of Systems:

☐ See attached Review of Systems **OR**

☐ I have reviewed the ROS completed by _____(name)

on _____(date) and considered the relevant findings. Pertinent findings in current review:
_____
_____

Past (Patient Psychiatric), Family, and Social History: Level 1 = 1 item. Levels 2 & 3 = 1 item from all 3 areas.

☐ See attached PFSH **OR**   ☐ I have reviewed the PFSH completed by _____(name) on _____

(date) and considered the relevant findings.

Pertinent findings in current review:
_____

Patient Past Medical History:
_____
_____
_____

Current Medications:_____
_____
_____

OUTPATIENT RECORD

Patient ID #:

NAME:

DOB:

Psychiatric/Mental Status Examination:

Physical Appearance:	Behavior/Activity level	Speech:	Affect:
☐ unremarkable	☐ cooperative/normal	☐ unremarkable	☐ normal
☐ distressed	☐ guarded	☐ loud/rapid rate	☐ blunted
☐ bizarre	☐ withdrawn/slowed	☐ slurred/inarticulate	☐ flat
☐ poor hygiene	☐ hostile/erratic	☐ pressured	☐ labile
☐ well groomed	☐ fidgety	☐ quiet/slowed rate	☐ congruent
☐ other:_____	☐ other:_____	☐ other:_____	☐ incongruent

Thought Form:	Mood:	Thought Content:
☐ organized/intact	☐ angry	☐ no concerns observed or reported
☐ blocking	☐ anxious	☐ obsessions: _____
☐ flight of ideas	☐ apathetic	☐ compulsions:_____
☐ evasive	☐ depressed	☐ delusions: _____
☐ latency of response	☐ euphoric	☐ hallucinations: _____
☐ perseveration	☐ excitable	☐ magical thinking:_____
☐ poor memory	☐ irritable	☐ suicidal ideation: _____
☐ tangential	☐ sad	☐ homicidal ideation: _____
☐ other:_____	☐ other:_____	☐ loose associations:_____

Orientation:	Abstraction:	Long Term Memory:	Short-Term Memory:
☐ oriented	☐ age appropriate	☐ age appropriate	☐ age appropriate
☐ confused	☐ impaired	☐ impaired	☐ impaired
☐ distorted	☐ unknown	☐ unknown	☐ unknown

Judgment/Insight:	Intellectual Functioning:	Attention/Concentration:	Fund of Knowledge:
☐ age appropriate	☐ above average	☐ attentive/good concentration	☐ age appropriate
☐ impaired	☐ average	☐ inattentive/poor concentration	☐ impaired
☐ unknown	☐ below average	☐ unknown	☐ unknown

Ancillary Physical Examination Findings:

☐ HEENT:_____

☐ GI:_____

☐ GU:_____

☐ CV:_____

☐ MS:_____

☐ NEU:_____

Comments_____

_____

Medical Decision Making (level based on combination of documented diagnosis or management options, amount and complexity of data reviewed, and overall risk to patient):

Clinical Assessment: _____

_____

_____

Data Reviewed:

☐ Laboratory/other tests reviewed" _____

_____

_____

☐ Tests ordered/results reviewed: significant results include: _____

_____

_____

OUTPATIENT RECORD	Patient ID #:
	NAME:
	DOB:

Differential Diagnosis (list diagnosis name for all ICD-9 diagnoses that are being ruled-out or considered):
Axis I: _____
Axis II: _____
Axis III: _____
Axis IV:_____ _____
Axis V: CGAS = _____ (1–17 years of age); GAF = _____ (18+ years of age)
Assessment of treatment options (i.e. all options considered and declined):
_____
_____
_____

Treatment Plan (list all current interventions):
☐ Assessment of behavior/functioning:_____
☐ Medication trial of:_____
☐ Referral for ☐ individual ☐ family therapy to focus on:_____
☐ Medical planning (i.e. tests, consultations, records to review):_____
Other issues/comments on treatment plan (must be specific):_____
Morbidity/Mortality Assessment: Patient is at risk for:
☐ suicidal ideation/self-harm activities:_____
☐ aggressive or ☐ sexual behavior towards others:_____
☐ medication toxicity requiring ongoing medical supervision:_____
☐ school suspension/expulsion_____
☐ drug/alcohol abuse_____
☐ criminal activity/legal problems_____
Other issues/comments regarding risk factors (must be specific):_____
☐ **Counseling and coordination of care** activities were greater than 50% of the total session and included:
  ☐ patient counseling _____
  ☐ phone call to PCP _____
  ☐ phone call: other mental health provider_____
  ☐ review of outside records/labs:_____
  ☐ counseling with parent/guardian:_____
  ☐ other:_____
E&M Code: ☐ 99201 ☐ 99202 ☐ 99203 ☐ 99204 ☐ 99205 **All levels require 3 of 3 key components.**
99201/Level 1: 10 minutes with patient/family; problem focused history and exam; straightforward decision-making
99202/Level 2: 20 minutes with patient/family; expanded problem focused history and exam; straightforward decision-making.
99203/Level 3: 30 minutes with patient/family; detailed history (cc, extended hpi, extended problem pertinent ROS [2–9 systems], pertinent PFSH [1 item from any area]); detailed exam; low-complexity medical decision-making (limited dx/treatment options, limited data, low risk).
99204/Level 4: 45 minutes with patient/family; comprehensive history (cc, extended hpi, comprehensive ROS [10+ systems]); pertinent PFSH [1 item from any area]); comprehensive exam; moderate-complexity medical decision-making (multiple dx/treatment options, moderate data, moderate risk).
99205/Level 5: 60 minutes with patient/family; comprehensive history (cc, extended hpi, comprehensive ROS [10+ systems]), complete PFSH; comprehensive exam; high-complexity medical decision-making (extensive dx/treatment options, extensive data, high risk).

Provider Signature:_____ Billing #:_____

Date of Documentation:_____ Time of Documentation:_____am/pm

Outpatient Record	**Patient ID #:** **Name:** **DOB:**

Appendix E.
Template for Documentation of Established Outpatient
Using Evaluation and Management Codes
(Billing Codes 99211- 99215 --- add "gt modifier" to code)

Date:____/____/____ Time:_____ a.m./p.m.
Total time spent with patient and/or family and caregivers:_____ minutes

Interval History/Subjective: *Chief Complaint (required for all levels):*
_____
_____

History of Presenting Illness/Concerns (required for all levels): _____
_____
_____
_____
_____

Review of Systems
Constitutional • Fever, fatigue, weight loss/gain, swollen glands, other
Allergic/immunologic: • Allergies, immunological disorders, other
Endocrine • Diabetes, hormnal problems, other
Musculoskeletal • Joint pain, swelling, weakness, other
Neurologic • Headache, lethargy, seizures, loss of consciousness, other
Integumentary (skin and breast) • Rashes, lumps, swelling, water retention, other

Updated Review of Systems: 99213 = 1 system; 99214 = 2–9 systems; 99215 = 10+ systems
I have reviewed the ROS completed by _____(name) on
_____(date) and considered the relevant findings. Pertinent findings in current review:
_____

Updated (Patient Psychiatric), Family, and Social History (PFSH): 99214 = 1 item; 99215 = 1
item from all 3 areas: _____
I have reviewed the PFSH completed by _____(name) on
_____(date) and considered the relevant findings. Pertinent findings in current review:
□ No new histories □ New histories _____
_____

Outpatient Record	Patient ID #:
	Name:
	DOB:

Psychiatric/Mental Status Examination:

Physical Appearance:	Behavior/Activity level	Speech:	Affect:
☐ unremarkable	☐ cooperative/normal	☐ unremarkable	☐ normal
☐ distressed	☐ guarded	☐ loud/rapid rate	☐ blunted
☐ bizarre	☐ withdrawn/slowed	☐ slurred/inarticulate	☐ flat
☐ poor hygiene	☐ hostile/erratic	☐ pressured	☐ labile
☐ well groomed	☐ fidgety	☐ quiet/slowed rate	☐ congruent
☐ other:_____	☐ other:_____	☐ other:_____	☐ incongruent

Thought Form:	Mood:	Thought Content:
☐ organized/intact	☐ angry	☐ no concerns observed or reported
☐ blocking	☐ anxious	☐ obsessions: _____
☐ flight of ideas	☐ apathetic	☐ compulsions: _____
☐ evasive	☐ depressed	☐ delusions: _____
☐ latency of response	☐ euphoric	☐ hallucinations: _____
☐ perseveration	☐ excitable	☐ magical thinking: _____
☐ poor memory	☐ irritable	☐ suicidal ideation: _____
☐ tangential	☐ sad	☐ homicidal ideation: _____
☐ other:_____	☐ other:_____	☐ loose associations:_____

Orientation:	Abstraction:	Long-Term Memory:	Short-Term Memory:
☐ oriented	☐ age appropriate	☐ age appropriate	☐ age appropriate
☐ confused	☐ impaired	☐ impaired	☐ impaired
☐ distorted	☐ unknown	☐ unknown	☐ unknown

Judgment/Insight:	Intellectual Functioning:	Attention/Concentration:	Fund of Knowledge:
☐ age appropriate	☐ above average	☐ attentive/good concentration	☐ age appropriate
☐ impaired	☐ average	☐ inattentive/poor concentration	☐ impaired
☐ unknown	☐ below average	☐ unknown	☐ unknown

Any further mental status issues:

_____

_____

Medical Decision-Making:

Current Assessment (e.g. pt stability, any new problems, any complications): _____

_____

_____

_____

Differential Diagnosis (especially any changes): _____

:_____

_____

Records reviewed/outside informants/tests and orders reviewed: _____

_____

_____

_____

OUTPATIENT RECORD	Patient ID #:
	NAME:
	DOB:

Treatment Plan (list all current interventions):
☐ Assessment of behavior/functioning:_____
☐ Medication trial of:_____
☐ Referral for ☐ individual ☐ family therapy to focus on:_____
☐ Medical planning (i.e. tests, consultations, records to review):_____
☐ Further records to obtain/review: _____

Other issues/comments on treatment plan (must be specific):_____

Morbidity/Mortality Assessment: Patient is at risk for:
☐ suicidal ideation/self-harm activities:_____
☐ aggressive or ☐ sexual behavior towards others:_____
☐ medication toxicity requiring ongoing medical supervision:_____
☐ school suspension/expulsion_____
☐ drug/alcohol abuse_____
☐ criminal activity/legal problems_____
Other issues/comments regarding risk factors (must be specific):_____

Counseling and coordination of care activities were greater than 50% of the total session and included:
☐ patient counseling _____
☐ phone call to PCP _____
☐ phone call: other mental health provider_____
☐ review of outside records/labs:_____
☐ counseling with parent/guardian:_____
☐ other

E&M Code: ☐ 99211 ☐ 99212 ☐ 99213 ☐ 99214 ☐ 99215 **All levels require 2 of 3 key components.**

99211/Level 1: 5 minutes with patient/family; minimal presenting issues
99212/Level 2: 10 minutes with patient/family; problem focused history (cc, brief hpi); problem focused exam; straightforward medical decision-making (minimal dx, and treatment options, limited data and low risk).
99213/Level 3: 15 minutes with patient/family; expanded problem focused history (cc, brief hpi, problem pertinent ROS [2–9 systems]); expanded problem focused exam; low-complexity medical decision-making (limited dx/treatment options, limited data, low risk).
99214/Level 4: 25 minutes with patient/family; detailed history (cc, extended hpi, extended problem pertinent ROS [2–9 systems], pertinent PFSH [1 item from any area]); detailed exam; moderate-complexity medical decision-making (multiple dx/treatment options, moderate data, moderate risk).
99215/Level 5: 40 minutes with patient/family; comprehensive history (cc, extended hpi, comprehensive ROS [10+ systems], complete PFSH); comprehensive exam; high-complexity medical decision-making (extensive dx/treatment options, extensive data, high risk).

Provider Signature:_____   Billing #:_____

Date of Documentation:_____   Time of Documentation:_____am/pm

---

OUTPATIENT RECORD

Patient ID #:
NAME:
DOB:

Appendix F.
Template to Document Patient Review of Systems:
For use with all Evaluation and Management Codes
(New Patient Codes: 99201 to 99205 ; or Established Patient Codes 99211 to 99215
(add "gt modifier" to codes)

Date:____/____/____   Time:_____ a.m./p.m.

Person(s) interviewed:_____

Problem Pertinent = 1 system; **Extended** = 2–9 systems; **Complete** = 10+ systems

Body System	Problems/concerns
Constitutional • Fever, fatigue, weight loss/gain, swollen glands	☐ no current problems reported or identified
Endocrine • Weight loss/gain, diabetes, hormone problems	☐ no current problems reported or identified
Eyes • Pain, double vision, redness, drainage	☐ no current problems reported or identified
Ear, Nose, Mouth, Throat • Ear pain, drainage, hearing loss; nasal/ sinus problems; tooth pain, sore throat, hoarse voice	☐ no current problems reported or identified
Respiratory • Wheezing, cough, asthma, breathing problems	☐ no current problems reported or identified
Cardiovascular • Heart problems, chest pains	☐ no current problems reported or identified
Gastrointestinal • Nausea, vomiting, diarrhea, constipation, appetite changes	☐ no current problems reported or identified
Genitourinary • Menstrual problems, discharge, difficulty with urination	☐ no current problems reported or identified
Musculoskeletal • Joint pain, swelling, weakness	☐ no current problems reported or identified
Neurologic • Headaches, lethargy, seizures, loss of consciousness	☐ no current problems reported or identified
Hematologic/Lymphatic • Anemia, bleeding, jaundice, swollen glands	☐ no current problems reported or identified
Allergic/Immunologic • Allergies, immunological disorders	☐ no current problems reported or identified
Integumentary (skin and/or breast) • Rashes, lumps, swelling, water retention	☐ no current problems reported or identified

Provider Signature:_____   Billing #:_____

Date: _____   Time: _____

OUTPATIENT RECORD

Patient ID #:
NAME:
DOB:

Appendix G.
Template to Document Past (Patient Psychiatric), Family, and Social History [PFSH]
For use with all Evaluation and Management Codes
(New Patient Codes: 99201 to 99205 ; or Established Patient Codes -99211 to 99215
(add "gt modifier" to codes)

Date:____/____/____ Time:_____ a.m./p.m.

Person(s) interviewed:_____

Pertinent = 1 item from any of the 3 areas; **Complete** = 1 item from all 3 areas

Past (Patient Psychiatric) History:

Prior inpatient psychiatric or partial hospitalization or psychiatric residential treatment:

☐ None reported

_____
_____

Prior outpatient psychiatric treatment: ☐ None reported

_____
_____

Prior and current psychiatric medications: ☐ None reported

_____
_____

Family History:

Medical history of family members: ☐ None reported

_____

Psychiatric history of family members: ☐ None reported

_____
_____

Social History:

Family constellation and living situation:_____

_____

Parent/caregiver marital status, employment and educational history:_____

_____

Familial substance abuse, domestic violence history: ☐ None reported

_____
_____

Provider Signature:_____   Billing #:_____

Date: _____   Time:_____ am/pm

OUTPATIENT RECORD	Patient ID #:
	NAME:
	DOB:

References

Abramson, E. L., Barrón, Y., Quaresimo, J., & Kaushal, R. (2011). Electronic prescribing within an electronic health record reduces ambulatory prescribing errors. *Joint Commission Journal on Quality and Patient Safety, 37,* 470–478.

Alicata, D., Guerrero, A., & Else, I. (2009). Clinical perspectives: Rural primary care and behavioral health access for children and adolescents through telepsychiatry in Hawaii. *Paper presented at the 56th annual meeting of the American Academy of Child and Adolescent Psychiatry.* Honolulu, HI.

American Academy of Child and Adolescent Psychiatry. Practice parameters for childand adolescent psychiatry. (2011). <http://www.aacap.org/cs/root/publication_store/practice_parameters_and_guidelines> Accessed 8.10.12.

American Psychiatric Association. Psychiatry online: AmericanPsychiatric Association practice guidelines: Psychiatric evaluation of adults. (2011). <http://psychiatryonline.org/guidelines.aspx> Accessed 8.10.12.

Appel, P. R., Bleiberg, J., & Noiseuz, J. (2002). Self-regulation training for chronic pain: Can it be done effectively by telemedicine? *Telemedicine Journal and e-Health, 8,* 361–368.

Bishop, J. E., O'Reilly, R. L., Maddox, K., & Hutchinson, L. J. (2002). Client satisfaction in a feasibility study comparing face-to-face interviews with telepsychiatry. *Journal of Telemedicine and Telecare, 8,* 217–221.

Blackmon, L. A., Kaak, H. O., & Ranseen, J. (1997). Consumer satisfaction with telemedicine child psychiatry consultation in rural Kentucky. *Psychiatric Services, 48,* 1461–1466.

Cain, S., Nelson, E., & Khanna, P. (2009). Diagnostic efficacy of child telepsychiatry services for a school population. *Telemedicine Journal and e-Health, 15,* S71–S72.

Cain, S., & Spaulding, R. (2006). Telepsychiatry: Lessons learned from two models of care. Clinical perspectives. *Paper presented at the 53rd annual meeting for the American Academy of Child and Adolescent Psychiatry.* San Diego, CA.

Coleman, J. J., Nwulu, U., & Ferner, R. E. (2011). Decision support for sensible dosing in electronic prescribing systems. *Journal of Clinical Pharmacy and Therapeutics, 37,* 415–419. doi:10.1111/j.1365-2710.2011.01310.x.

Elford, R., White, H., Bowering, R., Ghandi, A., Maddiggan, B., St, & John, K., et al. (2000). A randomized, controlled trial of child psychiatric assessments conducted using videoconferencing. *Journal of Telemedicine and Telecare, 6,* 73–82.

Fortney, J. C., Pyne, J. M., Edlund, M. J., Williams, D. K., Robinson, D. E., Mittal, D., et al. (2007). A randomized trial of telemedicine-based collaborative care for depression. *Society of General Internal Medicine, 22,* 1086–1093.

Frueh, B. C., Monnier, J., Yim, E., Grubaugh, A. L., Hamner, M. B., & Knapp, R. G. (2007). A randomized trial of telepsychiatry for post-traumatic stress disorder. *Journal of Telemedicine and Telecare, 13,* 142–147.

Gabel, S. (2009). Telepsychiatry, public mental health, and the workforce shortage in child and adolescent psychiatry. *Journal of the American Academy of Child and Adolescent Psychiatry, 48,* 1127–1128.

Grady, B., Myers, K. M., Nelson, E. L., Belz, N., Bennett, L., Carnahan, L., et al. (2011). Evidence-based practice for telemental health. *Telemedicine Journal and e-Health, 17,* 131–148.

Gros, D. F., Strachan, M., Ruggiero, K. J., Knapp, R. B., Frueh, B. C., Egede, L. E., et al. (2011). Innovative service delivery for secondary prevention of PTSD in at-risk OIF-OEF service men and women. *Contemporary Clinical Trials, 32,* 122–128.

Grossman, J. M., Boukus, E. R., Cross, D. A., & Cohen, G. R. (2011). Physician practices, e-prescribing and accessing information to improve prescribing decisions. *Research Briefs*, *20*, 1−10.

Harper, R. A. (2009). Clinical perspectives: Experience with urban and rural telepsychiatry consultations in Texas. *Paper presented at the 56th annual meeting of the American Academy of Child and Adolescent Psychiatry*. Honolulu, HI.

Hilty, D. M., Cobb, H. C., Neufeld, J. D., Bourgeois, J. A., & Yellowlees, P. M. (2008). Telepsychiatry reduces geographic physician disparity in rural settings, but is it financially feasible because of reimbursement? *Psychiatric Clinics of North America*, *31*, 85−94.

Hilty, D. M., Nesbit, T. S., Marks, S. L., & Callahan, E. J. (2002). Effects of telepsychiatry on the doctor-patient relationship: Communication, satisfaction, and relevant issues. *Primary Psychiatry*, *9*, 29−34.

Hilty, D. M., Sison, J. I., Nesbitt, T. S., & Hales, R. E. (2000). Telepsychiatric consultation for ADHD in the primary care setting. *Journal of the American Academy of Child and Adolescent Psychiatry*, *39*, 15−16.

Hilty, D. M., Yellowlees, P. M., Cobb, H. C., Bourgeois, J. A., Neufeld, J. D., & Nesbitt, T. S. (2006). Models of telepsychiatric consultation-liaison service to rural primary care. *Psychosomatics*, *47*, 152−157.

Institute of Medicine (IOM) (2004). *Rural health care in the digital age*. Washington, DC: National Academic Press.

Institute of Medicine and the National Research Council (IOM/NRC) (2004). *Children's health, the nation's wealth: Assessing and improving child health*. Washington, DC: National Academic Press.

Kannry, J. (2011). Effect of e-prescribing systems on patient safety. *Mount Sinai Journal of Medicine*, *78*, 827−833.

Lopez, A. M., Avery, D., Krupinski, E., Lazarus, S., & Weinstein, D. S. (2005). Increasing access to care via tele-health: The Arizona experience. *Journal of Ambulatory Care Management*, *28*, 16−23.

MacDowell, M., Glasser, M., Fitts, M., Nielsen, K., & Hunsaker, M. (2010). A national view of rural workforce issues in the USA. *Rural Remote Health*, *10*, 1531−1534.

McCormick, M. C., Flores, G., Freed, G. L., Homer, C. J., Johnson, K. B., & De Friese, G. H. (2011). Challenge to child health services research: Report from the committee on pediatric health and health care quality measures. *Academic Pediatrics*, *11*, 257−259.

Mitchell, J. E., Crosby, R. D., Wonderlich, S. A., Crow, S., Lancaster, K., Simonich, H., et al. (2008). A randomized trial comparing the efficacy of cognitive-behavioral therapy for bulimia nervosa delivered via telemedicine versus face-to-face. *Behaviour Research and Therapy*, *46*, 581−592.

Morland, L. A., Greene, C. J., Rosen, C. S., Foy, D., Reilly, P., Shore, J., et al. (2010). Telemedicine for anger management therapy in a rural population of combat veterans with posttraumatic stress disorder: A randomized noninferiority trial. *Journal of Clinical Psychiatry*, *71*, 855−863.

Mucic, D. (2010). Transcultural telepsychiatry and its impact on patient satisfaction. *Journal of Telemedicine and Telecare*, *16*, 237−242.

Myers, K. M., & Cain, S. (2008). Practice parameter for telepsychiatry with children and adolescents. *Journal of the American Academy of Child and Adolescent Psychiatry*, *47*, 1468−1483.

Myers, K. M., Sulzbacher, S., & Melzer, S. M. (2004). Telepsychiatry with children and adolescents: Are patients comparable to those evaluated in usual outpatient care? *Telemedicine Journal and e-Health*, *10*, 278−285.

Myers, K. M., Valentine, J. M., & Melzer, S. M. (2007). Feasibility, acceptability, and sustainability of telepsychiatry for children and adolescents. *Psychiatric Services*, *58*, 1493−1496.

Myers, K. M., Valentine, J. M., Morganthaler, R., & Melzer, S. (2006). Telepsychiatry with incarcerated youth. *Journal of Adolescent Health*, *38*, 643−648.

NARBHA web site, Northern Arizona Regional Medical Health Authority (NARBHA). (2012). <http://www.narbha.org/> Accessed 27.02.12.

National Institutes of Mental Health. Abnormal involuntary movement scale (AIMS). (2011). <http://www.atlantapsychiatry.com/forms/AIMS.pdf> Accessed 8.10.12.

Nelson, E., Barnard, M., & Cain, S. (2003). Treating childhood depression over teleconferencing. *Telemedicine Journal and e-Health*, *9*, 49−55.

Nelson, E., Bui, T. N., & Velasquez, S. E. (2011). Telepsychology: Research and practice overview. *Child and Adolescent Psychiatric Clinic of North America*, *20*, 67−79.

Neufeld, J., Yellowlees, P., Hilty, D., Cobb, H., & Bourgeois, J. A. (2004). The e-Mental health consultation service: Providing enhanced primary care mental health services through telemedicine. *Psychosomatics*, *48*, 135−141.

O'Reilly, R., Bishop, J., Maddox, K., Hutchinson, L., Fisman, M., & Takhar, J. (2007). Is telepsychiatry equivalent to face-to-face psychiatry? Results from a randomized controlled equivalence trial. *Psychiatric Services*, *58*, 836−843.

Power, A. K. (2009). Focus on transformation: A public health model of mental health for the 21st century. *Psychiatric Services*, *60*, 580−584.

Reed, G. M., McLaughlin, C. J., & Millholland, K. (2000). Ten interdisciplinary principles for professional practice in telehealth: Implications for psychology. *Professional Psychology, Research and Practice*, *31*, 170−178.

Ruskin, P. E., Silver-Aylaian, M., Kling, M. A., Reed, S. A., Bradham, D. D., Hebel, J. R., et al. (2004). Treatment outcomes in depression: Comparison of remote treatment through telepsychiatry to in-person treatment. *American Journal of Psychiatry*, *161*, 1471−1476.

Saeed, S., Diamond, J., & Bloch, R. (2011). Use of telepsychiatry to improve care for people with mental illness in rural North Carolina. *North Carolina Medical Journal*, *72*, 219−222.

Savin, D., Garry, M. T., Zuccaro, P., & Novins, D. (2006). Telepsychiatry for treating rural American Indian youth. *Journal of the American Academy of Child and Adolescent Psychiatry*, *45*, 484−488.

Shore, J. H., Brooks, E., Savin, D., Orton, H., Grigsby, J., & Manson, S. M. (2008). Acceptability of telepsychiatry in American Indians. *Telemedicine Journal and e-Health*, *14*, 461−466.

Singh, S. P., Arya, D., & Peters, T. (2007). Accuracy of telepsychiatric assessment of new routine outpatient referrals. *BMC Psychiatry*, *7*, 55−68.

Thomas, C. P., Kim, M., McDonald, A., Kreiner, P., Kelleher, S. J., Blackman, M. B., et al. (2012). Prescribers' expectations and barriers to electronic prescribing of controlled substances. *Journal of American Medical Informatics*, *19*, 375−381. doi:10.1136/amiajnl-2011-000209.

Thomas, K. C., Ellis, A. R., Konrad, T. R., Holzer, C. E., & Morrissey, J. P. (2009). County-level estimates of mental health professional shortage in the United States. *Psychiatric Services*, *60*, 1323−1328.

United States Department of Health and Human Services. (2003). *President's new freedom commission. Transforming mental health care in America.* Rockville, MD: Pub no SMA-03-3832.

United States Department of Health and Human Services (USDHHS), National Advisory Committee on Rural Health and Human Services. 2004 Report to the secretary: Rural health and human service issues. (2004). <http://www.hrsa.gov/advisorycommittees/rural/publications/index.html> Accessed 20.04.12.

Yeung, A., Hails, K., Chang, T., Trinh, N., & Fava, M. (2011). A study of the effectiveness of telepsychiatry-based culturally sensitive collaborative treatment of depressed Chinese Americans. *BMC Psychiatry, 11,* 154–161.

Zarate, C. A., Weinstock, L., Cukor, P., Morabito, C., Leahy, L., Burns, C., et al. (1997). Applicability of telemedicine for assessing patients with schizophrenia: Acceptance and reliability. *Journal of Clinical Psychiatry, 58,* 22–25.

Zaylor, C. (1999). Clinical outcomes in telepsychiatry. *Journal of Telemedicine and Telecare, 5,* S59–S60.

Section Six

Next Steps in Disseminating Telemental Health and Establishing an Evidence Base

17 Clinically Informed Telemental Health in Post-Disaster Areas

Eugene F. Augusterfer

Harvard Global Mental Health: Trauma and Recovery Program, Cambridge, MA

Introduction

Disasters, both natural and man-made, seem to be on the rise and affect millions of people around the world every year (Figure 17.1) (RED, The Centre for Research on the Epidemiology of Disasters, A World Health Organization Collaborating Agency, 2011). With disasters seemingly on the rise, humanitarian, health, and mental health needs for postdisaster relief are on the rise as well. The need for mental health services to address the problems caused by disasters is well documented. Telemental health has the potential to be an important component in meeting critical mental health needs of those who have suffered a natural disaster or armed conflict. Though telemedicine has been implemented successfully in disaster relief, the potential of telemental health specifically has yet to be realized. Telemental health provides a virtual surge capacity, enabling mental health professionals from around the world to assist overwhelmed local health and medical personnel with the increased demand for services postdisaster (Simmons, Alverson, Poropatich, Di'Orio, & Doarn, 2008).

This chapter aims to discuss the impact of disasters, both natural and man-made, on the mental health of survivors and the role telemental health could provide for sustainable care to survivors. Note that the terms telemedicine, telehealth, and telemental health are used by various authors to describe the delivery of health and mental health services via an electronically mediated secure-encrypted network. In this chapter, the term telemental health is used to refer specifically to the real-time delivery of direct mental health services or mental health consultation to other health-care providers that would usually be delivered in-person. Exceptions include direct quotations by cited references.

As will be discussed, telemedicine has been deployed successfully in disaster response both in the United States and globally. In a careful review of the published literature on telemedicine in disaster response, mental health is a topic that is often mentioned. This then helps document the need for development of telemental health in disaster response. As such, this chapter will review (i) the use

Telemental Health. DOI: http://dx.doi.org/10.1016/B978-0-12-416048-4.00017-8

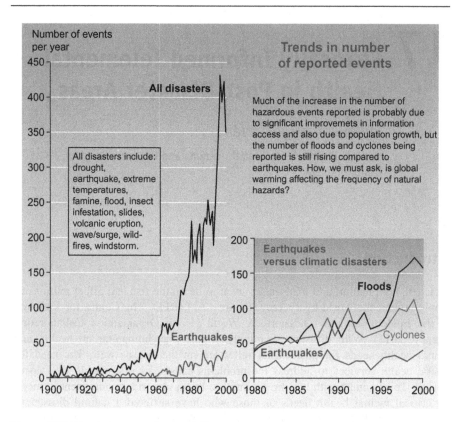

Figure 17.1 Trends in reported natural disasters.
Source: Centre for Research on the Epidemiology of Disasters (2011).

of telemedicine and telemental health in disaster response, (ii) the need for expanded use of telemental health in disaster response, (iii) barriers to implementation of telemental health, and (iv) the predicted future needs for telemental health in disaster response.

Literature Review and Background

Overview

"Over 1 billion persons (1 in 6) worldwide have been affected by violence and natural disaster" (R. Mollica, 2007). In the United States, about 1.5 million households experience injury or suffer property damage each year as a result of floods, tornadoes, hurricanes, or earthquakes (Rossi, Wright, Weber-Burdin, & Pereira, 1983). Although temporary symptoms are more common than severe long-term reactions (Freedy, Saladin, Kilpatrick, Resnick, & Saunders, 1994), the psychological sequelae can persist for up to 3–5 years after a natural disaster (Lima et al., 1993). In the United States, over 8 million people suffer from posttraumatic stress disorder (PTSD) (National Institute of Mental Health, 2012). Many of these people go on to develop depression and physical health problems related to trauma (Kohn, Levav, & Donaire Garcia, 2005). In fact, mental health is an issue of global importance; an estimated 450 million people worldwide have mental or behavioral disorders, accounting for 12% of the global disease burden. One of the tragic consequences of disasters, both natural and man-made, is the large numbers of internally displaced persons (IDPs). IDPs often live in temporary camps for months and years without permanent housing, education, and health care. The Internal Displacement Monitoring Centre estimates that there are approximately 27.5 million IDPs worldwide (Internal Displacement Monitoring Centre, 2011). A major issue for IDPs is the lack of adequate health and mental health services. It is the opinion of the author that both telemedicine and telemental health can, and should, play an important role in bringing needed services to this often neglected population.

Impact of Disasters on Mental Health

The impact of disasters on mental health has been well documented. In this section, the author will review some of the published literature.

"Disasters, terrorism, and traumatic events, whatever their source or scale, bring with them the potential to cause distress. Every person who is directly or indirectly involved in such an event may be affected and many may need psychosocial support" (NATO Joint Medical Committee, 2008). In addition to the medical care that might be needed for physical injuries, it is not surprising that great numbers of survivors develop acute reactions that need mental health attention. In fact, the definition of PTSD, reads, in part: "The essential feature of PTSD is the development of characteristic symptoms following exposure to an extreme traumatic stressor involving direct personal experience of an event that involves actual or threatened death or serious injury, or other threat to one's physical integrity" (Diagnostic and Statistical Manual of Mental Disorders (DSM-IV), 1994).

A study by Rodriguez and Kohn (2008) found that "some disasters do result in severe, lasting, and pervasive psychological consequences. Such disasters are frequently caused by human intent rather than by a natural event, and there is a high prevalence of injuries, threat to life, and loss of life." Similarly, Simmons et al. found that "injuries are those caused by the disaster event and are dependent on the nature of the disaster" (Simmons et al., 2008). The New York City terrorist attack on September 11, 2001, is another example of a man-made disaster that had significant impact on the mental health of survivors. Perlman et al. (2011) found "strong evidence is provided for associations between experiencing or witnessing events related to 9/11 and posttraumatic stress disorder."

These reports match the experience of the author, in that disasters caused by human intent appear to cause significant and long-lasting impact on the mental health of survivors.

However, natural disasters can have significant impact on the mental health of survivors as well. An example reported by Harvey, Smith, Abraham, Hood, and Tannenbaum (2007) is the natural disaster that struck the coast of southern Louisiana, Mississippi, and Texas in 2005. They found that "typically, postdisaster stress symptoms include (among others) recurrent nightmares, intrusive memories, hypervigilant arousal, impaired concentration, depression, emotional detachment from others, and disengagement from parts of life that were previously rewarding." Tracy, Norris, and Galea (2011) found similar results when they examined the survivors of Hurricane Ike that struck the gulf coast of Texas in 2008. They found that specific hurricane-related stressors, loss, or damage of sentimental possessions were associated with both PTSD and depression. They concluded that PTSD is indeed a disorder of event exposure, whereas risk of depression is more clearly driven by personal vulnerability and exposure to stressors. The role of nontraumatic stressors in shaping the risk of both pathologies suggests that alleviating stressors after disasters has clear potential to mitigate the psychological impact of these events.

Based on a review of the literature and this author's personal experience, it is clear that disasters leave in their path not only deaths, destructions, physical injuries, and sufferings but also hidden scars of psychological/emotional trauma (R. F. Mollica, 2006). Treating these hidden scars is as important to recovery as treating the physical injuries.

The Importance of Sustainable Care

In the immediate postdisaster chaos, dedicated international relief organizations such as the United Nations Development Programme, the International Committee of the Red Cross (ICRC), and Medecine Sans Frontieres (also known as Doctors without Borders) and others perform heroic efforts to save lives, treat the injured, and to provide safety, shelter, and food. Mental health issues are not a primary focus, yet failure to address these needs may impede recovery, possibly in the acute stage but certainly over the longer term.

Individuals who survive disasters require sustainable health care. Olsen (1998) defined sustainable health care as "a health service operated by an organizational system with the long-term ability to mobilize and allocate sufficient resources for activities that meet individual or public health needs." In the context of disaster response, sustainable care can be defined, in part, by responders staying to provide needed care during the emergency phase and the early stages of recovery, until the affected population has stabilized to the point of relative self-sufficiency.

Sustainability of mental health care is particularly relevant to disasters. While mental health problems may surface during or shortly after the acute phase of response, Olteanu et al. (2011) found that mental health service needs may continue unabated for extended periods. For example, following Hurricane Katrina, 29% of pediatric primary care patients presented with mental health or developmental/ learning problems, including the need for intensive case management, nearly for 2–4 years. As the acute postdisaster phase is winding down and emergency responders are often being asked to move to the next disaster, mental health problems tend to surface. Thus, mental health issues should be addressed as soon as they emerge and for as long as needed. As Dr. Shekhar Saxena of the World Health Organization noted in a recent seminar at Johns Hopkins Bloomberg School of Public Health, *"Can the developing world ignore mental health any longer?"* "Sustainable care is an ethical mandate!" (Saxena, Patel, Baingana, & Knapp, 2010).

The Role of Telemental Health in Sustainable Care

As noted above, relief and recovery efforts are followed by the emergence of mental health problems, a time during which there is often a gap in the provision of needed services. Since there is no published evidence-base that supports a specific approach to filling this gap, I will attempt to make the case that telemental health comprises a feasible component to developing sustainable mental health care in disaster areas. First, I will review the literature on telemedicine and telemental health that suggests and supports the critical factors to consider prior to implementation of a telemental health program in such an environment. Then, I will present case examples from Hurricane Katrina in New Orleans, the earthquake in Haiti, and the postconflict situation in Kenya—examples, respectively, of a US-based natural disaster, an international natural disaster, and international armed conflict. In so doing, I will draw from experience with telemental health programs that were deployed, and at other times I will suggest how a telemental health program might have benefited the response effort.

Because of the paucity of the empirical evidence-base, impressions and suggestions made here will be "clinically informed," i.e., based on an assessment of clinical needs conducted with the target population while understanding and respecting the cultural norms and expression of wellness and illness within that culture. Furthermore, "clinically informed" implies that recommended interventions will be based on best practices with clinical outcomes and impact on the population monitored and reported.

The Literature Supporting Telemental Health in Disaster Response

As mentioned earlier in this chapter, to date, telemedicine has a wider use in disaster response than telemental health; therefore, the review will reflect that reality.

One of the first documented uses of telemedicine in disaster response was the 1988 earthquake in Soviet Armenia. Nicogossian and Doarn (2011) looked at lessons learned following the earthquake in Soviet Armenia and found that "psychological, physical, and social sequelae persist years after the events." The authors went on to report that telemedicine is useful in response to the needs of survivors. They further added that telemental health would be helpful in targeting the psychological sequelae noted in the report. Another report by Porcari et al. (2009) looked at the use of telemental health for individuals with a history of trauma exposure and found that telemental health as delivered by videoteleconferencing (VTC) yielded comparable results to face-to-face methods in the assessment of PTSD, and patients expressed satisfaction with the VTC approach.

Simmons et al. (2008) examined the use of telehealth (telemental health) in natural and anthropogenic disasters and found that telehealth would play primarily a support role in the acute phase following a disaster and then continues to fill gaps in primary and specialty care, such as mental health. Taking a look more specifically at telemental health in natural or man-made emergencies and mass disasters, Yellowlees, Burke, Marks, Hilty, and Shore (2008) further noted that telepsychiatry can be especially useful in increasing access to psychiatric care for one-time clinical events and public health situations associated with mass disasters.

In a study that looked at a natural disaster, Hurricane Katrina, and a man-made disaster, the terrorist attacks of September 11, 2001, Rodriguez and Kohn found that nonavailability of mental health treatment was a factor in the reported low use of mental health services. They concluded that mental health services provided by professionals from outside-affected areas "could be utilized to remotely deliver services such as cognitive–behavioral therapy by telephone, Internet, or telecommunications" (Rodriguez & Kohn, 2008). Without using the term telemental health, Rodriguez and Kohn have endorsed telemental health as a means to bring distant mental health resources to the disaster site.

In an interesting and somewhat unique study, Johnson (2011) used a simulated earthquake in San Francisco Bay/Oakland, California, to compare the current disaster response approaches with a telemedicine-enhanced model. Using major, medium, and minor earthquake simulations, the study found that a telecommunication hub linking medical personnel at the scene with remote medical specialists could reduce mortality by 5.4%, 36.5%, and 27.3%, respectively, compared with current disaster response systems. Telemedicine improved survival rates in the three scenarios because it "augmented triage," increasing local treatment capacity. The telemedicine triage model assumed that remote generalist emergency medical providers could be connected to local care centers and, therefore, patients at the local care site who require more advanced treatment could access specialists via the telemedicine link.

Overall, given the acute surge in needed medical and mental health services following a disaster, there is considerable support indicating that telemedicine and telemental health have an important role in supplementing on-the-ground medical and mental health care during acute phases of disaster response and can take on a larger role in sustaining mental health care following the acute phase (Rodriguez & Kohn, 2008).

Case Examples of Disaster and a Potential Role for Telemental Health

Areas or countries that have suffered natural disasters, often referred to as fragile states in the international literature, are states that have suffered disasters such as floods, earthquakes, hurricanes, or droughts to the extent that their security, economic, health, and welfare systems are damaged or destroyed. A recent extreme and poignant example of the impact of a natural disaster in the United States is Hurricane Katrina, August 2005, which caused loss of life, massive destruction of property, and displacement of hundreds of thousands of people. Recent international examples include the earthquake in Haiti, 2010, which caused loss of life, massive destruction, and displacement of over a million people. Survivors of both of these natural disasters faced numerous obstacles to recovery, including health and mental health problems.

Postconflict states are states that have suffered armed conflict leading to loss of life, physical destruction, the displacement of people, the collapse of the systems such as security, economic, health, and welfare institutions that make a stable society. While similar to natural disasters, postconflict states are unique in some respects. Survivors of armed conflict have many of the problems as those who suffered a natural disaster including loss of life, sometimes a family member or friend, destruction of property, but most importantly, the knowledge that someone inflected the harm (disaster) on them by choice. As we will discuss later, this has significant implications for mental health and recovery.

Case Example I: Hurricane Katrina, Natural Disaster

Hurricane Katrina, one of the five deadliest hurricanes in US history, hit the southern United States on August 29, 2005. Katrina caused loss of life (1836 reported deaths) and significant damage (estimated at US$108 billion) from Florida to Texas. See Figure 17.2 showing the immense size of Katrina. However, the focus of this case discussion will be on New Orleans, the epicenter of loss of life and displacement of people.

When Katrina hit, the force of the wind and storm surge overwhelmed the levees and flooded the city causing loss of life, devastating damage, and massive displacement of people (Warner & Scott, 2005). Eighty percent of New Orleans was flooded and uninhabitable causing the displacement of the majority of the city population. Katrina caused the largest single displacement of people from a natural disaster in US history (Ladd, Marszalek, & Gill, 2006).

Following Katrina making landfall as a category 5 hurricane, New Orleans was declared an emergency site by local and federal authorities. Although there were various sites used as evacuation centers, the focus of this discussion will be on the three major evacuation centers: the Superdome in New Orleans; the Astrodome in Houston, Texas, and the Reunion Arena in Dallas, Texas. Furthermore, the discussion will briefly describe the conditions and mental health care provided, as reported, in each of these major evacuation centers. The discussion will be based on both published literature/reports and the author's personal experience as part of the Distributed Medical Intelligence (DMI) Conference Team: Disaster Response and Preparedness from Hurricanes to Infectious Disease, held in New Orleans, April 2006, hereafter referred to by the DMI Conference. The DMI Conference had as its primary focus to examine the impact of Hurricane Katrina on New Orleans.

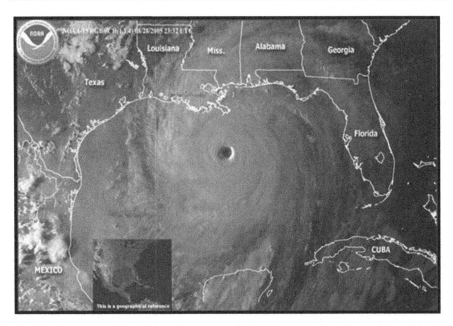

Figure 17.2 NOAA satellite image of Hurricane Katrina.
Source: Photos.orr.noaa.gov.

As such, there was a tour of the devastated areas and meetings with local medical and business leaders as they addressed the impact on the population, hospitals, clinics, and businesses. There were also speakers addressing the medical situation from the Superdome, the Astrodome, and the Reunion Arena.

From a medical and mental health standpoint, it appears all the three evacuation centers provided the best level of care possible given the circumstances, but there were some notable differences. The Superdome, being in New Orleans, was the most chaotic, understandably. As with most postdisaster situations, the closer to the actual disaster, the more chaotic the scene. There was however a system for triage that worked to identify those in the most critical need. The Astrodome, approximately 350 miles from New Orleans, was the next site that was examined. It appears that the time and distance from the disaster probably aided the planners in Houston to set up a more organized structure for identification of needs, medical and other needs, and to plan a system not only for triage but also for referral of those in need of more intense medical care. The Reunion Arena in Dallas, approximately 520 miles from New Orleans, was the third site examined. Being the most distant from the disaster, the Reunion Arena staff probably benefited from not only time and distance from the disaster but also had the advantage of hearing and seeing reports from the other two evacuation sites. As a result, the staff at the Reunion Arena were better prepared and, therefore, were the most organized and had the most functional triage and referral center. Specifically, the Dallas, TX, medical community, including the Reunion Arena, set up an excellent telecommunications network to handle the surge of patients that were to be evaluated at the Reunion Arena. Additionally, the Reunion Arena prepared by setting up segregated areas for screening/triage, emergency care, pediatrics, infectious disease, dental care, and mental health. This allowed for an organized flow which worked well for both staff efficiency and good patient care.

Another question worth asking is whether adding specialty telemental health care would actually improve overall efficiency of the primary-care-based evacuation centers. It is the opinion of the author that both telemedicine and telemental health could have been used to improve both staff efficiency and patient care. Whereas it is admirable that many people make the journey to assist in the recovery effort following a disaster, there continues to be more need than can be addressed. Therefore, the on-site medical and mental health professionals are working very long shifts in a chaotic atmosphere. All of the evacuation centers stated a relative lack of specialists, including mental health. Telemental health and telemedicine could bring not only specialty expertise but also could allow for needed support for evaluations and treatment, second opinions, case management, and possibly support to first responders to name a few of the services that could be provided.

Medical and Mental Health Impact

As with most disasters, much of the attention of medical professionals was devoted to emergency and first-aid care, treatment of acute physical injuries, and evaluation of need for more intense care. However, there were a notable number of mental health related issues in need of attention.

Those who were in mental health treatment prior to the hurricane often needed some level of care including medication. Additionally, there was a large population who had not been receiving any form of mental health care prior to the disaster, but upon interview reported heightened fear and/or stress and anxiety. The triage desk at the Reunion Arena reported that approximately 50% of the population had symptoms of stress, fear, and/or anxiety. Additionally, many of those closest in time to the disaster often suffer shock reactions, such as mental disorientation. While the staff and volunteers performed remarkably, there was a shortage of trained medical and mental health personnel. Again, the staffing situation was improved with each site as it was more distant from the disaster in terms of miles and time. As we will see below, telemental health could be of assistance in providing the much needed care.

The Role of Telemedicine and Telemental Health

To understand the lack of telemedicine and telemental health in response to Katrina, one must look at a number of factors. Simmons et al. (2008) found that in postdisaster situations, response is complicated by infrastructure that is overwhelmed by the surge in demand, damaged, or destroyed. However, if the infrastructure is not damaged or is repaired, telemental health could support specialty care services as well as address disaster-unique health-care needs, such as mental health and other needed services. Other impediments to the use of telemedicine are legal and ethical issues. As current laws in the United States generally state that the provider of care must be licensed in the state where the patient is receiving care. In the case of Katrina, telemedicine providers would have to have been licensed in either Louisiana or Texas, which would indeed limit the positive impact that telemedicine and telemental health could have made. Most, if not all, of these laws were written before the advent of telemedicine and were designed to protect patients/citizens from abusive practices. While well-meaning and probably appropriate during the times they were enacted into law, they seem outdated and in need of updating given the current capabilities of telemedicine, especially during disaster relief. However, consultation to on-site providers does not require a license in the state where the provider practices, as implementation of any recommendations resulting from the consultation remains the responsibility of the primary provider. Thus, if state laws preclude direct services to victims of disaster, consultation to on-site front line providers is possible and is highly recommended. Based on the experience of the author in other postdisaster situations, it would be legal and ethical to implement a telemedicine/telemental health program to provide teleconsultations to on-the-ground providers. Hopefully, legal barriers will be eventually surmounted to also allow needed specialty expertise to be provided directly to their patients. Telemental health could include a full range of services including coordination with pharmacies to bring medications to the disaster site, as often medications are destroyed in the disaster.

Case Example II: Haiti, International Disaster

"At 4:53 PM on January 12, 2010, a 7.0 magnitude earthquake shook Haiti. The epicenter of the earthquake was only 10 miles from Port-au-Prince, the bustling capital city of the Caribbean country. One of the most destructive natural disasters in history, the quake reduced buildings to rubble, instantly taking lives, and destroying homes. The Government of Haiti estimates that nearly 230,000 people died, 300,000 were injured, and over 1.5 million were displaced after their homes were damaged or destroyed." (US Geological Survey. National Earthquake Information Center). This devastating event also destroyed clinics and hospitals (Figure 17.3). However, health-care personnel from all over the world joined forces to treat the wounded. Shortly after the disaster struck, first-aid posts were set up by the Haitian Red Cross and the ICRC, providing basic health care to tens of thousands living in makeshift camps. Field hospitals and operating theaters were set up for the most severe cases (International Committee of the Red Cross, 2012).

Challenges in International Disaster Response

Before going further with discussion of the Haiti Earthquake and the response effort, it is important to discuss some of the challenges in international disaster response work. First, international actors need to be aware that they are entering

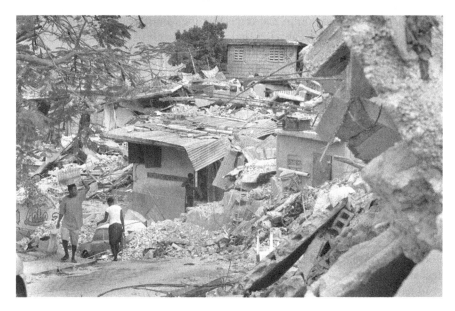

Figure 17.3 Haiti earthquake.
Source: NOAA/NGDC, Red Cross.

another country and must adhere to international laws, specific country laws, and customs, and be aware that they are guest in the country. To paraphrase an old saying *"having good intentions is not enough!"* One of the first documents to be aware of and to adhere to is the Inter-Agency Standing Committee (IASC) Guidelines on Mental Health and Psychosocial Support in Emergency Settings (Inter-Agency Standing Committee, 2007). It is imperative that relief agencies and individuals be aware of and adhere to these guidelines. This should include those who would provide care via telemental health and/or telemedicine.

In the chaos that followed the earthquake in Haiti, it was clear that many agencies and individuals were not aware of these guidelines and, therefore, some guidelines were violated. Additionally, when entering another country, it is important to be aware of local laws and customs. Without awareness of customs and norms, one could easily err in judgments and decisions. Lastly, when working in an international environment, providers must be aware of and respect each country's Ministry of Health as the local authority on health concerns, including relief efforts and telemedicine and telemental health interventions. Many relief agencies and/or workers in Haiti seemed to be unaware of this principle. Unfortunately, this led to several incidents that attracted international attention. The most published incident, as reported by Reuters on January 30, 2010, was the arrest of 10 American missionaries for attempting to take 33 Haitian children out of Haiti without parental permission or proper papers (Delva, 2010). To simply put, being aware of international guidelines and standards such as the IASC guidelines, being informed about local laws, customs, and norms, and respecting the Ministry of Health of a country are imperative in international relief and recovery work. Additionally, this author recommends maintaining a respectful and cooperative attitude when working with locals as they are indeed the experts in their culture.

Medical and Mental Health Impact

The needs in postdisaster Haiti were tremendous. Rahn Kennedy Bailey, M.D., Chairman of the Department of Psychiatry and Behavioral Sciences, and Executive Director of the Lloyd Elam Mental Health Center, at the School of Medicine, Meharry Medical College, headed a team that arrived in Haiti on January 28, 2010, just 2 weeks after the devastating earthquake. Dr. Bailey reported that the need for food, shelter, health care, and psychological support among these displaced and devastated people was brutally obvious. There is a need to better understand the full impact of this type psychological assault on an individual's psychological defense mechanisms. It stands to reason that any individual who has been so affected has fewer emotional reserves available to be able to address the primary day-to-day struggles to which they are exposed. Depressive and anxiety disorders can be very debilitating, especially in individuals with poor premorbid functioning (Bailey, Bailey, & Akpudo, 2010). Kathleen Molly McShane, M.D., writes about her experience as a psychiatric resident serving in the field hospital that was created by Project Medishare and the University of Miami, Miller School of Medicine's Global Institute. She reports that in addition to the loss of life and the destruction of property, Haiti lacked a coordinated mental health-care system and that "hundreds of patients presented to triage and emergency rooms daily with symptoms related to psychiatric disorders, such as heart palpitations, sweats, head-aches, and memory problems. The symptoms usually started after the disaster and were often due to anxiety, depression, posttraumatic stress disorder (PTSD), or other syndromal psychiatric disorders" (McShane, 2011). Additionally, the author would add from discussions with those providing direct mental health care in Haiti that depressive symptoms such as sadness, crying spells, sleep disturbances, feelings of helplessness, and hopelessness were common among survivors.

As seen in these reports, identification and treatment of mental health problems are significant in postdisaster recovery efforts. Based on first-hand interviews with several international agency leaders, the author would add that while the over-whelming loss of life, injuries to survivors, and destruction of properties are what impacted aid workers initially, mental health related problems such as depression, anxiety, and PTSD were also significant in the relief effort. Or, as Safran, Chorba, Schreiber, Archer, and Cookson (2011) stated "As in most disasters, attention to mental health after the earthquake was overridden initially by basic survival needs such as food, water, shelter, acute medical care for traumatic injuries, and concern for dead and missing people. Shortly after a disaster, a range of psychological symptoms are common. Resilience is common for many people, yet for some, symptom severity, persistence, and associated impairment progress to mental illness (e.g., PTSD, depression, other anxiety disorders)."

The Role of Telemedicine and Telemental Health

Just days after the devastating earthquake struck Haiti on January 12, medical volunteers from the University of Miami in Florida arrived and set up a tent hospital in Port-au-Prince. Antonio Marttos Jr M.D., assistant professor of surgery at the University of Miami School of Medicine and director of trauma telemedicine at Jackson Memorial Medical Center's William Lehman Injury Research Center in Miami, Florida, reported to the *Medscape Medical News* "Everything was destroyed over there, and in the first days there was no Internet in Port-au-Prince," "But we were able to connect to our trauma center in Miami." "Team members also used the satellites for triage and video consultations." Marttos went on to say "What's most exciting is that we are building an entire health system in Haiti. That's where telemedicine and technology will come in. I think Haiti is finally going to be connected to the rest of the world." (Louden, 2010).

Haiti, like many disaster areas, lost much of the communications infrastructure that is so crucial for telemedicine. Reports vary about the length of time it took for the communications network to be repaired and/or replaced; however, most reports suggest that the capital, Port-au-Prince, communications was functional within 2−4 weeks. As discussed earlier, mental health problems often surface after the emergency phase of postdisaster relief work. Therefore, the communications infrastructure that telemedicine depends on was functional as mental health problems began to surface. As such, a number of telemedicine programs, mostly linked to US-based medical centers and universities, began to develop.

This brings into focus the central point regarding the use of telemedicine in postdisaster environments, i.e., while there are numerous medical needs in such an environment, one of the needs repeatedly articulated is the need for specialized expertise, including mental health expertise. A telemedicine network linking a postdisaster area, like Haiti, to a hub consisting of specialists, including mental health, can serve as a case consultation and/or mentoring network for those on the front lines in need of specialty expertise. Haiti continues to suffer postdisaster needs for medical expertise, including mental health, to support the dedicated on-the-ground providers of care. Telemedicine, including telemental health, can be important in meeting those needs.

Case Example III: Kenya, Armed Conflict

General Elections were held in December 2007. "While Kenya has remained fairly stable and peaceful during most of the postindependence period, violence between ethnic groups has tended to erupt around elections since the introduction of competitive multiparty politics. More recently, violence and general lawlessness escalated to unprecedented levels following the General Elections in December 2007. The conflict resulted in loss of hundreds of lives, exodus of a quarter of a million people, and widespread destruction of property" (Kimenyi et al., 2010).

The reports of the number of killed and displaced in Kenya are varied with some reports claiming "that around 1100 people were killed and up to 600,000 people were displaced" (International Crime Court Press Release, 2010).

What we do know is that the elections of 2007 led to ethnic violence that killed many innocent people, including women and children, and led to displacement of hundreds of thousands of people. We also know that conflict and war are unfortunately common in many sub-Saharan countries. Blattman (2012) reports that "Development in Africa is inseparable from warfare. In the mid-1990s alone, a third of sub-Saharan African countries had an active civil war; many lasted a decade or more. Mass violence has afflicted nearly every African nation since Independence. These conflicts are epic events in each nation's history, destroying life, skills, wealth, and infrastructure, and potentially damaging a society's social bonds and institutions".

Mental Health Impact

Published articles on the mental health impact of the postelection violence in Kenya are limited. However, Ndetei et al. (2007) looked at the impact of postelection traumatic experiences on secondary school students and found that in a cross-sectional study of 1110 students (629 men and 481 women), aged 12—26 years, PTSD symptoms were common; avoidance and reexperiencing occurred in 75% of the students and hyperarousal was reported by over 50%. Furthermore, Kenya has little provision for mental health services. Jenkins et al. (2010) report that there are only 75 active psychiatrists in Kenya to serve a population of more than 38 million. Only a third of these psychiatrists work in the public sector. The Kenyan budget allocates less than 0.5% of financial resources to mental health (W'Atwoli, 2011).

The author personally interviewed those providing direct care after the conflict in Kenya and suggested that the mental health impact is difficult to estimate due to underreporting. Much of the underreporting appears to be due, in part, to the embarrassment of survivors to answer surveys and/or the stigma associated with "mental illness." However, it seems that once a relationship was formed through some nonthreatening activity, such as task groups, women and children were more likely to tell their story and admit to suffering. Once expressed, the most prevalent problems appeared to be a combination of depressive and anxiety symptoms, including social withdrawal and isolation, shame, hopelessness, helplessness, fear, numbing, and anxiety. Of course, it takes time and commitment to work with survivors to build the relationships that allow for the disclosure of such information. Additionally, it takes awareness and appreciation of cultural differences in the expression of emotions and suffering to effectively adapt best practices to the host culture.

The Role of Telemedicine and Telemental Health

Can telemental health play a role in the response to armed conflict disasters like the situation in Kenya? Considering the reported scarcity of mental health professionals and the large number of those in need, telemental health can, and should, be a major part of disaster response in such instances. As stated above, there are telecommunication challenges in many areas of the developing world, but with coordination with groups such as Telecoms Sans Frontières (also known as

Telecoms without Borders—www.tsfi.org/en); telemental health can be operational as soon as the telecommunications infrastructure is functional. So, this brings us to the question was telemental health used in the postelection situation in Kenya?

While Kenya did not suffer the destruction of its communications infrastructure like Haiti and New Orleans in their disasters, Kenya has many rural areas that have unreliable communications. Therefore, this must be taken into consideration when planning any telemedicine and/or telemental health program. However, as stated above, there are dedicated telecommunication professionals and programs that can provide needed assistance. As an example, the University of Texas Medical Branch (UTMB) has an excellent program in Kenya. Dr. Summerpal Kahlon, a UTMB postdoctoral fellow and resident in the Infectious Disease division of UTMB's Internal Medicine department, worked with local doctors in Kenya using telemedicine to confirm his diagnosis of Rift Valley fever, a mosquito-borne infection, with one of his patients. Additionally, Dr. Kahlon and his mentor, Dr. C. J. Peters, were able to advise a local physician via telemedicine on other important medical issues, proper public health measures, and protection of hospital staff (Wireless Healthcare, 2011).

Since the UTMB telemedicine program was so effective in Kenya, were there telemental health programs having impact in Kenya? Unfortunately, a review of the literature does not report any published data on telemental health programs in Kenya. Given the absence of published data, the author will report on his personal experience with the Harvard Program in Refugee Trauma (HPRT) in Kenya. The HPRT program is a telemental health program that blends face-to-face education, training and mentoring of providers in the identifica and treatment of postdisaster trauma care with a continuing process of education, training, mentoring and case supervision via a secure-encrypted telemental health network. In the world of telemedicine, the HPRT program is known as a "blended program." Programs like the UTMB and the HPRT are, in the opinion of the author, one of the most effective ways to meet both the medical and the mental health needs of the global population regardless of location.

Since the election violence in Kenya, the HPRT faculty has collaborated with a number of doctors, nurses, social workers, and community workers in Kenya. A common refrain of those providing care in Kenya has been the need for support for those providing on-the-ground mental health services, second opinions, and current best practices for mental health trauma care.

While the HPRT model focuses on providing support to those providing direct care via a telemental health program, direct patient care is possible as well. One of the important factors regarding the philosophy of the HPRT program is that the on-site providers are an integral part of the host culture and therefore understand the local culture and the expression of illness and wellness. Local providers in Kenya, as well as others in 70 different countries, have stated that the HPRT telemental health program is a "lifeline" that allows them to provide current best practices regardless of their location, which is often quite remote.

In the process of case discussions, consultations, and mentoring of the on-the-ground providers, it is clear that a large segment of the Kenyan population, especially women and children, have suffered significant trauma; physical, sexual, and emotional. As such, the need for evidence-based, culturally relevant, best practice focused on trauma care is imperative. The results of this blended telemental health program have been excellent. The HPRT program is proud to be functioning as a blended telemental health program in Kenya and over 70 other countries at this time.

It is the opinion of the author that the experience of the HPRT program in Kenya is an example of how telemental health can provide help to those suffering from the consequences of disaster regardless of location—globally!

Lessons Learned

The discussions of man-made and natural disasters and the subsequent needs of survivors, to include mental health, led to both lessons learned and opportunities to use telemental health to provide needed sustainable care and support, as summarized below.

- The literature on the use of telemental health for interventions after disasters is lacking and needs to be addressed. Therefore, we must extrapolate from the literature on trauma-focused mental health care, international care, cross-cultural mental health care, and telemedicine for physical disorders.
- Telemental health programs should report their implementation, applications, successes, and failures. Only then can others learn and adapt to their own needs—the Kenya experience is an example of this issue.
- The nature of most disasters is that they are not predictable; therefore, local, national, and international groups, and government and nongovernmental organizations, must coordinate and plan effective disaster response, including telemental health. Both acute response and longer term sustainability should be included in planning.
- Telemental health services must be tailored to the disaster site, including issues such as the nature of the disaster, infrastructure, and personnel available. The stage of disaster response is important as efforts must be sustainable over the longer term as posttraumatic symptoms, depression, and anxiety may manifest after the acute trauma after many relief and recovery health-care professionals have departed the disaster area,
- In the initial stages of disaster response, mental health care is often deemed secondary to other care creating a gap in mental health services; therefore, telemental health can, and should, play an important role in providing needed services early in the disaster response.
- Globally, especially in the developing world, primary care is the standard of health-care delivery. This includes primary care medical professionals and paraprofessionals. Therefore, the need for specialty expertise is critical. Telemental health can help bridge this gap by providing a full range of needed mental health expertise, including trauma informed care, in consultation to primary care providers and/or in providing direct service to individuals in need.
- Additionally, our experience at HPRT is that mental health expertise is one of the most requested areas of specialty care by those working is postdisaster areas, including nongovernmental organizations and other international agencies.
- As noted in the Kenya case study, there is often an absence of data reported on the use of telemental health in disaster response. Frontlines disaster responders are often too

overwhelmed with caring for survivors to take time for organized data collection. Yet, the collection, analysis, and reporting of such data are crucial for documentation and future program development, including development of telemental health programs. Some of the expertise provided through telemental health should be allocated to the systematic assessment of the challenges, successes, and failures of such efforts in disaster response.

* The telecommunications equipment and telemental health programs deployed in a postdisaster environment should be as simple as possible and designed for the local communications network and infrastructure as well as for the circumstances of the specific disaster. An important aspect of a telemedicine program is the training of rescue and relief workers in the use of telemedicine equipment and sustainability of the equipment and services after other programs have moved out of the area.

Future Directions

One of the most promising areas of telemental health and telemedicine is the use of mobile devices such as notepads and smart phones that can be used in the delivery of health care. Mobile Health, or *m*Health, is a particularly important method of delivery in the developing world. Much of the developing world has skipped the wire generation and moved into the wireless generation with force. In fact, Africa is reported to be one of the most rapidly developing mobile phone markets in the world. This allows populations that heretofore were isolated from specialty medical care to gain access to a level of care not previously available. In areas that have suffered disasters, communications infrastructure is often damaged or destroyed; however, repair or replacement of communications infrastructure is often a priority in the immediate postdisaster phase. Therefore, wireless connectivity for telemedicine and telemental health is often an option early in relief and recovery efforts. The author's experience with international populations and disaster events suggests that telemental health through the use of mobile technology for delivery of mental health care will continue to increase the reach of best practices to global populations in need. An example of this occurred during the "Arab Spring" uprising in Libya. During the height of the armed conflict, HPRT was able to provide on-going mental health support and provide valuable second opinions from Cambridge, MA, to the main hospital in Benghazi, Libya. Because of problems with connectivity, most of the consultations were via teleconference calls. This critical link was a clear demonstration of the value of bringing outside specialty mental health consultation during the height of war.

Conclusion

Disasters, natural and/or man-made, often cause significant loss of life, injuries, and sufferings, destruction of properties, and displacement of people. The need for humanitarian groups to step in and provide medical and mental health care is critical. The mental health needs of survivors impact recovery and their emergence is phasic: fear, anxiety, and mild disorientation in the early phase of postdisaster care, while depression and/or posttrauma problems emerge after weeks or months. Yet, mental health is not a priority in most countries. One of the major issues reported in postdisaster work is the lack of specialist in many fields, including mental health, particularly over the longer term after rescue and relief workers have left. This brings the issue of sustainable care into crisp focus, i.e. specialty care, including mental health, are in demand following the acute phase of disaster response. It is the experience of the author that telemental health is the most efficient means of bringing sustained mental health best practices to those in need following a disaster. Telemental health should have a role in providing needed mental health services to survivors as well as supervision, mentoring, and case consultation to those providing care in the field. Many studies now support the feasibility, acceptability, and effectiveness of telemental health in underserved communities. These data lay the foundation for further work in implementing telemental health in disaster areas and examining best practices for working in such areas with highly traumatized populations. Challenges will be great, available and acceptable technologies will vary with geography or political situations and not all telemental health clinicians will be able to work across cultural barriers or with interpreters; therefore, tolerance for the vicissitudes of such work must be high. Collaboration with providers in the field must be a core principle. Telemental health can, and should, be a major component in meeting the mandate for sustainable world-class health care to those in need regardless of location.

Despite these challenges, the author would like to restate the importance, and great satisfaction, of disaster response work and the role that telemedicine and telemental health do play to help ensure the delivery of evidence-based care and best practices to those in critical need. To paraphrase the title of Thomas Friedman's best seller, *The World is Flat* (Friedman, 2005), the author would like to suggest that with the assistance of telemedicine and telemental health, *The Telemental Health World is Flat!*

References

Bailey, R. K., Bailey, T., & Akpudo, H. (2010). On the ground in Haiti: A psychiatrist's evaluation of post earthquake Haiti. *Journal of Health Care for the Poor and Underserved, 21*, 417−421.

Blattman, C. (2012). Post-conflict recovery in Africa: The micro level. In E. Aryeetey, S. Devarajan, R. Kanbur, & L. Kasekende (Eds.), *The Oxford companion to the economics of Africa*. New York, NY: Oxford University Press.

Delva, J. G. (2010). Americans arrested taking children out of Haiti, Reuters. <http://www.reuters.com/article/2010/01/30/us-quake-haiti-arrests-idUSTRE60T23I20100130> Accessed 22.02.12.

Diagnostic and Statistical Manual of Mental Disorders (DSM-IV). (1994). The American Psychiatric Association, Washington, DC.

Freedy, J. R., Saladin, M. E., Kilpatrick, D. G., Resnick, H. S., & Saunders, B. E. (1994). Understanding acute psychological distress following natural disasters. *Journal of Traumatic Stress, 7*, 257–273.

Friedman, T. (2005). *The world is flat.* New York, NY: Farrar, Straus and Giroux.

Harvey, R., Smith, M., Abraham, N., Hood, S., & Tannenbaum, D. (2007). The Hurricane choir: Remote mental health monitoring of participants in a community-based intervention in the post Katrina period. *Journal of Health Care for the Poor and Underserved, 18*, 356–361.

Inter-Agency Standing Committee (IASC). (2007). *IASC guidelines on mental health and psychosocial support in emergency settings.* Geneva: IASC.

International Committee of the Red Cross. *Haiti earthquake: Medical aid for the survivors..* (2012). <http://www.icrc.org/eng/resources/documents/film/haiti-medical-aid-video-010210.htm>. Accessed 22.02.12.

International Crime Court Press Release. *Kenya's post election violence: ICC Prosecutor presents cases against six individuals for crimes against humanity.* (2010). <http://www.icc-cpi.int/NR/exeres/BA2041D8-3F30-4531-8850-431B5B2F4416.htm> Accessed 22.02.12.

Internal Displacement Monitoring Centre. (2011). Colombia. <http://www.internal-displacement.org/> Accessed 24.02.12.

Jenkins, R., Kiima, D., Njenga, F., Okonji, M., Kingora, J., Kathuku, D., et al. (2010). Integration of mental health into primary care in Kenya. *World Psychiatry, 9*, 118–120.

Johnson, K. (2011). Telemedicine could reduce earthquake mortality. *Medscape Today News.* <http://www.medscape.com/viewarticle/739744> Accessed 22.02.12.

Kimenyi, K. S., Gutierrez Romero, R., Dercon, S., Bratton, M., Vicente, P., & Bold, T. (2010). Elections, ethnic polarization and managing post-electoral conflict in Kenya. Improving Institutions. <http://www.iig.ox.ac.uk/research/09-elections-ethnic-polarization-kenya.htm> Accessed 22.02.12.

Kohn, R., Levav, I., & Donaire Garcia, I. (2005). Psychological and psychopathological reactions following Hurricane Mitch in Honduras: Implications for service planning. *Pan American Journal of Public Health, 18*, 287–295.

Ladd, A. E., Marszalek, J., & Gill, D. A. (2006). The other dispora: New Orleans student evacuations impacts and responses surrounding Hurricane Katrina. Paper presented at the annual meeting of the Southern Sociological Society. New Orleans, LA, March.

Lima, B. R., Pai, S., Toledo, V., Caris, L., Haro, J. M., Lozano, J., et al. (1993). Emotional distress in disaster victims: A follow-up study. *Journal of Nervous and Mental Disease, 181*, 388–393.

Louden, K.. (2010). Telemedicine connects earthquake ravaged Haiti to the world. *Medscape Medical News.* <http://www.medscape.com/viewarticle/717232> Accessed 22.02.12.

McShane, K. M. (2011). Mental health in Haiti: A resident's perspective. *Academic Psychiatry, 35*, 8–10.

Mollica, R. (2007). Harvard global mental health: Trauma and recovery program. Presented at the Harvard Global Mental Health Program. Orvieto, Italy, November.

Mollica, R. F. (2006). *Healing invisible wounds: Paths to hope and recovery in a violent world.* Orlando, FL: Harcourt.

NATO Joint Medical Committee. *Psychosocial care for people affected by disasters and major incidents.* (2008). <http://www.coe.int/t/dg4/majorhazards/ressources/virtuallibrary/materials/Others/NATO_Guidance_Psychosocial_Care_for_People_Affected_by_Disasters_and_Major_Incidents.pdf> Accessed 22.02.12.

National Institute of Mental Health. Anxiety disorders. (2012). <http://www.nimh.nih.gov/health/topics/anxiety-disorders/index.shtml> Accessed 24.02.12.

Ndetei, D. M., Ongecha-Owuor, F. A., Khasakhala, L., Mutiso, V., Odhiambo, G., & Kokonya, D. A. (2007). Traumatic experiences of Kenyan secondary school students. *Journal of Child and Adolescent Mental Health, 19*, 147–155.

Nicogossian, A. E., & Doarn, C. R. (2011). Armenia 1988 earthquake and telemedicine: Lessons learned and forgotten. *Telemedicine Journal and e-Health, 17*, 741–745.

Olsen, I. T. (1998). Sustainability of health care: A framework for analysis. *Health Policy and Planning, 13*, 287–295.

Olteanu, A., Arnberger, R., Grant, R., Davis, C., Abramson, D., & Asola, J. (2011). Persistence of mental health needs among children affected by Hurricane Katrina in New Orleans. *Prehospital and Disaster Medicine, 26*, 3–6.

Perlman, S. E., Friedman, S., Galea, S., Nair, H. P., Eros-Sarnyai, M., Stellman, S. D., et al. (2011). Short-term and medium-term health effects of 9/11. *Lancet, 378*, 925–934.

Porcari, C. E., Amdur, R. L., Koch, E. L., Richard, D. C., Favorite, T., Martis, B., et al. (2009). Assessment of post-traumatic stress disorder in veterans by videoconferencing and by face-to-face methods. *Journal of Telemedicine and Telecare, 15*, 89–94.

RED, the Centre for Research on the Epidemiology of Disasters, A World Health Organization Collaborating Agency. (2011). <http://maps.grida.no/go/graphic/trends-in-natural-disasters> Accessed 22.02.12.

Rodriguez, J., & Kohn, R. (2008). Use of mental health services among disaster survivors. *Current Opinion in Psychiatry, 21*, 370–378.

Rossi, P. H., Wright, J. D., Weber-Burdin, E., & Pereira, J. (1983). Victimization by natural hazards in the United States, 1970–1980: Survey estimates. *International Journal of Mass Emergencies and Disasters, 1*, 467–482.

Safran, M. A., Chorba, T., Schreiber, M., Archer, W. R., & Cookson, S. T. (2011). Evaluating mental health after the 2010 Haitian earthquake. *Disaster Medicine and Public Health Preparedness, 5*, 154–157.

Saxena, S., Patel, V., Baingana, F., & Knapp, M. (2010). Can developing economies afford to ignore mental health? Presented at the Johns Hopkins University, Bloomberg School of Public Health, Baltimore MD, March.

Simmons, S., Alverson, D., Poropatich, R., Di'Orio, J., & Doarn, C. (2008). Applying telehealth in natural and anthropogenic disasters. *Telemedicine Journal and e-Health, 14*, 968–971.

Tracy, M., Norris, F. H., & Galea, S. (2011). Differences in the determinants of posttraumatic stress disorder and depression after a mass traumatic event. *Depression and Anxiety, 28*, 666–675.

US Geological Survey. National Earthquake Information Center. <http://earthquake.usgs.gov/regional/neic/> Accessed 24.02.12.

Warner, C., & Scott, R. T. (2005). Where they died. *The Times-Picayune.* <http://www.nola.com> Accessed 24.02.12.

W'Atwoli, L. (2011). Why budgeting for mental health care is crucial. <http://allafrica.com/stories/201110100776.html> Accessed 22.02.12.

Wireless Healthcare. *Telemedicine system links doctors in Texas with patients in East Africa.* (2011). <http://www.wirelesshealthcare.co.uk/wh/news/wk05-07-0003.htm> Accessed 22.02.12.

Yellowlees, P., Burke, M. M., Marks, S. L., Hilty, D. M., & Shore, J. H. (2008). Emergency telepsychiatry. *Journal of Telemedicine and Telecare, 14*, 277–281.

18 Social Networking and Mental Health

Benjamin Hidy, Emily Porch, Sarah Reed,
*Michelle Burke Parish and Peter Yellowlees**

Department of Psychiatry, UC Davis School of Medicine, Sacramento, CA

Introduction and History of Social Networks

During 2010, in the United States, there was a cluster of adolescent and young adult suicides that were highly publicized on national news media outlets. This caught the nation's attention. It prompted an outpouring of grief, support, and inspired millions to try to end bullying and change the future of America's youth. It also inspired a new generation of young Americans to rise to the challenge of trying to enact change in their communities and government. Jennifer Hewlett from Kentucky.com profiled one such young American.

> *Matthew Vanderpool, a 26-year-old man in Lexington, KY, was running for a seat in the Kentucky House of Representatives with a dream of equality and the wish to improve the lives of millions in his state. As far as his friends knew he was a very happy and emotionally stable man, and he happened to be openly gay. However, on the night of Tuesday July 12, 2011, Matthew wrote a public message to his friends on the social networking site he used, Facebook. These are his messages that he posted at 7:36 p.m. that night:*
>
> *"I have friends that are by my side like security at a presidential debate...They protect me from not only others, but from myself. We have shared some crazy times, happy times, sad times and times that we will never forget ... one because the video camera won't let us and two because that is who we are as friends. My friends are my family...I've just been looking back today at some of the things I have done and started a list of the things I want to do! Just writing thoughts I guess."*

At 9:40 p.m. that night the Lexington, KY, police were called by this man's father, from out of state, stating that his son had a gun and was having thoughts of wanting to end his life.

Although Matthew's statement is lacking in obvious intention to end his life, this subtle method is often how emotional states are conveyed online. Social Media networking has changed how people reach out emotionally to their friends and

Telemental Health. DOI: http://dx.doi.org/10.1016/B978-0-12-416048-4.00018-X

loved ones (Hewlett, 2011). It is uncommon for social media users to explicitly state their "mood" or whether they are having "thoughts of self-harm." Therefore, reading between the lines and determining the tone of the written comment is important. In Matthew's case, it is possible that someone who knew him well may have read the post and seen darker undertones or would have recognized that such a post was out of character for him. Communications on social networks can be automatic in that a person may often write impulsively without giving much thought to what it means, or how it will be interpreted by others. Such posts may provide clues to an individual's underlying emotional state and level of functioning. A trained mental health professional who is familiar with a patient may be able to recognize deeper meaning in a post and intervene in whatever way may be necessary. To understand the dynamics of cases like Matthew's and the implications of social networking in health care and the field of mental health, a little history of the development of social networking sites, such as Facebook, and how they are used is needed.

The Development of Facebook and Twitter

Current research demonstrates a sharp increase in the usage of social networking sites as well as an increase in the development of health-care platforms in this media form. This communication technology is rapidly evolving and adapting to increasing social pressure and demand from patients and society. It presents concrete as well as abstract ethical and legal complications clinicians must navigate. The impact it will have upon care provision, rapport building, and even personal quality of life is thought to be profound.

This is a new frontier for mental health. It is a pivotal time of development and exciting change, especially in the realm of telemental health. Patients are providing critical and useful information freely in the public web domain. Physicians and other health-care professionals have an obligation to decide how, and if, to use this information for the good of their patients. If not, health-care professionals may find themselves in the future having to adapt to an online health-care system that is already established, instead of being an integral part of the development process.

Although a relatively recent development, the concept of social networking has had a dramatic and profound impact on the way mankind interacts. The basic function of communication remains unchanged, that is to say that people still talk about and share ideas in much the same manner, but the method of communication delivery has been vastly altered. Anecdotally, an informal developmental history of social networking sites began in the 1970s when the concept of electronic mail, commonly referred to today as e-mail, was introduced to the world. This innovation began to replace voice communication over a telephone or face-to-face contact allowing for instantaneous communication in written form over long distances. As a result of technologies limitations preventing the ability to "scan" documents, such as copying a hand-signed document into electronic media form, the regular postal service remained intact, but eventually attained the slightly humorous pseudonym of "snail mail."

In the ensuing decades, technology was developed that led to the introduction in 1994 of one of the world's first social networking sites, or social media sites, named Geocities. This networking tool allowed users to create personal web sites and index them in locations referred to as "cities," according to their focus of content. It is important to note, however, that the major boom for social networking did not occur until the early 1990s and increased access for most people to the "information super highway" (Rucker, 2011).

Many initial online service providers, such as CompuServe, Prodigy, and America Online (AOL), quickly became household names. These services offered easy-to-use "interfaces" or visual displays on the computer screen that allowed personal computer users to access the Internet. With this development, web sites began to offer message boards, similar to an online bulletin board or forum that users could write on or "post" personal responses to stories and other content.

The year 1997 marked a critical development that changed the way that individuals used the Internet and perhaps began a generational shift in Internet users as well. The introduction of AOL Instant Messaging began an entire Internet culture of instant textual communication that has grown and persisted in various forms ever since and has culminated in modern day cellular telephone text messaging (Rucker, 2011). Similar to e-mail, the communication occurred instantaneously; however, the model of communication mirrored common casual conversation in that the interface displayed an easy-to-read record of the communications.

Quickly following this, the development of "chat rooms" allowed multiple users to communicate instantly in an online group forum, even if those individuals were on different continents. "Blogs" were formed as individual personal web sites became more common. Blogs function to allow for an individual to post focused news articles, opinions, information, advice, instructions, or just about any other form of communication one can think of. Sometimes they take the form of a daily diary, such as with Xanga, which was a company that made individual blogs widely available. Some "bloggers," or individuals who develop and maintain a blog, have become so well known that they have been able to make large sums of money from their work. Often, message boards will be used on blog sites as well, so readers can post about their personal experience or reaction to the information provided on the blog.

Following trends in information technology, the development of Internet communication continued to take on a more social tone. In 2002, the world was introduced to Friendster, one of the first "social-networking sites". This site allowed users to create online personal "profiles" or personal webpages with their photograph, biographical information, and other details the user wanted to publish publicly. It also allowed the users to share media content and play games (Bloomberg Businessweek, 2011; Perdu, 2008). In 2003, a similar company called MySpace was released that focused more on the social aspect of social networking. It chiefly focused on the creation of personal profiles, with lists of friends (other users who have profiles that can be connected to the primary user's profile), the ability of one user to post messages on other users' profiles and sharing of photographs and other media (Myspace, 2011).

In 2004, the preeminent social networking site, Thefacebook (now known as Facebook), was released (Wyld, 2012). This site allowed the user all of the above tools, but differed in the way the site was perceived by the public. Facebook was not open initially to everyone; it started at Harvard University and was only available to Harvard students. Slowly the company allowed expansion to other universities in the United States and then internationally. This gave the site an element of exclusivity, which greatly enhanced its desirability to users.

After Facebook had established itself, it opened to high-school students, businesses, and later to anyone with an active e-mail account over the age of 13 years (Wyld, 2012). In 2009, Compete.com ranked Facebook as the world's most active social networking site, and in July 2011, the company was noted to have over 800 million worldwide users (Kazeniac, 2009; Olivarez-Giles, 2011). The company's popularity even prompted the creation of a blockbuster movie, entitled "The Social Network," in which the company's history is detailed. Another quality adding to the site's popularity is the relative ease of joining as a member. All interested persons needs to do is go online to the web site, www.facebook.com, and they will be immediately offered the opportunity to join. First, the site will prompt individuals for their name, a valid e-mail address, and birth date. Then, further prompting will allow individuals to search for other people they know who might be using the site, generally by e-mail address or name. They will also be able to fill out their biographical information as well as place their photograph on their main profile page, as described below. All of this is designed to guide the user through the setup process with as little confusion as possible (Wyld, 2012).

Facebook, Myspace, and various other profile-based social networking sites share the commonality of the personal profile and list of friends. Users can "friend" others on the site, which by definition is a request for other site users to acknowledge their shared friendship, which will then link their two profile pages; this process is also commonly referred to as "friending." After this, the new friend's profile picture will be displayed on the user's profile, and a link between the two profiles will be displayed on a "news-feed" and "wall." A news-feed is a running list of all events that a user has completed on the site that is available to be viewed by all other "friends." A wall is similar to a news-feed, except that it is localized only to the person's profile page, and "friends" can comment on it with a "status update," i.e., any information that "friends" want the Internet world to know.

Users can also "post," or add, pictures to their wall or even to their friends' walls. This can be taken using a mobile smartphone from a phone application connected to Facebook or uploaded to the Internet social networking site from a computer hard drive. This same process of posting a picture can be applied to posting a video on a wall or even a hyperlink to a web site. Another unique feature is the ability of users to add their personal interests, including movies, books, celebrities, and even their gender and sexual orientation, to their profile. In addition, users will often post their educational and employment history and even contact information.

These sites offer many options in terms of security and do not require this information to be listed and even can be restricted from view for certain persons.

A slightly different approach to social networking soon followed the aforementioned sites. Twitter was launched in 2006. It allows users to form smaller profiles, in which they can "microblog," meaning to send short messages about various topics usually consisting of less than 140 characters (Twitter, 2010). This message is commonly referred to as a "tweet." These messages are directed to other users who are subscribed to each others' profiles. This is also known as "following" a user. This company has been very successful in capturing celebrities, politicians, and news media, which often use "tweets" as a form of communication to the public. This company has also found a niche in the ability to rapidly spread real-time news updates, such as that occurred during the Arab Spring revolutions in the Middle East and with acts of terrorism (Lipsman, 2009).

Broad and Diverse Applications of Networking Sites

With this complicated developmental history of social media sites and their various functions, who is using them anyway and for what purposes? The answer is most everybody. People from all age groups, different countries, men, women, students, professionals, celebrities, companies are using these online communication tools. What started out mainly in the professional Internet technology world has quickly spread to the average American house, office, and dorm room, and even across generations. Recently, more involvement has been seen with users over 65 years of age.

It is estimated that there are millions of Facebook users under the age of 13, who thus are breaking terms of registration on the site (Computers and Internet, 2011). This is important to note because of issues regarding legal consent; frequently governmental laws require a citizen to be over 13 years in order to enter into a contract of use with an online entity. This has implications for mental health-care providers who operate an online forum as they may need to confirm young patients' age through face-to-face contact before allowing them to use their online site. Of course, the issue of consent to medical treatment for persons under the age of 18 would still apply in an online situation as it does in the clinical office setting.

The total percentage of persons with a social media site profile doubled between 2008 and 2010 from 24% to 48% (Saint, 2010). A breakdown of American user demographics was provided by Edison Research and published by Business Insider in June 2010. These data revealed that between the sexes, women were more likely to use social networking sites on a regular basis than men, by a margin of 57−43%. It was also notable from research trends that social networking sites are more frequently accessed by regular Internet users and by those who identify themselves as likely to adopt new electronic gadgets more quickly than the average person. The age group most likely to use these social media sites is the

18–25-year-old group, standing at 25% of all users. This is followed by the 25–34-year-old group at 23%, 12–17-year-old group at 18%, 35–44-year-old group at 16%, 45–54-year-old group at 9%, and finally the 55 + group at 9%. By racial demographic data, those identifying themselves as Caucasian are most likely to use these sites with 66% reporting frequent usage, followed by self-identifying African-American participants at 14%, Hispanic-identifying participants at 10%, Asian-identifying participants at 2%, and other race at 8%. On a final note, students and full-time employed persons were the most likely of all occupations to use social networking sites.

It is clear that the use of social media is omnipresent in American culture, but how are individuals utilizing these applications? More specifically, how are these applications influencing how users communicate emotional information and, by extension, how are they influencing the field of mental health care?

Use and Effectiveness of Social Networking in Health-Related Behaviors

In December 2010, AOL News launched a story out of Sacred Heart Hospital in Eau Claire, Wisconsin. A 56-year-old woman had arrived at the emergency department complaining of chest pain and shortly thereafter had become comatose. It was determined by the hospital physicians that this patient has sustained a stroke, and efforts were made to contact her family. However, the only available family member was her son who was of limited help in determining her medical history. The rest of her family lived far away, but it was discovered that the patient had an active Facebook profile. After accessing her account in the public domain, the physicians found that she had listed all of her symptoms and medications as well as past medical history and procedures. She had even put the dates that certain symptoms and procedures had occurred. From this information, the medical team determined that this patient had a cardiac septal defect allowing for thromboemboli to pass into her systemic blood flow to her brain, leading to multiple cerebral infarctions. Neurosurgery was consulted. At the time of publication on AOL News, the woman had recovered from the coma and was progressing through rehabilitation (Gingritch & Thapar, 2010).

This case underscores the potential of social networking as a powerful tool in the field of health care and mental health care. However, the future of social networking in medicine and mental health care presents many dilemmas for patients and providers in sharing personal information, as well as new opportunities for health-care providers to interact with, provide information to, and care for patients. While there is a substantial amount of research examining how health-care consumers and providers are utilizing social networking, the rapidly evolving nature of Internet interactions makes it difficult to establish a definitive evidence-based guide to incorporating social networking into practice. While gaps in current research will be discussed later in this chapter, a review of the current literature provides insight into the possibilities and pitfalls of using social networking in clinical practice.

As social networking profiles become increasingly popular, more people are disclosing potentially health-relevant information on their social profiles, prompting many researchers to examine these sites as an important source of collateral information about social risk factors and mental health symptoms. These studies suggest that not only clinically significant behavioral patterns in a person's life are mirrored in their social network interactions but also that cumulative postings can be themselves diagnostic of both Axis I and Axis II disorders (Mikami, Szwedo, Allen, Evans, & Hare, 2010). Furthermore, as the aforementioned case of Matthew Vanderpool indicates, the online community's response to posts can prompt disclosure of personal mental health status and influence a person's help-seeking or self-harming behaviors (Moreno, Jelenchick et al., 2011). Additionally, research has found that online profiles reveal a wealth of information about social risk factors including risk taking and substance-use behavior (Moreno, Briner, Williams, Walker, & Christakis, 2009; Ridout, Campbell, & Ellis, 2011). These findings are particularly relevant to adolescents.

As of March 2011, the United Kingdom established a task force with Facebook to try to and minimize suicide attempts. This project stems from the multiple suicidal comments made on social networking sites, which were seen by others, but no action was made to contact the person or local governmental authorities. This task force acts to get the word out to Facebook users and alert them to the ongoing problem. For a person who suspects a friend of being in danger, a Help Desk icon visible on the webpage allows the user to be directed immediately to services that then obtain more information about the person at risk. The information is then passed to police and to a local psychological and emotional support organization that act to intervene. In December 2011, Facebook opened a similar initiative in the United States, letting users who view suicidal statements to alert Facebook staff through a link available next to each user comment. This link directs Facebook to send an e-mail to the poster with a link to National Suicide Prevention hotline counselors, who are available through Facebook's chat system.

Consumer Health Social Networks

By definition, all types of social networking sites provide a platform for users to interact with each other; however among these, a subset of sites called "Consumer Health Social Networks" (CHSN) provide a place specifically for patients to network and share information. These sites are increasingly popular and are often sponsored by health organizations (such as the Centers for Disease Control (CDC), National Alliance on Mental Illness (NAMI), or American Cancer Society) for patients to interact with each other and their providers, including posting questions, experiences, and knowledge about health issues. A popular example where patients can create profiles, learn more about symptoms and treatments, and meet others with the same medical issues is the site "Patients Like Me" (www. patientslikeme.com), an online patient community. Multiple studies show the popularity of these sites and reveal that a large percentage of the population now use the Internet to look up mental health information whether they have a mental health problem or not, often within these patient-driven CHSNs (Burns, Davenport, Durkin, Luscombe, & Hickie, 2010; McMullan, 2006). This new way of learning about health-care issues is affecting the ways that patients and their providers interact.

As much as these sites facilitate patient participation in and learning about their care, they also are problematic when seen as authorities on illness course or treatment. Nearly every provider today has experienced the patient who brings in a printout of some health-care-related "fact" they found on the Internet. Recent analyses of social networking sites highlight the problems with socializing medical knowledge (Tsai, Tsai, Zeng-Treitler, & Liang, 2007; Vance, Howe, & Dellavalle, 2009). In reviews of information shared between users both on social networking sites specific to health care and within more generalized social networks, such as Twitter and Facebook, the authors found that the medical information posted by users was often inaccurate, with errors in greater than 50% of the posts that contained medical knowledge (Vance et al., 2009). The dissemination of misinformation is fostered by problematic blind authorship common in Internet postings, lack of source citation, and a forum which facilitates presenting opinions as medical facts. Furthermore, research has not yet developed generalizable instruments to measure the quality of information on health sites (Breckons, Jones, Morris, & Richardson, 2007).

Instant linking between sites makes the Internet a wealth of easily accessible misinformation, and patients armed with false knowledge can make even the most patient provider cringe. However, while the possibility for the propagation of incorrect information on the Internet is endless, the prevalence of health information sharing through social networking sites suggests that this method of health education is here to stay. Providers need to be aware of how patients are using these site and the ways these social networks can be used to enhance patient care.

Involvement of Health-Care Systems with Social Networking

As the public's comfort with social networking has grown, many health-care organizations are exploring social media to interact with their patients, utilizing everything from Twitter feeds to post clinic updates to broad spectrum social networking allowing patients bidirectional interaction with their providers (Hawker, 2010). Some boutique practices have developed entirely paperless systems of health-care delivery using CHSNs, weblogs, instant messaging, video chat, and patient profiles to facilitate cost-effective patient care (Hawker, 2010; Hawn, 2009). One review of over 80 web sites focused on diabetes care showed that many web sites are falling short of comprehensive, interactive chronic care models of care, offering instead didactic-style information. However, this same review noted that sites which mimicked behavioral change models, including interactive assessments, social support, or problem-solving assistance, had the potential for greater patient benefit, especially for those dealing with chronic illness information (Bull, Gaglio, Mckay, & Glasgow, 2005).

A trial of a model CHSN focused on HIV care offered comprehensive health information as well as forums for networking with both experts and other patients. In this trial, patients using these sites reported at 3 and 6 month mark increased feelings of social support, decreased negative emotions, and increased participation in health care. Furthermore, it showed that patients engaged in this CHSN spent 15% less time during ambulatory care visits, made 47% more phone calls to providers, and experienced 35% fewer hospitalizations (Gustafson et al., 1999).

While both mainstream social networking sites and specialized CHSNs can provide innovative ways of delivering health care in all fields, the interactive nature of social networking lends itself especially well to providing cost-effective mental health care and Web-based therapy. CHSNs are ideal for hosting supportive therapy groups, especially for patients going through similar experiences, and participation in these groups can significantly improve outcomes in chronic disease (Kash, Mago, & Kunkel, 2005). Several studies have also shown that these Internet-support groups provide normalization, reassurance, and emotional support, and provide therapeutic community for isolated individuals going through crisis. Additionally the online format can be ideal for maintaining anonymity, reducing the stigma barrier for a patient seeking treatment (Fleischmann, 2005).

Online groups are also being used successfully for behavioral change intervention, including groups for substance-use cessation (Etter, 2006). In addition to engaging a therapeutic community, participants often use their social networking group site to expand social awareness, fundraise, and further research (Bender, Jimenez-Marroquin, & Jadad, 2011). The ease of this transition from group support to public outreach makes social networking an ideal system for actively engaging participants in recovery.

As social networking quickly brings together groups with common experiences or interests, some of the same features that make these sites ideal for connecting people therapeutically can also be utilized to propagate unhealthy habits. Social networking has seen an upswing in the formation of anti-therapeutic groups, where participants with similar troubles seek each other to normalize and encourage pathological coping. These groups are probably best exemplified by the "pro-ana" and "pro-mia" (sometimes written "proanamia") sites, which support and promote anorexia and bulimia and post "thinspiration" photos and techniques to further encourage pathological weight loss. Studies have found concerning trends where even healthy individuals visiting these sites have lower self-esteem, perceived themselves as heavier, and engaged in more image comparison after browsing these groups (Bardone-Cone & Cass, 2007). More troubling, these sites have become increasingly prevalent and accessed by a significant percentage of adolescents (Custers & Van den Bulck, 2009).

Unfortunately this model for propagating unhealthy behaviors through social networking is not limited to one disorder. Online groups have also created forums to discuss effective ways to complete suicide and form suicide pacts between members. This trend has been especially widespread in Japan, which has seen hundreds of people complete suicide in groups formed through online communities (Ozawa-De Silva, 2010). Similarly, there have been several instances in which users have committed cyber-public suicides, publishing their suicide intent on Facebook and inviting comments (where online "friends" often encourage the person to continue with their plans) or even streaming their self-harm live for viewers (http://www.dailymail.co.uk/news/article-1344281/Facebook-suicide-None-Simone-Backs-1-082-online-friends-helped-her.htm). Mental health providers need to be aware of these trends in social networking and screen for potential unhealthy networking activities in Internet-using patients.

Potential Benefits of Social Networks for Both Patients and Providers

While the full range of applications for social networking in mental health care has not been fully developed, it has the potential to save an outpatient, or even inpatient, physician valuable time and money. For example, a pediatrician performing adolescent well-visit assessments may find that it is much more efficient and accurate to gather information about risky behavior, home life, and school performance from a patient's Facebook page instead of verbally probing for this information from a shy or guarded adolescent. Similarly, a psychiatrist may use Facebook posts to obtain quick "collateral" information to sway a disposition decision on a noncooperative patient who is at high risk for suicidal behavior.

Providers who have concerns about individual patient–provider "friendships" may find financial benefit in creating patient-centered or diagnosis-themed social networking groups on a general social networking site or even developing a CHSN of their own. Instead of spending valuable time on the phone answering the same question from 10 different patients, a provider may simply log on to a group page and quickly respond to a variety of patient "posts." A provider can also save office time by preemptively posting up-to-date answers to frequently asked questions about office policies and current health-care related topics. A provider can cut back on patient phone calls and possibly appointment length by posting links to recommended, provider-approved Internet reading in order to divert patients away from anxiety-provoking and misguided Internet health-care sites.

Face-to-face medication management groups are a regular component of many psychiatric outpatient services but the structure of these groups often suffers from poor or unwieldy attendance. By conducting these groups through convenient online networking, a physician may improve attendance and find it easier to manage difficult group dynamics. In addition, patients who have transportation issues or physical disabilities may be excited for the opportunity to participate.

Physicians can have greater personal freedom by conducting medication management sessions or therapy groups from their own office or home using individualized or video chat services. If desired, providers may charge online fees for these sessions, thereby eliminating the need to for an in-person office assistant.

Social networking also allows for the easy creation of multidisciplinary groups, which are otherwise nearly impossible to arrange. Local pharmacists, physicians, therapists, and other care providers can log into a single social networking group to post and discuss detailed and specialized information. Patients with complex disorders may be willing to pay additional fees to join an online social networking group composed of specialized physicians, social workers, and therapists. Practice-specific CHSNs would be an efficient and effective means of providing patients with up-to-date clinical information. However, it should be noted that most current social networks, such as Facebook groups and user comment boards, lack the privacy and security that are required in health-care practices. Despite all the advances in technology, further work and time are needed to make these innovations compatible with the Health Insurance Portability and Accountability Act (HIPAA).

With recent advances in technologies, many companies have allowed their employees to pursue work-from-home options. By and large, physicians and mental health providers have not been able to take advantage of this growing trend. However, the future of social networking and telemedicine may allow some providers to "work-from-home," while continuing to meet patient needs. Mental health providers are in a unique position to take advantage of such an option, as psychiatric assessments focus primarily on verbal communication and visual observation. Many mental health providers are already using social networking to augment and prolong benefits of traditional therapy.

Engaging patients in ongoing therapeutic social networking following a psychiatric hospitalization can reduce relapse rates and extend treatment gains following discharge from acute hospitalization. One study examined the course of 186 patients after inpatient hospitalization. Following discharge, half of these patients continued to receive weekly 90 min therapist-conducted Internet chat therapy sessions in groups of 8−10 years old. After a year, those engaged in the Internet therapy groups were less than half as likely as controls to experience relapse in symptoms (22% vs 46%). These gains were increased by the use of Internet chat therapy groups (Bauer, Wolf, Haug, & Kordy, 2011). Such studies offer a model of how mental health consumers can access low cost and accessible ways to continue care and grant mental health providers opportunities to provide quality care from a distance.

Comparisons between online groups and traditional groups show similar gains in participant self-image, social relations, and well-being, with similar rates of patient satisfaction. Many traditional group dynamics including cohesion, forming group norms, transference, and scapegoating are also frequently seen in Internet therapy groups. The online therapy group culture differs somewhat, however, in regard to contract, boundaries, leaving the group, and extra-group socialization. Internet groups also can develop higher levels of aggression, action orientation, and therapist support and control than traditional group therapy (Barak & Wander-Schwartz, 1999;

Weinberg, 2001). As social networking sites become an increasingly popular platform for hosting online support and therapy groups, further research is being conducted to examine the applicability of traditional group theory to online psychology, as well as ethical concerns (Childress, 2000).

The ubiquity of smartphones is making these benefits even more accessible. Several CBT and substance-use applications have been developed for smartphones and are available to allow patients to track thoughts, emotions, and behaviors in real time on their smartphone. This digitalization of therapy techniques may facilitate ease of engagement in groups and ongoing therapy homework for the tech-savvy patient.

Providers may also use social networking sites to deal with after-hours patient questions. For example, a provider may prefer that nonemergent, after-hours questions be "messaged" or "posted" to a social networking page, instead of waking up the provider with a phone call. A provider may also be able to easily extend his or her hours, offering special online services to patients who want evening or weekend sessions. A psychiatrist who wants to offer "home visits" can increase a patient load and decrease transportation costs by offering weekly video chat services in lieu of traveling. A family member who is unsure if a situation is emergent (such as a stroke, seizure, or wrist cutting) may post a picture or send a video message to a physician via an online service. The physician can immediately triage the patient by video and determine if the condition necessitates hospitalization.

Clinical and Ethical Dilemmas of Professional Social Networking Sites

Before embarking on a mass professional "friending" expedition, providers and patients must have clear expectations about the benefits and limitations of online professional social networking relationships. First and foremost, providers should determine whether their patient demographic is willing to partake in health-care-related social networking. To date, there have been no validated methods for determining which patient populations would benefit from social networking health-care services. Based on general findings for social networking use, it is reasonable to assume that younger, educated patients are more apt to use this technology, and patients with higher economic means are more likely to have access to these services. Therefore, a provider who primarily works with geriatric or cognitively impaired patients would naturally have more barriers to cross before providing regular professional social networking services. A geriatric specialist may need to spend additional time and money training his patients on how to use these services, while a provider working with adolescents may find it easy to immediately offer social networking health care.

Research is needed to determine whether specific psychological traits or mental health diagnoses are associated with a greater acceptance of professional social networking relationships. Research on this topic would likely reveal that mental health social networking may be valuable for certain subgroups of patients but contraindicated for others. For example, severely depressed or suicidal patients who cannot muster the energy to attend a clinician's appointment could seek life-saving help by "posting" on a provider's wall. If a provider has concerns about a depressed patient who missed an appointment, he or she may log on to a professional social networking site and find that this patient posted a revealing "status update" earlier that morning. A patient with a history of self-mutilation may avert crisis and self-harm behavior by instantly accessing a social networking group about dialectical or cognitive behavior therapy. Anxious patients who require a great deal of personal attention and reassurance may find quicker relief if they use online social networking services instead of waiting for a provider's return phone call.

In other circumstances, a provider may be inclined to dissuade Internet use among certain subgroups of patients. For example, a patient with social phobia or avoidant personality disorder may be excited to converse with a clinician or other peers through an internet-based professional service, in order to evade the embarrassment of face-to-face contact. However, with these patients, social networking may be detrimental to care because it can reinforce the exact behavior that is causing functional impairment. Similarly, computer use and personal profile pages may trigger or worsen psychotic symptoms, particularly in patients who have paranoia or technology related delusions.

Patients who are financially and cognitively able to use professional social networking sites may be resistant to "friend" their provider for various other reasons, particularly when patients are required to connect with their provider through their own personal site. Many patients may view such a provider–patient online "friendship" as invasive and paternalistic, even if this "friendship" is made in the context of a professional social networking site. Individuals' Facebook profile typically include more than just identifying information, and profile owners are not solely responsible for the content on their profile page. If profile owners are concerned with their online image, they must continually monitor these "posts" from other friends and "de-tag" potentially defamatory material, such as photographs. A patient who strives to appear mentally and physically healthy may be uncomfortable with inadvertently sharing these personal details with a mental health provider. Patients who regularly update their Facebook profiles may simply be overwhelmed by the idea that their provider can use social networking to monitor their daily activities. This may incite patients to modify or falsify their profiles just to appear socially acceptable to their providers. In essence, "friending" a provider may take the fun out of social networking. Further research is necessary to address these potential patient concerns.

Since certain groups of patients may gravitate toward or away from social networking services, providers must avoid selectively spending more cumulative time or energy on patients who are willing to access these services. For example, with the advent of smartphones, many providers now have unlimited and unrestricted access to Internet services, which offers the freedom of logging into a professional social networking site from nearly anywhere. A provider can, therefore, quickly and quietly respond to patient posts on professional social networking sites, even if the provider is in a public setting. Clinicians can also engage in a quick online dialogue with patients and send patients useful links to other informative Internet sites. If patients are unable or unwilling to utilize social networking services, they may contact their clinicians via more traditional routes, by leaving a voice message or by scheduling an emergency appointment. Since verbal interaction is required with these patients, time constraints and privacy concerns limit when and where a provider can return a patient phone call. Similarly, emergency appointments are typically limited to regular working hours which impose stricter limitations on the patient−provider interaction. As a result, providers may unintentionally delay contact with patients who choose more traditional routes of communication. These patients may also not receive supplemental materials, including resources available on health-related web sites, simply because a provider is unable or unwilling to print out a hard copy of this information.

Conversely, providers must also be careful not to subconsciously decrease face-to-face time with patients who are taking advantage of online services. It would be easy to discourage a patient from making a face-to-face appointment if a patient's needs can be addressed through social networking services. However, if a clinician does not carefully monitor this behavior, patients who are willing to communicate through social networking may receive an inadequate, inappropriate and, at times, unsafe level of care.

Incorporating social networking into a clinical practice creates yet another level of care, and with it, the possibility of creating even more work for a mental health professional. Running an effective and profitable clinical practice requires providers to balance thoughtful and thorough patient-centered care with high-demand clinical requirements. In order to successfully incorporate this tool into a provider's practice, major concerns regarding finances and time must be addressed as providers must have incentives for using these services. At present, there are no studies addressing the potential financial advantages or disadvantages of incorporating social networking into a clinical practice. There is also no precedent to help clinicians determine whether they can, or should, charge additional fees for social networking services.

As technology advances, the multiple possibilities for enhancing patient convenience must be balanced with the increased demand for providers' time. Many business employees now complain that although they can use their smartphone to e-mail from virtually any place in the country, they are also now responsible for answering e-mails 24 hrs a day, 7 days per week. Technology has made 8 hour workdays largely obsolete. If social networking and advanced technology become incorporated into mental health care, providers may face these same pressures from patients who may expect extended access to their clinicians. Of course, clinicians can set limits on this type of access, yet face professional consequences if patients start to choose clinicians based on their availability after hours. Providers who choose not to incorporate these services into their practice could be less competitive and risk losing their patients to a more technologically savvy and accessible mental health provider.

Even more worrisome, a provider could suffer a loss of his or her privacy and personal time, as patient encounters intrude on personal spaces. Professional social networking may allow clinicians to provide more intensive services for at-risk mental health patients, but the inherent question that needs to be answered is whether or not telemental health social networking will create more work and little reward for providers. If done correctly, this technology does have the potential to improve clinicians' time management as well as care, but more experience in the field and research is needed to determine the optimal use of technology to improve patient–provider communication and access.

Confidentiality, Privacy, and Setting Boundaries

Unfortunately, the immediate use of social networking in clinical practice is also limited by unanswered legal and ethical questions regarding privacy. As Internet laws play catch-up to technological advances, the ability to maintain patient anonymity is at the forefront of these concerns. HIPAA (1996) provides "federal protections for personal health information held by covered entities and gives patients an array of rights with respect to that information." With the advent of electronic medical records, HIPAA has expanded to address legal requirements for electronic communication of patient information. For example, HIPAA does allow for provider-to-provider e-mail exchange of confidential patient information provided that appropriate security measures are in place to prevent breaches of confidentiality. HIPAA has not yet developed guidelines specifically targeting patient confidentiality in social networking settings, which leaves providers susceptible to unknowingly violating broad parameters. HIPAA violations result in severe monetary and professional penalties (Ewing, 2005). Providers must, therefore, use the most conservative interpretations of these laws to protect themselves from professional and legal consequences.

Thousands of hospitals in the United States advertise their services through professional social networking pages and individual providers are increasingly seeing the value in this marketing environment. By and large, providers use these professional social networking sites to supplement or support advertising web sites. The sites typically provide one-way, dry informational content about office policies or, at most, information on broad patient-care topics such as flu shots or guidelines issued by the Food and Drug Administration. These pages rarely support specific patient–physician relationships or allow for active two-way conversation. Nonetheless, legal and ethical questions arise even in this setting.

For instance, if a patient "friends" a provider's advertising page, the patient's name and picture and the provider's "friendship" with the patient become a part of the public domain. Per Facebook terms of use, Facebook has "a nonexclusive, transferable, sublicensable, royalty-free, worldwide license to use any Internet content that users post in connection with Facebook (IP License)." In essence, the owners of Facebook not only are aware of online relationships, but they can also disseminate this "friendship" to wider sources. Furthermore, if any applications are added to a Facebook page, the users' "friendships" are also shared with these applications. If privacy settings are not carefully updated, and multiple patients "friend" a provider, these "friends" can view all of the names and faces of the provider's various other "friends." An online "friend" may, therefore, make an educated guess that the majority of a provider's "friends" are, in fact, existing patients.

One can easily argue that patient-to-provider "friending" is not a HIPAA violation because patients are knowingly disclosing their names and faces and assuming the risks and responsibilities of this relationship. However, despite the Web site's disclaimer, patients may not be aware of what they are consenting to when they initiate an online professional relationship with a provider. By "friending" a clinician, a patient may naively reveal private information to neighbors, friends, insurance companies, and employers. With the stigmatization of mental illness, patients could face discrimination by peers and employers simply by revealing an association with a mental health provider. Even if these relationships are legally allowed, providers have an ethical obligation to protect their patients from harm.

Unintentional face-to-face disclosures can also occur in mental health waiting rooms, as patients assume the risks of running into acquaintances while awaiting appointments. However, most office personnel minimize this risk by referring to a patient by first name only to ensure complete protection of patient identity. Unfortunately, Facebook has a policy that prohibits users from providing "false personal information" or "creating more than one personal profile." Therefore, to be legally compliant with Facebook terms, a patient cannot avoid disclosing personally identifying information, which can then legally be disseminated to the public. Providers who manage patients with sensitive and stigmatized illnesses should strongly consider how these seemingly legal but unforeseen disclosures may be detrimental to their patients.

An alternative approach would involve having all patients remain anonymous on a provider's professional social networking page in order to avoid HIPAA violations. This practice, of course, violates Facebook policies but may be permitted on other networking services in the future. However, this solution would limit the provider's ability to provide patient-specific care and could also introduce liability issues and if an anonymous patient "friend" makes suicidal or violent statements. Even so, if all privacy settings are carefully selected and a patient's posts are not authorized for public viewing, the owners of social networking sites still have access to these posts and this, in itself, can violate confidentiality.

The singular distinguishing feature of social networking lies in the ease of its two-way communication. Static web sites and blogs allow a writer to disseminate information to the masses but these services generally do not support public replies or ongoing conversations. On the other hand, social networking sites thrive on relationships, which are exemplified through public wall "posting." Providers who choose to use a professional social networking site instead of a web site or blog should be selecting this service because they see value in two-way online relationships. Thus, providers should be prepared and excited to have patients "post" on these professional pages. However, patient "posts" also pose legal and ethical questions.

At present, patients can post an unlimited range of content on a provider's professional social networking page. These posts can share private, harmful, discriminatory, and otherwise negative opinions with the general public. Fortunately, Section 240 of The Communications Decency Act of 1996 provides "immunity from liability for providers and users of an 'interactive computer service' who publish information provided by others." Based on this law, a provider may not be held legally responsible for inappropriate postings by patients or other "friends." Yet, even if providers are legally protected, they can be held to other ethical standards if they do not address and monitor inappropriate wall posts. Providers who do not remove unwanted posts may appear to endorse these negative statements. If a patient posts personal identifying information on a provider's public wall, that provider may be in violation of HIPAA laws by responding to this post with identifying information. Editing a patient post is also not recommended because an editor may assume responsibility for the content of the original post. Providers who maintain professional social networking sites must monitor and manage postings on a regular, preferably daily, basis to avoid the consequences of publishing unwanted content on their pages.

Special Considerations for "High Risk" Patients

Mental health professionals must be particularly cautious when providing mentally ill patients with unlimited "posting" opportunities. If privacy settings allow, a "friend" can post a public suicidal, homicidal, of life-threatening statement on a provider's professional page. In addition, patient "friends" can also post serious allegations of abuse or neglect. These hypothetical situations set off major medical-legal and ethical alarms for many providers. Is a provider liable for acting on these posts? If so, what are the appropriate actions to take and how can a clinician verify that this post was not written by an imposter? Public posts are not only written records but they are also read and, therefore, witnessed by other "friends." Failing to act on these statements in a timely manner can result in serious legal, professional, and emotional consequences.

Response delay is a concern with all emergent phone calls and social networking posts, as providers cannot be continuously monitoring messaging services while also meeting clinical requirements and engaging in their private lives. A suicidal or homicidal act may therefore be completed by the time a provider is able to respond to a message or post. However, this situation becomes even more complex on a professional social networking site because threatening posts on a community forum are not necessarily a direct communication with a provider. Unlike a professional voicemail service, a provider may not know to check these community posts and there is currently no way to alert a provider when a patient posts these threats on a professional page. The law has not yet resolved the legal responsibilities for managing these threats in a social networking setting. Before starting patient-to-provider social networking relationships, mental health professionals must carefully consider how to prevent and address these complicated legal situations.

Developing strategies to handle these written pleas is a complex task for mental health providers, as therapists are bound by law to act on suicidal intent or statements of intent to harm. In 1976, the California Supreme Court upheld the commonly known "Tarasoff rule," which mandates that mental health professionals have a "duty to warn" and a "duty to protect" a third party who is being threatened with bodily harm by a patient. The professional may "discharge the duty" by notifying police, warning the intended victim, and/or taking other reasonable steps to protect the threatened individual. Current California law has expanded this rule by upholding that the "duty to protect" must be enacted if a psychotherapist "believes or predicts" that the patient poses a serious risk of inflicting serious injury upon a reasonably identifiable victim, even if the statements of threat were divulged from a third party and not directly from the patient. Prior to enacting a "duty to protect," a mental health provider must act quickly to conduct a thoughtful violence risk assessment, in order to prevent public harm and avoid serious legal penalties (Ewing, 2005).

There is no precedent for how to manage statements of harm posted on a provider's social networking site. It must be conservatively assumed that the Tarasoff rule applies to threats "posted" to professional social networking sites, yet acting on these threats may be extremely complex. A mental health provider must first confirm that the posted threat was indeed made by the patient himself and not by an imposter. A provider must then determine how to quickly conduct a violence risk assessment on a patient who may or may not be willing to verbally discuss these statements or participate in an evaluation. If unable to efficiently perform a complete violence risk assessment, the provider must choose to either enact the duty to warn without sufficient evidence, placing the patient at risk if the threat was not credible, or ignore the threatening post, placing the provider at serious legal risk and the public in harm's way.

These issues arise when determining how to address patient "posts" that threaten self-harm. Mental health providers regularly manage patients with active, passive, acute, and chronic suicidal ideation. These providers are trained to conduct suicide risk assessments, which involve detailed consideration of multiple risk factors, including, but not limited to, assessing suicidal intent, suicidal plan, access to suicidal means and examination of previous suicidal behaviors. If a patient publically posts a suicidal statement or death-themed message on a provider's professional social networking page, a provider must determine how to act on this statement. In an ideal situation, a provider would immediately see the post, contact the patient, and advise the patient to make an immediate appointment with the provider or seek emergency care. However, like homicidal posts, a provider must determine how to properly conduct a suicide risk assessment, if a patient cannot be verbally contacted. Suicidal statements do not always equate to immediate suicidal intent. For example, dependent or attention-seeking patients with no true suicidal intent may post dramatic and self-destructive statements on a provider's social networking site, with the primary aim of seeking comfort from a provider or other social networking "friends." If a patient who posted a suicidal statement cannot be contacted, a provider must, once again, determine the patient's intentions and the level of care needed based on a single written "post."

Other patients who view this post online may also be inclined to preemptively contact authorities, a situation which must be considered by the provider and the owner of the professional social networking page. Providers who choose to act aggressively on all self-harm posts run the risk of overwhelming emergency psychiatric services and alienating attention-seeking patients. Yet, choosing to ignore even one suicidal post may result in serious preventable injury to a patient as well as emotional, professional, and legal harm to a provider.

Concerns about managing alarming patient "posts" become even more complex when these statements are only posted on the patient's personal social networking page to which the provider has been "friended." Providers with professional social networking sites cannot reasonably be expected to regularly view and monitor all of their patients' personal social networking pages. However, social network users typically post thoughts and views on their own pages before posting comments on other sites. If patients post concerning statements or pictures on their own social networking pages, are their providers liable or ethically bound to act on these statements? If these posts were not directly sent to a provider, how should this content be addressed with patients?

A patient or family member may also post statements or tag pictures that suggest physical, sexual, or emotional abuse. Providers who already have suspicions that a patient is being abused may use these images or statements to justify reporting their concerns to authorities. However, it is less clear how a provider, who has never held these concerns before, should respond to alarming abuse-related content on a patient's personal page. These hypothetical discussions can expand exponentially when considering all of the mandated reporting required of both health-care providers. Reporting requirements and ethical practices must be updated to include these complicated social networking situations.

These outstanding ethical and legal considerations will hopefully be answered by future laws and practice protocols. However, professional social networking guidelines will not protect a clinician from the awkwardness of online relationships. Typically, patients who are engaged in therapy and other treatments develop verbal rapport with their providers and, with this growing connection, patients choose to reveal more and more about their personal histories and beliefs. If a provider has access to a patient's online identity and uncovers information that a patient has previously denied or not yet disclosed in therapy sessions, this can have a significant and potentially damaging impact on the therapeutic process. For example, a patient who struggles with alcohol abuse may be very embarrassed or angry to realize his provider viewed an online "tagged" picture of alcohol-related content. This therapeutic breech may force the patient and provider into an uncomfortable and ill-timed confrontation.

Mental health providers are trained to manage patient transference, which can negatively or positively enhance patient care. Yet few training programs prepare providers for the challenges of online patient transference. A patient who is subconsciously angry with a provider may "de-friend" his clinician in a passive-aggressive, hostile attempt to punish the provider. How does a provider appropriately address this behavior—should it be done in person or online? What if a provider does not even notice? Alternatively, a patient may use an online relationship to grow close to a provider. This patient may cross boundaries that force the provider to consider "de-friending" the patient or, at the very least, minimize online communication. Managing transference is complex in any setting but it becomes even more complicated when a patient has unlimited online access to a provider. Future research and expert opinions are needed to address these inevitable questions.

Like most other areas of medicine, telemental health-care providers must be exquisitely careful to prevent difficult legal and ethical issues that may arise in the absence of firm regulations on professional social networking sites. One strategy is to post appropriate legal disclaimers and mandate that patients are thoroughly consented before they agree to a professional social networking relationship. A provider should post an easily viewed policy section that stipulates the voluntary nature of the online relationship and lists caveats that eliminate provider liability. In this process, it is absolutely critical that providers publicize how often they reasonably expect to view and update their professional social networking pages. In doing so, clinicians should also excuse themselves from liability if they do not monitor the page during vacations or other extended periods of time. Clinicians should post their expectations for managing "at-risk" patients and document how they will respond to threats publically posted on their web site. Consents and disclaimers must also discuss the risk of unforeseen dissemination of information if a provider's page is subjected to a computer virus or is victimized by "hacking." For the utmost protection, it is recommended that a provider consult with an attorney and/or have patients physically sign consent paperwork, in the presence of a witness, before online relationships are initiated.

Special Considerations for the Use of Personal Social Network Sites: Dual Relationships, Inadvertent Disclosure, and Nonmalfeasance

With the increasing popularity of social networking sites for personal as well as professional use, ethical dilemmas may also arise for mental health clinicians engaging in their personal social networks that are not developed specifically for patient care. Ethical issues regarding dual relationships, boundaries, and the clinician—patient relationship have been debated; however, research in this area is limited. Ethics codes established to guide mental health professionals ethical practice address ethical guidelines for mental health professionals "scientific, educational, and/or professional roles," but do not largely address the intersection of private and professional roles (American Psychological Association, 2002). With the development and widespread use of technology, there may be a greater risk for personal information intended for a private audience to cross over into the professional arena (Behnke, 2008). This is of particular concern with social networking sites where mental health-care professionals may intentionally or unintentionally share personal information publically, which may become visible to patients, colleagues or students.

Intentional or unintentional self-disclosure online runs the risk of breaching relationship boundaries or otherwise adversely influencing providers' relationships with clients, students, or colleagues. Boundary and ethical violations that may occur through the sharing of information online are of concern as are the development of dual relationships between the provider and patient or a person close to the patient. Ethical standards for addressing issues such as mental health professionals' responsibility to conceal private information, professional conduct online, and appropriate clinician–patient interactions through social networking must be considered.

Studies suggest that mental health and medical providers are accessing personal social networking sites and sharing information that may become visible to those in their professional lives. Reports indicate that a majority of recent medical graduates (MacDonald, Sohn, & Ellis, 2010) and early career psychologists (Lehavot, Barnett, & Powers, 2010; Taylor, McMinn, Bufford, & Chang, 2010) are members of online social network sites. In a national survey of over 600 psychologists, the majority (77%) of participants reported maintaining a personal social networking site. A large majority of these participants (85%) reported implementing privacy controls in an effort to protect their personal information. It is not surprising that age was a factor in the use of social networks with the largest reported users of social networks being respondents under the age of 30 (86%) who comprised the majority of the sample (76%) (Taylor et al., 2010). While studies indicate that the majority of psychologists (> 60%) participating in personal social networks take measures to protect privacy, a substantial portion (15–40%) may not (Lehavot et al., 2010; Taylor et al., 2010).

In one study, many psychology graduate students surveyed reported that their social network sites contained personal information that they would not want their colleagues (6%), professors (13%), or particularly their clients (37%) to access. When asked about experiences of client contact on personal social networks, a small percent (7%) of the student sample reported that clients had directly reported to them that they had researched them online. A surprisingly large portion of the students (27%) reported seeking out information about their clients online (Lehavot et al., 2010). The lack of privacy precautions reported in these studies illustrates that there is reasonable potential for clients to access personal information shared by mental health professionals which may in turn lead to boundary violations, potentially damaging disclosures or engagement in dual relationship concerns. There may be even greater potential for online exposure of providers' private information, taking into consideration that providers may not be fully aware of the limits of social networking privacy controls. Privacy on social networks varies by site, and the privacy settings within the same site may change periodically as the site upgrades and evolves.

The acceptability of self-disclosure between a mental health provider and client is a complex ethical issue that is widely debated. Psychologists recognize that unintentional self-disclosure is bound to occur and should be addressed directly with clients (Taylor et al., 2010). However, this issue becomes further complicated with the increasing popularity of social networking applications. Self-disclosures online may be more personal, damaging, and may be more likely to be unknown to the provider than other instances of unintentional self-disclosures.

Studies evaluating publically available content of medical graduates illuminate further concern on this issue. Chretien, Greysen, Chretien, and Kind (2009) found reports of medical student misconduct online in medical schools across the United States. Of the participating medical schools, 60% reported incidents of students posting unprofessional content online, including use of profanity (52%), discriminatory language (48%), description of intoxication (39%), and sexually suggestive material (38%), and 13% of these schools reported incidents of violations of patient confidentiality online. One study evaluating the use of the social network Facebook in recent medical graduates found that 37% had settings allowing public access (MacDonald et al., 2010). These public accounts shared information including sexual orientation, religious views, relationship status, and showed photographs of the users drinking alcohol, images of the users intoxicated, and photographs of the users engaged in unhealthy behaviors (MacDonald et al., 2010).

Because patients may be motivated to research their providers online, even if primarily to evaluate their credentials, stumbling upon personal information could impact patients, particularly for those actively engaged in therapy. While an unintentional disclosure may not effect a patient or therapy at all, depending on the content of the information and the patient-therapist relationship, it may hinder the patient's relationship with the therapist. Ethics codes do not directly address the issue of self-disclosure; however, the overarching ethical principles of benevolence and nonmalfeasance (requiring providers to be of greater benefit than harm to their patients or to "do no harm") are in place to guide providers in the protection of patients from both intentional and unintentional harm.

Due to the confidential nature of information shared in a mental health setting, mental health clinicians operate under stringent ethics codes and confidentiality requirements, and considerable attention is paid to the patient–provider relationship as it is often thought to be the vehicle for therapy and thus has a have positive or negative influence on a patient's success in therapy. These codes and requirements are designed to protect the patient's confidential information and well-being throughout the therapeutic relationship and beyond. The American Psychiatric Association ethics code states that "A psychiatrist shall not gratify his or her own needs by exploiting the patient. The psychiatrist shall be ever vigilant about the impact that his or her conduct has upon the boundaries of the doctor–patient relationship, and thus upon the well-being of the patient. These requirements become particularly important because of the essentially private, highly personal, and sometimes intensely emotional nature of the relationship established with the psychiatrist" (American Psychiatric Association, 2010). Similarly, the American

Psychological Association is clear about the importance of the clinician–patient relationship and maintaining appropriate boundaries to protect the patient's well-being and to avoid exploitation. The American Psychological Association's ethics code addresses the issue of multiple relationships and defines it as: "A multiple relationship occurs when a psychologist is in a professional role with a person and (1) at the same time is in another role with the same person, (2) at the same time is in a relationship with a person closely associated with or related to the person with whom the psychologist has the professional relationship, or (3) promises to enter into another relationship in the future with the person or a person closely associated with or related to the person." The code advises that "A psychologist refrains from entering into a multiple relationship if the multiple relationship could reasonably be expected to impair the psychologist's objectivity, competence, or effectiveness in performing his or her functions as a psychologist, or otherwise risks exploitation or harm to the person with whom the professional relationship exists" (American Psychological Association, 2002). Such standards apply to interactions that are "in person, postal, telephone, Internet, and other electronic transmissions" (American Psychological Association, 2002).

Ethics codes are clear about the dangers of multiple relationships; however, it may be difficult to determine if a relationship with a client or a person close to a client through a personal social network site is a potentially harmful multiple relationship. One experience that many mental health professionals may soon be faced with is a client or clients family member "friending" them on their personal social networking web site. "Friending," as previously described, is when a person asks to be added to another's social networking webpage. While most social networking sites have privacy controls which can be put in place to prevent viewing of the webpage content by anyone but "friends," most allow anyone to send friend requests.

Requests by patients to be added to their providers' personal page may bring up a variety of concerns. If providers accept the "friend" request, the patients will have access to their personal information, friends, and contact information, at which point, an inappropriate dual relationship may be established. Depending on the content that providers post, their patients become privy to a large part of the providers' private lives and experiences that are largely outside the value of therapy. Decisions about accepting or not accepting such requests from patients are difficult and important ethical questions arise. If requests are accepted, when and if does the social networking relationship cross the line into a dual relationship? How will it affect the patient and the therapeutic relationship if a request is denied? How should a provider address this issue as it arises with patients? Is it appropriate to accept "friend" requests from a family member of a patient, the mother of a pediatric patient for example? Is it ethical to accept "friend" requests from some patients but not others? What are the clinical implications of doing so?

Ethics codes are clear that relationships with patients are not unethical if they are not exploitive (i.e., in the case of a sexual relationship with a patient), and providers' ability to operate in their professional role with patients is not otherwise impaired. However, it can be difficult to determine when these relationships might cross the line into a dual relationship. Therefore, it is generally recommended that providers avoid engaging in significant personal relationships with patients until considerable time has passed following termination of treatment (Barnett, 2008; Pipes, 1997). Guidelines are yet to be developed to address these issues directly, and research in this area is new and very limited.

Taylor et al. (2010) evaluated attitudes and ethical concerns with the use of social networks in a sample of psychologists. They noted that psychologists were aware of the ethical and professional risks to using these sites and took privacy precautions; however, several issues were raised including dilemmas about addressing "friend" requests by clients or relatives of clients, discovering shared "friends" with clients, and addressing suicidal ideation or intent to harm shared by clients over the Web. They report that psychologists' surveys overall were ambivalent about the need for the development of ethics codes in this area; however, the authors note that graduate ethics education should include training on this issue. Guidance in this area for graduate students and early career psychologists may be of utmost importance as this group is more likely than their older colleagues to access social networks and thereby more likely to face these dilemmas (Taylor et al., 2010). Furthermore, this group may be the most vulnerable to more serious ethical violations such as breaches of confidentiality.

Providers must take heed to ensure that all communications over social networking sites conform to appropriate professional boundaries, existing ethics codes, and HIPAA (Hader & Brown, 2010). Studies evaluating medical residents' social network sites found that patient privacy violations did occur over social networking sites (Chretien et al., 2009; Thompson et al., 2011). Instances of medical professionals sharing patient information over social networking sites have been widely documented in other health-care fields. Cases of intentional exposure of patient information are considered to be egregious legal ethical violations and have resulted in severe punishments including fines and loss of licensure. However, it may be difficult for young mental health professionals to differentiate between appropriate and inappropriate disclosure of patient information.

Fledgling mental health clinicians are likely to consult on cases and are encouraged by mentors to obtain supervision for challenging cases. However, if clinicians seek consultation with colleagues via their private social network, their discussions may become exposed to others in their social network and risk violating patient confidentiality. Such ethical issues should be addressed in graduate education and continuing education courses to ensure that mental health providers are armed with the best tools possible to protect their clients and themselves in this ever changing technological world.

In the face of limited guidelines for mental health providers practicing in the midst of this social media paradigm shift, several clinicians and researchers have established blogs and discussion forums to offer advice and guidelines to assist providers in avoiding ethical debacles. One such blog makes several recommendation including that clinicians avoid "friending" clients on personal sites, become educated about privacy controls and their limitations on these sites, develop a social media policy to share with patients, be up front with patients about Internet and social networking policies and any intent that a clinician may have to research them online, and set clear boundaries regarding any communication with clients in any form and stick to them (Grohol, 2010). Furthermore, others suggest using considerable caution before accepting "friends" and joining groups as any information shared with patients on their pages may be visible to their entire social network. Providers should adjust their privacy to be as secure as possible, consider making their profiles unsearchable for the public, not accept "friendship" requests from unknown persons, and never discuss patient information or any confidential professional issues with "friends" on social networking sites (Parish & Friedman, 2011). Further, we advise that mental health clinicians participating in social networking sites should review the public view of their online profiles to evaluate what information would be available to patients or colleagues who access their profile in a public search, evaluate the appropriateness of patients or colleagues having access to this information, and adjust their privacy settings accordingly.

Another issue to consider is the existence of old social networking site accounts that are no longer used, but may still contain personal information, and may be accessible to patients, colleagues, and students. Social networking accounts can be difficult to delete. Changes in the ever-evolving privacy controls for these sites may accidentally allow for private information to become public. Providers must always consider that public postings can be viewed by anyone and could potentially be as public as if posted on the front page of the daily newspaper.

Conclusion

While specific sites may come and go with the inherent trendiness of Internet fads, social networking is now a permanent part of the society and already is transforming the way people disclose and discuss their mental health. Contemporary mental health providers must be aware of the prevalence of social networking, for it is not only a wealth of mental health information but also influences the way its users think about themselves and access health information. While these can be forums to enhance patient care, the frequency of misinformation, as well as the opportunities for users to encourage self-harm behaviors, needs to be acknowledged by mental health providers. Health-care systems are starting to establish patient-friendly sites for interacting with their health-care providers, and early models have shown benefits to both patients and providers. This will likely become standard practice within mental health services and is particularly adapted for the telemental health provider. The availability of an Internet connection rather than geographic location determines access to these services. With this new interface for interacting with clients, guidelines for effective and ethical professional boundaries around social networking relationships need to be integrated into mental health training. There is potential for dual relationships and privacy violations within online interaction. As we move into the cyber century, social networking provides a platform for delivering traditional mental health therapy through the Internet and also offers an opportunity to expand and develop novel Internet-based avenues for care.

References

American Psychiatric Association. (2010). *The principles of medical ethics with annotations especially applicable to psychiatry*. 2010 Edition (pp. 1–38).

(2002). American Psychological Association. Ethical principles of psychologists and code of conduct *American Psychologist* 57, 1060–1073.

Barak, A., & Wander-Schwartz, M. (1999). Empirical evaluation of brief group therapy conducted in an internet chat room. *American Psychological Association annual convention* August.

Bardone-Cone, A. M., & Cass, K. M. (2007). What does viewing a pro-anorexia website do? An experimental examination of website exposure and moderating effects. *International Journal of Eating Disorders, 40*, 537–548.

Barnett, J. E. (2008). Online 'sharing' demands caution. *The National Psychologist, 17*, 10–11.

Bauer, S., Wolf, M., Haug, S., & Kordy, H. (2011). The effectiveness of internet chat groups in relapse prevention after inpatient psychotherapy. *Journal of Psychotherapy Practice and Research, 21*, 219–226.

Behnke, S. (2008). Ethics rounds- Ethics in the age of the internet: in narrowing the gap between our personal and professional lives, the internet raises challenging ethical questions. *Monitor on Psychology, 39*(7), 74. Retrieved October 27,2011 from http://www.apa.org/monitor/2008/07-08/ethics.aspx.

Bender, J. L., Jimenez-Marroquin, M. C., & Jadad, A. R. (2011). Seeking support on facebook: A content analysis of breast cancer groups. *Journal of Medical Internet Research, 13*, e16.

Breckons, A., Jones, R., Morris, J., & Richardson, J. (2007). What do evaluation instruments tell us about the quality of complementary medicine information on the Internet? *Focus on Alternative and Complementary Therapies, 12*, 9–19.

Bull, S. S., Gaglio, B., Mckay, H. G., & Glasgow, R. E. (2005). Harnessing the potential of the internet to promote chronic illness self-management: Diabetes as an example of how well we are doing. *Chronic Illness, 1*, 143–155.

Burns, J. M., Davenport, T. A., Durkin, L. A., Luscombe, G. M., & Hickie, I. B. (2010). The internet as a setting for mental health service utilisation by young people. *The Medical Journal of Australia, 192*, S22–S26.

Childress, C. A. (2000). Ethical issues in providing online psychotherapeutic interventions. *Journal of Medical Internet Research, 2*, e5. Retrieved January 25, 2012 from http://www.jmir.org/2000/1/e5.

Chretien, K. C., Greysen, S. R., Chretien, J. -P., & Kind, T. (2009). Online posting of unprofessional content by medical students. *Journal of the American Medical Association, 302*, 1309–1315.

Computers and Internet. *Five million facebook users are 10 or younger.* (2011) *Consumer News.* Retrieved January 25, 2012 from http://news.consumerreports.org/electronics/2011/05/five-million-facebook-users-are-10-or-younger.html.

Custers, K., & Van den Bulck, J. (2009). Viewership of pro-anorexia websites in seventh, ninth and eleventh graders. *European Eating Disorders Review, 17,* 214−219.

Etter, J. (2006). Internet-based smoking cessation programs. *International Journal of Medical Informatics, 75,* 110−116.

Ewing, C. P. (2005). Tarasoff reconsidered: The tarasoff rule has been extended to include threats disclosed by family members. *Judicial Notebook, 36,* 112.

Fleischmann, A. (2005). The hero's story and autism. Grounded theory study of websites for parents of children with autism. *Autism: The International Journal of Research and Practice, 9,* 299−316.

Gingritch, N., & Thapar, K. (2010). Facebook is—literally—a lifesaver. *AOL News.* Retrieved January 25, 2012 from http://www.aolnews.com/2010/12/06/facebook-is-literally-a-lifesaver/?a_dgi = aolshare_email.

Grohol, J. (2010). Google and facebook, therapists and clients. *PsychCentral,* Retrieved January 25, 2012 from http://psychcentral.com/blog/archives/2010/03/31/google-and-facebook-therapists-and-clients.

Gustafson, D. H., Hawkins, R., Boberg, E., Pingree, S., Serlin, R. E., Graziano, F., et al. (1999). Impact of a patient-centered, computer-based health information/support system. *American Journal of Preventive Medicine, 16,* 1−9.

Hader, A. L., & Brown, E. D. (2010). Patient privacy and social media. *American Association of Nurse Anesthetists Journal: Legal briefs, 78,* 270−274.

Hawker, M. D. (2010). Social networking in the national health service in England: A quantitative analysis of the online identities of 152 primary care trusts. *Studies in Health and Technology Informatics, 160,* 356−360.

Hawn, C. (2009). Take two aspirin and tweet me in the morning: How twitter, facebook, and other social media are reshaping health care. *Health Affairs, 28,* 361−368.

Health Insurance Portability and Accountability Act, 110 Stat. 1936 (1996).

Hewlett, J. (2011). *Politics and government.* Retrieved January 25, 2012 from http://www.kentucky.com/2011/07/14/1810483/former-political-candidate-found.html.

Internet Software and Services. Friendster, Inc. *Bloomberg Businessweek.* (2011). Retrieved January 25, 2012 from http://investing.businessweek.com/research/stocks/private/snapshot.asp?privcapId=6856690>.

Kash, K. M., Mago, R., & Kunkel, E. J. S. (2005). Psychosocial oncology: Supportive care for the cancer patient. *Seminars in Oncology, 32,* 211−218.

Kazeniac, A. (2009). *Social networks: Facebook takes over top spot, twitter climbs.* Compete pulse. Retrieved January 25, 2012 from http://blog.compete.com/2009/02/09/facebook-myspace-twitter-social-network.

Lehavot, K., Barnett, J., & Powers, D. (2010). Psychotherapy, professional relationships, and ethical considerations in the Myspace generation. *Professional Psychology: Research and Practice, 41,* 160−166.

Lipsman, A. (2009). *What Ashton vs. CNN foretold about the changing demographics of twitter.* comScore Voices. Retrieved January, 25, 2012 from http://blog.comscore.com/2009/09/changing_demographics_of_twitter.html.

MacDonald, J, Sohn, S, & Ellis, P. (2010). Privacy, professionalism and facebook: A dilemma for young doctors. *Medical Education, 44,* 805−813.

McMullan, M. (2006). Patients using the internet to obtain health information: How this affects the patient-health professional relationship. *Patient Education and Counseling*, *63*, 24–28.

Mikami, A. Y., Szwedo, D. E., Allen, J. P., Evans, M. A., & Hare, A. L. (2010). Adolescent peer relationships and behavior problems predict young adults' communication on social networking websites. *Developmental Psychology*, *46*, 46–56.

Moreno, M. A., Briner, L. R., Williams, A., Walker, L., & Christakis, D. A. (2009). Real use or "real cool": Adolescents speak out about displayed alcohol references on social networking websites. *The Journal of Adolescent Health*, *45*, 420–422.

Moreno, M. A., Jelenchick, L. A., Egan, K. G., Cox, E., Young, H., Gannon, K. E., et al. (2011). Feeling bad on facebook: Depression disclosures by college students on a social networking site. *Depression and Anxiety*, *28*, 447–455.

Myspace. (2011). *Mashable*. Retrieved January 25, 2012 from http://mashable.com/follow/topics/myspace.

Olivarez-Giles, N. (2011). Facebook f8: Redesigning and hitting 800 million users. *Los Angeles Times*. September 22, 2011. Retrieved January 25, 2012 from http://latimesblogs.latimes.com/technology/2011/09/facebook-f8-media-features.html.

Ozawa-De Silva, C. (2010). Shared death: Self, sociality and internet group suicide in japan. *Transcultural Psychiatry*, *47*, 392–418.

Parish, K., & Friedman, J. (2011). Counselors, clients and facebook. *Counselor: The Magazine for Addiction Professionals*, *12*, 2–5.

Perdu, A. (2008). The history of friendster: Myspace took over friendster's number one position in popular social networking sites when it was introduced in 2004. *WebUpon*. Retrieved January 25, 2012 from http://webupon.com/social-networks/the-history-of-friendster.

Pipes, R. B. (1997). Nonsexual relationships between psychotherapists and their former clients: Obligations of psychologists. *Ethics and Behavior*, *7*, 27–41.

Ridout, B., Campbell, A., & Ellis, L. (2011). "Off your face(book)": Alcohol in online social identity construction and its relation to problem drinking in university students. *Drug and Alcohol Review*, *31*, 20–26.

Rucker, J. (2011). The history of social networking. *Fast Company*. Retrieved January 25, 2012 from http://www.fastcompany.com/1720374/the-history-of-social-networking.

Saint, N. (2010). A comprehensive look at who uses social networks and how. *Business Insider*. Retrieved January 25, 2012 from http://www.businessinsider.com/a-comprehensive-look-at-who-uses-social-networks-and-how-2010-6#.

Taylor, L., McMinn, M. R., Bufford, R. K., & Chang, K. B. T. (2010). Psychologists' attitudes and ethical concerns regarding the use of social networking web sites. *Professional Psychology: Research and Practice*, *41*, 153–159.

Thompson, L. A., Black, E., Duff, W. P., Paradise Black, N., Saliba, H., & Dawson, K. (2011). Protected health information on social networking sites: Ethical and legal considerations. *Journal of Medical Internet Research*, *13*, e8 Retrieved January 25, 2012 from http://www.jmir.org/2011/1/e8.

Tsai, C. C., Tsai, S. H., Zeng-Treitler, Q., & Liang, B. A. (2007). Patient-centered consumer health social network websites: A pilot study of quality of user-generated health information. *AMIA annual symposium proceedings, October 11, 2007*.

Twitter. *Business Insider*. (2010). Retrieved January 25, 2012 from http://www.businessinsider.com/blackboard/twitter.

Vance, K., Howe, W., & Dellavalle, R. P. (2009). Social internet sites as a source of public health information. *Dermatologic Clinics, 27*, 133–136.

Weinberg, H. (2001). Group process and group phenomena on the internet. *International Journal of Group Psychotherapy, 51*, 361–378.

Wyld, A. (2012). Facebook. *The New York Times.* January 23, 2012. Retrieved January 25, 2012 from http://topics.nytimes.com/top/news/business/companies/facebook_inc/index.html.

19 Research in Telemental Health: Review and Synthesis[1]

Carolyn L. Turvey[a,b,] and Kathleen Myers[c]*

[a]Department of Psychiatry, University of Iowa Carver College of Medicine, Iowa City, IA, [b]Comprehensive Access and Delivery Research and Evaluation (CADRE) Center, Iowa City VA Healthcare System, Iowa City, IA, [c]Department of Psychiatry and Behavioral Sciences, University of Washington School of Medicine, Director, Telemental Health Service, Seattle Children's Hospital, Seattle, WA

Introduction

This chapter will review the evidence base for mental health practice conducted using real-time videoteleconferencing (VTC) to provide standard models of care such as psychiatric assessment, consultation, and ongoing direct care and psychotherapy. To date, the majority of the research in telemental health (TMH) has served primarily two main goals: (1) to demonstrate feasibility and satisfaction and (2) to demonstrate equivalency to same-room mental health care. Studies have demonstrated equivalence between same-room and TMH care in psychiatric diagnosis, psychological assessment, treatment plan development, and treatment outcome studies for both psychiatry and psychotherapy. The sophistication of research has improved more recently with the publication of large randomized controlled trials comparing treatment response for TMH to same-room care and more sophisticated economic analyses of TMH.

The results of these explorations are largely positive and are well reviewed in several articles (Andersson, 2009, 2010; Antonacci, Bloch, Saeed, Yildirim, & Talley, 2008; Frueh, Deitsch et al., 2000; Garcia-Lizana & Munoz-Mayorga, 2010; Grady et al., 2011; Hilty, Luo, Morache, Marcelo, & Nesbitt, 2002; Monnier, Knapp, & Frueh, 2003). Patients, their families, and clinicians endorse high levels of satisfaction with TMH. Assessments and care provided through VTC are largely comparable to that of same-room care. Large randomized controlled trials

---

[1]The views expressed in this article are those of the authors and do not necessarily reflect the position or policy of the Department of Veterans Affairs or the United States government.

*Corresponding Author: Carolyn Turvey, Department of Psychiatry, University of Iowa Carver College of Medicine, Iowa City, IA 52242. Tel.: +1-206-987-1663, Fax: +1-206-987-2246, E-mail: Carolyn-Turvey@uiowa.edu.

Telemental Health. DOI: http://dx.doi.org/10.1016/B978-0-12-416048-4.00019-1

demonstrate effectiveness. In discussing each of these topics, this chapter will provide a research agenda to address specific and persistent limitations of each area of research and potential solutions to such limitations.

This chapter will also discuss newer areas of research that are relevant to how recent technologic developments present new opportunities for delivering care. For example, there is a considerable and growing literature on the effectiveness of cognitive behavioral therapy (CBT) conducted through the Internet without real-time interaction with a therapist. This chapter will also discuss the need for research into the growing availability of technologic adjuncts to therapy such as web-based programs to support intersession behavioral practice or relaxation.

The context of most prior research in TMH is an effort by the telemedicine community to gain legitimacy in the eyes of clinicians, insurers, and policy makers. Therefore, most discussion sections of published studies emphasize TMH's benefits while understating any potential problems that may be evident in the results section. Though the thrust of this entire text is that there is adequate clinical and research evidence supporting integration of TMH into day-to-day clinical practice, there are sporadic findings that point to better ways that we could, and should, be conducting TMH. Ignoring potential drawbacks revealed by the research is short sighted. There is adequate research supporting the practice of TMH, so we can now move beyond the defensive stance of having to prove ourselves, to a more self-critical discussion of how we could improve TMH research and practice. The overarching aim of this chapter is to affirm the progress in demonstrating the overall efficacy of TMH while still acknowledging the less favorable results that illustrate the areas for continued development.

Satisfaction Research

Satisfaction research comprises the largest portion of empirical research in TMH. Satisfaction with TMH is extraordinarily high with average percentages of patients defined as "satisfied" ranging between 75% and 100% (Blackmon, Kaak, & Ranseen, 1997; Callahan, Hilty, & Nesbitt, 1998; Hilty, Yellowlees, & Nesbitt, 2006; Holden & Dew, 2008; Simpson, 2001; Williams, May, & Esmail, 2001). For example, Blackmon et al. (1997) reported 100% satisfaction overall for a child telepsychiatry service between a university and three primary care sites. Some studies even report patients, such as soldiers, preferring TMH to same-room care (Wilson, Onorati, Mishkind, Reger, & Gahm, 2008) or patients receiving intensified substance abuse counseling (King et al., 2009). Callahan et al. (1998) reported that 60% of their sample preferred TMH and the mean rating of satisfaction was 4.6 on a 5-point Likert-type scale. These findings are typical and support assertions that TMH is accepted and possibly even preferred by patients.

Though studies of feasibility and satisfaction are the first essential step in the evaluation of a new clinical service, research to date suffers some limitations.

General satisfaction scores based on general items presented in Likert-scale format to volunteer respondents tend to be biased upwards (Jenkinson, Coulter, Bruster, Richards, & Chandola, 2002). Jenkinson et al. (2002) found that 55% of patients who rated a recent inpatient episode as "excellent" on a 5-point Likert scale also indicated four or more problems with their stay on the Picker Survey (1999), a survey developed to capture specific aspects of patient experience such as Respect for Patient Preferences or Coordination of Care.

Patients are hesitant to criticize when they believe clinicians will see their ratings (Williams et al., 2001). Most satisfaction studies include patients who agreed to receive TMH to begin with and, therefore, self-selected into this type of treatment. It is uncertain whether their satisfaction scores would generalize to the entire population seeking care in any given clinic. In short, one may characterize most of the satisfaction research in TMH, and in health care in general, as tossing a pair of loaded dice. It is far more likely that satisfaction will be rated high than low.

In light of this potential for positive bias, it is important to explore satisfaction with a critical eye using methods most likely to yield candid responses from patients and providers. In a review of the measurement of satisfaction with health care, the United Kingdom's National Health Service Health Technology Assessment Programme described methods one could use to increase respondent candidness about potential areas of dissatisfaction (Crow et al., 2002). Impersonal and mail methods where anonymity is preserved yield lower ratings of satisfaction. In addition, qualitative assessments, though costly, can often provide more in-depth understanding of the respondent's experiences that provide a rich context for interpreting the quantitative scales. In a recent analysis of patient satisfaction with a telehealth intervention conducted by one of the chapter authors (Carolyn Turvey), patients consistently endorsed Likert satisfaction measures highly, with a mean of 4.6 on a 5-point Likert-type scale. However, when asked an open-ended question, two of the respondents openly stated they missed the personal contact of same-room therapy. This does not necessarily mean that the satisfaction ratings were false; it simply acknowledges that the patients are noticing a difference and investigators should not summarily conclude that patients' experience of TMH is equivalent to same-room care. In efforts to improve the provision of TMH, future studies may want to interview patients who do acknowledge a difference on quantitative satisfaction scales by using additional qualitative interviews to determine which aspects of same-room care are missed. It would also be important to determine if any of these missed features of same-room care have an impact on treatment alliance and effectiveness. Efforts can then be made to improve TMH care, which address these concerns.

When resources are not available for qualitative studies, more nuanced Likert-scale questions may provide added insight. Early studies of satisfaction tended to assess only one or two aspects of satisfaction such as a global rating of satisfaction and whether or not a patient would recommend telemedicine to others (Williams et al., 2001). More recent studies in TMH have explored therapeutic alliance in addition to satisfaction yielding a richer understanding of the therapeutic experience (Cook & Doyle, 2002; Ertelt et al., 2011; Frueh, Monnier, Grubaugh et al.,

2007; Frueh, Monnier, Yim et al., 2007; Morgan, Patrick, & Magaletta, 2008; Porcari et al., 2009). Fortunately, most studies find ratings of therapeutic alliance to be comparable between same-room and TMH care. However, Porcari et al. (2009) found that although patient ratings of alliance were similar and even slightly higher for TMH as compared with same-room care, participants stated they would prefer same-room care if the distance to care was the same as for TMH. Greene et al. (2010) examined therapy process ratings in a trial comparing mode of delivery for anger management in veterans. Most therapy process measures were comparable between same-room and TMH-delivered care. However, the same-room condition yielded higher ratings than the TMH condition on alliance between the participant and the group leader. This difference was found in spite of comparable effectiveness of the two treatments on the main outcome of interest, anger symptoms. Contrary to much of the therapeutic alliance research in same-room care, the difference in participant and group leader alliance did not mediate aggregate differences between treatment groups though alliance did predict better individual outcomes. This counterintuitive finding was also reported by Knaevelsrud and Maercker (2006) in an online CBT where correlations between alliance and outcomes were positive but low and did not reach statistical significance.

Though questions about general satisfaction are always helpful, the time has come for more in-depth exploration of both patient and clinician experience of TMH. Qualitative methods, more specific items about process on satisfaction rating scales, and methods to overcome response bias are likely to yield more informative results than simple satisfaction measures. Such information will tell us how to better provide mental health care through videoconferencing. The findings of Greene et al. (2010) that lower ratings of therapeutic alliance did not mediate differences between treatment groups support the continued use of TMH to conduct group therapy for anger management. However, the lower rating of therapeutic alliance in the VTC group calls for exploration of how this may be remedied.

Another potential area for increased understanding is a deeper exploration of the consistent difference between patients' and providers' levels of satisfaction with TMH (Day & Schneider, 2002; Ertelt et al., 2011; Ruskin et al., 2004; Williams et al., 2001). Though both patients and clinicians score high on satisfaction with TMH, clinicians' satisfactions ratings tend to be lower. Ruskin et al. (2004) found no difference in satisfaction between patients receiving in-person versus.

TMH care for depression; yet there was a statistically significant difference in providers with same-room care yielding higher provider satisfaction. The relatively lower ratings of satisfaction found in clinicians need to be understood better because it may provide insight into the widespread impression that adoption of TMH is hindered more by practitioners than by patients (Hilty, Luo et al., 2002). It is difficult to recruit and retain clinicians to conduct TMH than same-room care. Turnover is more frequent and it is difficult to find clinicians willing to conduct their entire practice through TMH.

One possible explanation for differences in satisfaction between patients and clinicians is that patients new to mental health care have nothing by which to compare their experience. In contrast, most clinicians will use same-room care as the referent for their satisfaction. The difference between patients and clinicians in satisfaction could also be attributed to the fact that telemedicine increases access and convenience for the patient but not necessarily for the doctor. However, the association between reduced travel time and satisfaction ratings is mixed (Grubaugh, Cain, Elhai, Patrick, & Frueh, 2008; Mekhjian, Turner, Gailiun, & McCain, 1999; L. Schopp, Johnstone, & Merrell, 2000; L. H. Schopp, Johnstone, & Merveille, 2000). In a more recent study with a large sample size, Grubaugh et al. (2008) did find that rural patients with posttraumatic stress disorder (PTSD) were more comfortable with TMH if it would save them a one hour drive to a clinic. Future studies of satisfaction need to continue efforts to tease apart whether the satisfaction is related to the actual quality of TMH care or to the reduced burden of receiving care for patients in poorly served areas.

To date, the provision of TMH may not reduce burden for clinicians and, in some instances, may increase burden relative to standard same-room consultation. TMH is often conducted in a special room, not the clinician's usual consultation room, and clinicians need to adapt their clinical style to the constraints associated with whatever form of VTC is adopted. For example, it is generally better for a clinician conducting VTC not to move too much in his or her seat. Though these are small discomforts compared to some of the travel burden of patients, they could add up to just enough inconvenience to put a clinician outside of his or her comfort zone.

However, the newer consumer-grade desktop technologies may provide one area of added convenience for clinicians that would increase adoption. The use of desktop computer or Internet-delivered VTC technologies may allow clinicians to work from home or at least from their regular clinical office using their personal computer. The impact of this development is already being observed in the growth of Internet-based TMH companies which serve as a conduit between clinicians providing care from their own office or home to patients at remote sites. Here, TMH is reducing burden for providers by facilitating patient recruitment and allowing clinicians to provide care from their preferred work spot, be it home or their clinical office. Satisfaction studies of these newer models of care are lacking and would provide greater insight into the mediating role of reduced clinician burden to general TMH satisfaction.

Comparability Between TMH and Same-Room Care

Similar to the research on satisfaction, the research on comparability between TMH and same-room care is overwhelmingly positive. Comparability has been examined for a range of interventions including, psychiatric and psychological assessment, consultation to primary care, and psychiatric treatment and psychotherapy. As stated in the American Telemedicine Association's Practice Guidelines for TMH and its accompanying Evidence Base for the Practice of TMH (Grady et al.,

2011; Yellowlees, Shore, Roberts, & American Telemedicine Association Guidelines Workgroup, 2010), there is no evidence suggesting a contraindication for use of VTC in mental health care. It has demonstrated comparability in children (Myers, Sulzbacher, & Melzer, 2004; Nelson, Barnard, & Cain, 2003), adults (Fortney, Pyne et al., 2007; Frueh, Monnier, Yim et al., 2007; Morland, Greene, Rosen, Foy et al., 2010; O'Reilly et al., 2007; Ruskin et al., 2004), geriatric (Egede et al., 2009; Holden & Dew, 2008; Rabinowitz et al., 2010; Sheeran et al., 2011), and even cognitively impaired patients (Rabinowitz et al., 2010; L. H. Schopp et al., 2000). It has been tested in mood disorders (Carlbring et al., 2011; Fortney, Pyne et al., 2007; Garcia-Lizana & Munoz-Mayorga, 2010; Kaltenthaler, Parry, Beverley, & Ferriter, 2008; Proudfoot et al., 2004; Ruskin et al., 2004), anxiety disorders (Bouchard et al., 2004; Frueh, Monnier, Yim et al., 2007; Gros, Yoder, Tuerk, Lozano, & Acierno, 2011), substance-use disorders (Frueh, Henderson, & Myrick, 2005; King et al., 2009), and psychosis (Sharp, Kobak, & Osman, 2011; Zarate et al., 1997). It is effective in outpatient, inpatient, institutionalized, and correctional settings (Antonacci et al., 2008; Doze, Simpson, Hailey, & Jacobs, 1999; Fortney, Pyne et al., 2007; Holden & Dew, 2008; Mekhjian et al., 1999; Morgan et al., 2008; Rabinowitz et al., 2010; Shores et al., 2004). Though the research in TMH is of relatively poorer quality than that of pharmaco- or psychotherapy, there are adequate numbers of well-designed studies in each of these areas to support the use of TMH to provide mental health care. The most frequently cited shortcomings for TMH occurred mainly in the earlier studies (pre-2000) and were due directly to low bandwidth. This type of problem is really no longer an issue as bandwidths of 128 kbps are rarely used today even in remote areas. Most current TMH applications rely on transmission of 384 kbps or higher.

Seasoned clinicians who have not practiced TMH continue to raise concerns based on their clinical understanding of how specific psychopathology may interact negatively with VTC care. For example, delusions of reference in psychotic patients can often involve the television and may thereby be exacerbated by actually talking with a television for TMH care. This concern has been well explored with no evidence that psychotic patients are vulnerable to an increase in symptoms in this treatment (Sharp et al., 2011). Assessment and treatment of schizophrenia through VTC is largely comparable to same-room care. APPAL-Link, a large project in Southwestern Virginia, found that remote management of chronically mentally ill lead to reduced hospitalization and no adverse events (Graham, 1996). Some earlier studies did find that the rating of negative symptoms or self-neglect common in schizophrenia was not as reliable when assessed through VTC, though this was only in conditions of low bandwidth (Zarate et al., 1997). This drawback was not found for transmission of 384 kbps or higher.

Similarly, concerns are raised that providing care through VTC may collude with the avoidance of travel often found in patients with anxiety disorders. Though VTC may reduce barriers to care for anxiety patients, both real-time VTC and therapist-guided Internet interventions have demonstrated effectiveness comparable to that of same-room care (Andrews, Davies, & Titov, 2011; Bouchard et al., 2004). In a guided Internet intervention, Andersson, Carlbring, and Grimund (2008) found agoraphobic avoidance negatively impacted the outcome assessed with the Agoraphobic Cognitions Questionnaire and the Body Sensations Questionnaire (Chambless, Caputo, Bright, & Gallagher, 1984) in the same-room condition but was not relevant to these outcomes for the Internet-delivered CBT. The authors speculate that Internet-delivered CBT for agoraphobia may be particularly well suited for patients in early stages of overcoming their anxieties.

Effectiveness Research and Noninferiority Statistical Methods

Recently, investigators of comparability between VTC and same-room care have adopted methods of comparative effectiveness research (Morland, Greene, Rosen, Mauldin, & Frueh, 2009). Comparative effectiveness research aims to demonstrate that one treatment is as good as the current state-of-the-art treatment for a specific clinical presentation. Therefore, the aim is to demonstrate noninferiority, not superiority. Though the actual conduct of noninferiority trials contains many of the same elements of a superiority trial (e.g., randomization, blind rating of outcomes, treatment protocol adherence, and fidelity), the statistical analysis is different. In noninferiority trials, investigators set an apriori, difference in both the final outcome and the change in outcome, based on expert consensus about what is a clinically meaningful difference on the main outcome measure. This is used to define a range of acceptable differences whereby the new treatment would be considered noninferior to the standard treatment. Though the range is anchored by the observed outcome mean in the standard treatment allowing for newer treatments to fall within the superior range on this measure, the primary interest is whether the novel treatment mean falls outside of the inferior range. This range is labeled the margin of inferiority. Most often, mixed effects linear models tailored to sampling and randomization structures specific to each study will be conducted to determine the magnitude of difference between the two interventions and whether or not this is large enough in favor of the state-of-the-art treatment to decide the novel treatment being tested is inferior.

One of the first to use these methods, Morland, Greene, Rosen, Foy et al. (2010) compared TMH group therapy for anger management in PTSD received via telemedicine versus same-room care. They will also apply such methods on a current study comparing VTC and in-person cognitive processing therapy for rural combat veterans with PTSD. The analysis of this trial will actually combine noninferiority analyses, to demonstrate comparability between TMH and same-room care, with tests of statistical significance on the main outcome, the Clinician Administered PTSD scale (Morland, Greene, Rosen, Mauldin et al., 2009). This combination is the most rigorous of methods as it examines noninferiority as well as whether or not the treatments were actually effective in reducing PTSD symptoms, thereby combining a noninferiority and effectiveness trial.

Another significant development in effectiveness research in TMH is the conduct of large full-scale randomized controlled trials. O'Reilly et al. (2007) conducted a randomized controlled trial comparing same-room to TMH psychiatric consultation for 495 adult patients in Canada referred by their primary care clinician. Consistent with much of the TMH research in psychiatry, the authors did not focus on a specific psychiatric disorder but recruited a general patient sample. The primary outcome was the proportion of patients moving from dysfunctional to functional on an a priori threshold for caseness on the Brief Symptom Inventory (BSI) 4 months after initial psychiatric consultation. The BSI was self-administered, so the ratings were not blind per se, but outcome assessment was within the generally accepted methods for clinical trials. At 4 months, 22% of patients receiving TMH improved as compared with 20% in the same-room care. The two groups were also comparable in the percentage hospitalized at 1-year follow-up with 6.6% hospitalized in the TMH group and 7.3% hospitalized in the same-room group. This carefully conducted study recruited until the projected samples size was obtained. However, only 58% of the participants initially randomized completed the 4-month follow-up assessments. Of note, study psychiatrists provided both remote and same-room care, the latter entailing traveling 1000 km by plane to a rural outpatient health-care center.

Ruskin et al. (2004) compared telepsychiatry to same-room care in 119 depressed veterans and found 49% of subjects in the TMH group responded as compared with 43% in the same-room condition. The intervention included psychotropic medication, psychoeducation, and brief supportive counseling. A unique aspect of this study relative to prior work in TMH is the focus on a specific patient group, depressed veterans, and the main outcome, defined as a decline of 50% or greater on the 24-item Hamilton Depression Rating Scale. This is one of the first studies in TMH that allows comparison of treatment response to standard trials of effectiveness conducted in pharmacotherapy trials. Though the response rate is somewhat lower that what one hopes for antidepressant trials, it is consistent with response rates found in primary care with patients suffering significant medical comorbidity. Results on the Beck Depression Inventory (BDI) also demonstrated effectiveness and comparability between remote and same-room psychiatric care.

TMH-facilitated collaborative care has also been explored because VTC addresses the geographic barriers to collaborative care models. Within the Department of Veterans Affairs (VA), Fortney, Pyne et al. (2007) randomized 395 veterans in primary care to receive the telemedicine-enhanced antidepressant management (TEAM) intervention or usual care. The TEAM intervention included provider education through interactive video and web site, depression screening, and a stepped care model where telepsychiatrists, pharmacists, and depression nurse care managers worked with the primary care team to optimally manage veterans with depression. Though the two treatment groups did not differ in the percentage with an active antidepressant prescription at 6 months, patients in the TEAM arm were twice as likely to be adherent to their antidepressant medications (OR = 2.1, $P = 0.04$) and were significantly more likely to respond to depression treatment at 6 months (OR = 1.9, $P = 0.02$).

In contrast with telepsychiatry, effectiveness research in psychotherapy conducted through VTC tends to focus on manualized treatment for a specific disorder such as PTSD or anxiety disorders and the sample sizes are considerably smaller. Gros et al. (2011) conducted a *nonrandomized* trial of veterans suffering PTSD to receive either telehealth-delivered exposure therapy ($N = 62$) or in-person exposure therapy ($N = 27$). The main outcome was decline on the military version of the PTSD checklist (PCL) (Blanchard, Jones-Alexander, Buckley, & Forneris, 1996). There was actually a statistically significant difference where in-person patients experienced greater decline than telehealth patients though both patient groups experienced statistically significant reduction in symptoms. The telehealth group's PCL score went from a mean of 63.2 (SD = 10.4) to 47.8 (SD = 15.0) while the same-room condition PCL scores went from 62.5 (SD = 10.1) to 31.6 (10.5). Similar findings were found for the BDI in which the telehealth mean decreased from 34.1 (SD = 9.7) to 22.4 (SD = 10.9) pre- to postintervention, while the same-room condition means declined from 28.7 (SD = 9.3) to 11.2 (SD = 7.0). The authors state that the uncommon finding of greater improvement in the same-room condition appears to be due to an unexpectedly robust treatment response that is inconsistent with response rates in prior studies. Moreover, treatment assignment was not randomized. This study's findings will need to be explored further for confirmation and the novel findings may be related to nonrandomized treatment assignment.

One recent study of therapist-delivered Internet psychotherapy (Kessler et al., 2009) has received a lot of attention as it was published in the Lancet and reported a 38% response rate for the TMH intervention as compared with the 24% response rate in the usual care group. This was a well-designed study with sophisticated randomization and analysis. Although it described a real-time psychotherapy intervention, the communication was entirely through secure messaging and entailed no video component. Though it reports a statistically significant difference between the intervention and comparison group, it was a usual care comparator whereas most of the prior psychotherapy studies reviewed herein were compared to an active same-room comparator.

Morland, Greene, Rosen, Foy et al. (2010) found comparable levels of decline on the State Trait Anger Expression Inventory-2 between TMH and same-room care in veterans receiving care for anger management in PTSD with an indication of a larger effect size for veterans in the TMH condition. This study is notable in two respects. It was one of the first TMH studies to use noninferiority statistical methods and it is one of the first randomized controlled trials of group therapy using TMH. The authors also found no group differences in decline on the PCL military version. The authors conducted noninferiority analyses determining the two treatments to be equally effective on all clinical outcomes.

Mitchell et al. (2008) compared TMH with same-room care in cognitive behavioral treatment for 128 adults suffering bulimia nervosa. Both groups experienced significant decline in binge eating and purging frequencies posttreatment and at 3 and 12-month follow-up. However, the same-room condition had slightly higher rates on many of the clinical outcomes, including abstinence, and decline in binge eating and purging frequencies with some of these comparisons reaching statistical significance.

Day and Schneider (2002) examined the effectiveness of CBT for participants suffering from a range of mild mental disorders, randomizing 107 patients to receive either same-room care, video TMH care, telephone delivered care, or no treatment. None of the treatments differed on the main outcome measures posttreatment including the Derogatis BSI, the Global Assessment of Functioning Scale, or the Target Complaints Method. However, standard clinical trial analyses were not conducted and the authors did not present data allowing for comparison in change from baseline.

In psychotherapy for children, a smaller study conducted by Nelson et al. (2003) found superior response to CBT for the VTC condition as compared with same-room therapy. Though the sample size was only 28 children randomized to two treatment arms, the study is notable because it was very well designed and conducted, using CONSORT criteria for both collecting and reporting of data (Altman et al., 2001). Using the Children's Depression Inventory as the main outcome, the VTC condition dropped from 14.36 to 6.71, while the same-room condition declined from 13.57 to 11.64. The group by time interaction was significant. These results are all the more impressive given that the technology used transmitted at 128 kbps.

In contrast to the research in telepsychiatry, telepsychology has more mixed results regarding the comparability between TMH and same-room care. Though the authors of the psychotherapy trials, where TMH yielded smaller declines in clinical outcomes, claim the two groups are equal, noninferiority methods such as those used by Morland, Greene, Rosen, Foy et al. (2010) are needed to substantiate these claims. Moreover, more research is needed with larger sample sizes to better discern if there is a difference in treatment response between these two modes of delivery.

The clinical tasks of psychotherapy as compared with psychiatry differ and it may be that the challenge of developing effective TMH applications for therapy will be more difficult. Medication management mainly involves assessment of symptoms and side effects. The quality of the relationship may play less of a role in psychiatry. However, the study of Ruskin et al. (2004) did include supportive counseling and psychoeducation, so the boundaries between psychiatry and psychotherapy are not always so firmly drawn. This large, well-designed study did not find evidence for low efficacy of the TMH arm.

Future Directions in Effectiveness Research

Though noninferiority trials are the appropriate model of TMH comparability research, it is not clear that they necessarily set a higher threshold for acceptance of the new treatment. Statistical significance in differences between means is often more easily detected than clinical significance particularly on continuous measures. Moreover, it is possible to demonstrate noninferiority; yet neither

treatment results in statistically significant decline in scores on the main outcome measure. Therefore, the hybrid statistical analysis that combines noninferiority with standard tests for improvement of clinical outcomes over time
between groups is needed.

Further studies in which the sole aim is to simply demonstrate noninferiority of
TMH compared with same-room care across two health-care centers will provide
little new information. It takes little additional effort to also evaluate the effectiveness of the TMH treatment as well as to explore other important issues such as
comparability of process measures, and cost-effectiveness or work-load burden.
Innovative hybrid models using both noninferiority statistical methods combined
with standard effectiveness analyses yield much needed evidence of actual effectiveness in VTC care. Process measures such as therapeutic alliance are easily
administered. Though slightly more complex to analyze, comparison of cost-
effectiveness and work-load issues provide critical information to assist in the
eventual implementation of TMH.

One new area of noninferiority research that does need to be explored is the provision of care from a health-care center or single provider to patients in clinically
unsupervised settings (Luxton, Sirotin, & Mishkind, 2010). P. Shore (2011) and
colleagues within the VA and the Department of Defense have developed a thorough Standard Operation Procedures for home based care. Provision of TMH to
clinically unsupervised settings is growing rapidly due to the general availability of
high-quality consumer-grade desktop technology or mobile technology. The issues
in these trials differ from that of the large established literature of TMH between
two health-care settings. Though there is much prior research comparing the difference in quality based on bandwidth transmission, few studies have examined the
issue of screen size. Though relatively new, TMH is being conducted where the
patient monitor is an iPad or even a smartphone. Does the size of the screen impact
alliance and patient comfort and engagement? Moreover, does receiving care in
nonclinical settings, such as the patient's home or office, increase or reduce patient
engagement? Are there certain patient subgroups, such as children or agitated
elderly, for whom the constriction of remaining on screen is counter-therapeutic or
simply not feasible? Do all of these factors impact actual effectiveness of the
TMH-delivered care?

Issues regarding screen size are just one of the many issues to be explored when
testing the effectiveness of providing care to clinically unsupervised settings. In
addition to the process issues listed above, safety management for potentially violent patients needs to be explored. This is an exciting area because it is difficult to
guess how delivering care directly to patients will impact effectiveness. Patients
may be more at ease talking with a clinician in the comfort of their own home or
they may be more easily distracted and take the whole process less seriously.
Exploration of effectiveness as well as these critical process variables is needed,
particularly as some hold this type of care may be so appealing to patients that it
will expand rapidly before an adequate evidence base has formed.

Though, like satisfaction research, the comparability between TMH and same-
room care has been well documented, several new areas of exploration continue to

develop mostly related to the ever-changing horizon of high-quality mobile video-technology. Advances in research methods, such as noninferiority trials and continuous development of appropriate therapeutic process measures, are needed. The field of TMH currently needs to replicate and expand its investigations of efficacy, particularly for psychotherapy interventions. The disconnect between the overwhelming evidence for satisfaction and the modest findings comparing effectiveness on treatment outcomes in psychotherapy highlights that more work needs to be done and patients would benefit from our learning more effective ways to deliver TMH.

Though TMH is slow to develop a solid evidence base of randomized controlled trials with large sample sizes, it should be noted that this is extraordinarily difficult research to conduct. A randomized controlled trial of psychiatric or psychological interventions where one arm uses TMH entails far more resources than standard clinical trials which are already quite labor intensive. For example, in the trial of O'Reilly et al. (2007), therapists had to fly 1000 km to provide the same-room care. Requiring the patients to travel that distance would reduce investigator burden but introduce such a significant confound related to patient burden and potential resentment that the results may be rendered uninterpretable. Day and Schneider (2002) addressed this issue by having all patients receive care in the same building, yet some received it through VTC, others by phone and others received same-room care. Though clever, it is not clear how well these results would generalize to genuine differences in outcomes between remote versus same-room provision of care in day-to-day practice. Randomized TMH trials also demand resources to purchase and distribute the VTC equipment. This is a major investment that is difficult to obtain, especially for pilot data collection which is a requirement before anyone can apply for funding of a major clinical trial. The difficulty in developing VTC infrastructure underlies why most of the current research in VTC TMH is conducted within the VA or the Department of Defense where the infrastructure is already in place as part of their clinical practice. It is hoped that the lower cost, more accessible desktop VTC software will reduce this burden and facilitate broader research in this area.

Future effectiveness trials, even when using noninferiority methods for comparison, may yield a more sobering evaluation of TMH than prior satisfaction research. Therefore, it is important to include sophisticated examination of mediators and moderators of treatment response to help clinicians committed to improving access through technology to develop more effective treatments (Kraemer, Wilson, Fairburn, & Agras, 2002). As discussed earlier, one strong mediator in same-room therapy, that of therapeutic alliance, does not appear to impact treatment response in the same way for TMH. This needs to be examined further and does not really warrant abandoning TMH; rather it calls for renewed efforts to improve ways to enhance alliance when using VTC. Examination of treatment mediators and moderators is relatively recent and has yet to reveal clear ways to improve our treatments. Gros et al. (2011) failed to find any predictors of treatment response in a sample of veterans suffering PTSD. Age, sex, race, service cohort, or disability status did not affect effectiveness on the intervention. More studies are needed that can examine how patients' and clinicians' comfort with technology relates to responsiveness to treatment.

The line of research that has best examined treatment mediators are investigations of effectiveness in using psychotherapy delivered entirely through the Internet with minimal or no therapist support. This research area has not been the main focus of this text and falls more clearly under the heading of *e*-Therapy. However, the research in this area is exemplary and serves as a good model of solid research in TMH.

Internet-Delivered Therapy with Little or No Real-Time Interaction

Evidence for effectiveness of psychotherapy delivered entirely through the Internet with little or no therapist contact has been well examined allowing for three comprehensive reviews (Andersson & Cuijpers, 2009; Barak, Hen, Boniel-Nissim, & Shapira, 2008; Kaltenthaler et al., 2008) Internet therapy is fairly heterogenous with some interventions consisting of a series of readings with regular corresponding guidance by a therapist through secure messaging or phone, real-time secure messaging between therapist and patient, and web-based self-help and instruction for patients who receive minimal but regular instruction and review by nonprofessionals. Internet therapy has been developed primarily for depression and anxiety and substance abuse (Gainsbury & Blaszczynski, 2011).

In a recent metaanalysis of Internet therapies for adult depression conducted by Andersson and Cuijpers (2009), 12 randomized controlled trials including 2446 participants were used to determine the estimates of effect size and correlates of strong impact. The mean effect size reported was 0.41 indicating moderate effect. Heterogeneity between studies was high and it was found that computerized interventions in which there was at least minimal therapist communication or support had an average between-group effect size of 0.61, while unsupported treatments yielded a 0.25 between-group effect size. These studies are typically well designed and use reasonable comparison groups such as scheduled online educational sessions with minimal therapist contact.

Internet-based treatments produce low to moderate effect sizes, and their potential to radically increase access to effective interventions supports further investigation of this medium. Christensen, Griffiths, Mackinnon, and Brittliffe (2006) conducted a randomized controlled trial of brief and longer term CBT on a web site entitled MoodGYM, which was openly accessible within Australia, the United Kingdom, the United States, Canada, and New Zealand. The MoodGYM program consists of five 20—40 min modules undertaken sequentially. It introduces patients to CBT concepts such as identification and modification of dysfunctional thoughts and behavioral strategies to improve mood. Six separate configurations of these modules were randomly assigned to 2794 participants—a sample size which was possible due to international access to the MoodGYM web site. The primary outcome was total score on the Goldberg

Depression Scale which correlates strongly with the Hamilton Rating Scale for Depression.

Combinations of the six versions were compared to completion of a single introduction module only. Those including an extended CBT component, problem-solving techniques, and behavioral strategies were most effective with effect sizes ranging from 0.34 to 0.40. This effect size is considerable in light of the fact that the intervention did not include therapist support. The effect size for reduction of anxiety symptoms in this sample was similar. However, as common in interventions delivered entirely through the Internet, attrition was high. Seventy percent of those who completed the baseline assessment for this study failed to complete even the first module of the intervention. Further investigation is needed to determine the potential public health impact of what amounts to essentially free care to anyone with Internet access, yet high likelihood of patient attrition. Christensen et al. (2006) report some of the largest effect sizes in unsupported treatments, indicating their program captures some of the critical components of pure self-help therapy options for the treatment of depression.

Investigators of Internet therapy have also examined mediators and moderators of treatment effectiveness more thoroughly that those conducting research in real-time VTC TMH. Kessler et al. (2009) tested whether baseline severity, marital status, adverse life stressors, depression history, education, or age, predicted treatment response to an online real-time secure messaging treatment for depression. Of these, only pretreatment severity and marital status moderated response, with more severely depressed patients responding less well to the intervention. Andersson, Carlbring, and Grimlund (2008) examined predictors of outcome in an online therapy versus same-room therapy. As mentioned earlier, agoraphobic avoidance was associated with outcome in same-room treatment but not with Internet treatment, while comorbid personality disorder predicted outcome in both modes though apparently more so for Internet treatment. Treatment credibility and cognitive capacity were not predictive of outcome for either group.

Once the online intervention is developed, the implementation of online therapies is far less labor intensive than a randomized controlled trial for real-time TMH interventions. This allows for large sample sizes with sophisticated dismantling designs (such as that conducted by Christensen et al. (2006)) or stepped interventions. Nonetheless, both the examination of critical components for effectiveness and moderators of treatment response should be adapted to real-time TMH research in order to increase insight into possible improvements in care.

e-Health Adjuncts to Same-Room and TMH Care

With the increased adoption of mobile technologies including smartphones, *e*-Health adjuncts to boost effectiveness of clinical care are developing rapidly. The evidence base for such adjuncts is too nascent to draw any initial conclusions about effectiveness. Nonetheless, a brief discussion of potential applications is warranted to begin the discussion of this exciting new chapter in TMH.

Grassi, Preziosa, Villani, and Riva (2007) used mobile phone applications to assist in relaxation exercises for nonpatient participants. The program facilitated imagination of calm environments and progressive muscular relaxation. Participants receiving both audio and visual components of this program experienced a significant reduction in anxiety and improvements in self-efficacy. The impact of such an intervention on psychiatric patients is unknown.

Case reports or small sample studies describe the use of mobile devices in developmentally delayed children, primarily children with Asperger's syndrome (Ferguson, Myles, & Hagiwara, 2005; Mechling, Gast, & Seid, 2009). The devices prompt participants to complete important tasks, such as self-care or homework, independently. The devices serve to compensate for participant deficits in organization or problem solving, yet the average to high intelligence of Asperger's patients allows them to make use of technological devices.

Web-based mobile applications designed to educate and guide people suffering mental health issues are rapidly proliferating. The United States Department of Defense, one of the most advanced in harnessing technology for TMH, has developed a mobile application called PTSD Coach (Mobile App: PTSD Coach). PTSD Coach is a mobile application free to download for anyone. The application contains four content areas: (1) information about PTSD, (2) self-assessment of PTSD symptoms and a function which allows tracking on this measure over time, (3) coping strategies for managing systems for which the user can set preferences, and (4) information on how to find support. The coping strategies module includes progressive relaxation exercises. The user can also integrate other features of his or her mobile device into PTSD Coach by linking to favorite mood enhancing or soothing songs or photographs.

Within the VA, a computer-based software program called *My Recovery Plan* will be made available to veterans through the VA personal health record portal termed "My Health*e*Vet" (Cucciare, Weingardt, & Humphreys, 2009). This program provides homework, monitoring sheets, and progress reports to be used in conjunction with recovery-based therapies provided by the VA. By connecting the program with "My Health*e*Vet", the veteran can readily access monitoring and homework sheets to complete and then share with his or her therapist at the next session.

Comparable to the studies examining *e*-Therapy, future research of these promising adjuncts to therapy should be evaluated using dismantling clinical trial designs where the added benefit of the technology to standard therapy is determined. There is growing excitement about the potential for mobile technologies to revolutionize medical and public health interventions. More technology is not always better, but it tends to fascinate. Once again, systematic investigation using a critical eye, comparable to the research conducted in *e*-Therapy, is needed to ensure that novelty does not override actual effectiveness in what is eventually adopted.

Cost-Effectiveness Studies in TMH

One of the most frequent questions asked of advocates of TMH is whether the organizational cost of starting a TMH service would be offset by a decrease in downstream costs of untreated mental health. To truly answer this question, sophisticated modeling by a trained health-care economist is needed, and even then, it is likely that the answer will not be a simple "yes" or "no" (Kennedy, 2005). Though research in cost in TMH studies is growing, most studies to date rely on straightforward calculations (Fortney, Maciejewski, Tripathi, Deen, & Pyne, 2011; Mair, Haycox, May, & Williams, 2000; McCrone et al., 2004; O'Reilly et al., 2007; Spaulding, Belz, DeLurgio, & Williams, 2010)

Ruskin et al. (2004) conducted one of the most complex cost-effects analyses in TMH literature which took into account a wide range of potential contributors to cost such as depreciated equipment expenses, cabling, access fees, and actual access charges. They estimated that the marginal costs to the institution were US$86.16 per telepsychiatry session and US$63.25 per in-person psychiatry session ($P < 0.0001$). They then added in cost of travel time of the psychiatrist to the patient's location and concluded that the cost of TMH was equal to in person if the psychiatrist had to travel 22 miles or more to a remote health-care site. There was no significant difference in health-care consumption over the 6-month period of the study between telepsychiatry and same-room patients.

Fortney, Maciejewski et al. (2011) conducted a cost analysis of their telepsychiatry collaborative care intervention described earlier. There were no significant differences in the total number of primary care encounters and their costs between the TEAM participants and the usual care group. The intervention group did have significantly more specialty physical health encounters than the usual care group leading to overall greater cost for the TEAM intervention group.

These results echo cost analyses of earlier studies where cost neutral or cost benefit aspects of TMH are not demonstrated until travel cost for either the patient or the clinician are entered into the equation. Though travel cost is relevant in determining societal cost of health care, many organizations are focused solely on the burden on their own financial resources. Therefore, saving the cost of travel, when that cost would most often be absorbed by the patient, may not be persuasive to health-care providers or insurers.

The studies which demonstrate cost-effectiveness are most often in contexts in which the provider of care or payer of care is under some obligation to make health-care accessible to its enrollees. Therefore, they assume some of the responsibility of travel to care. The study of Ruskin et al. (2004) was conducted within the VA which is under this obligation to some extent. Two studies conducted in other countries with universal health care, O'Reilly et al. (2007) in Canada and Trott and Blignault (1998) in Australia, actually demonstrate cost-savings though, again, travel cost was included in the analysis, most often psychiatrists' travel cost.

This work may become more relevant in the United States if reforms in health care make providers more responsible to a specific geographic area and community.

It is assumed that payers may feel more obligation to develop innovative ways to improve access to care. Therefore, it is essential that future cost-effectiveness studies for TMH harness state-of-the-art methods for health economic analysis and to engage health economists throughout the design and conduct of the study.

Another difficulty in calculating cost in TMH is the rapidly declining cost of conducting VTC. Granted, this is the type of difficulty one wants to have. J. H. Shore, Brooks, Savin, Manson, and Libby (2007) calculated the direct costs for new clinics of conducting psychiatric assessment, comparing VTC versus in-person. Costs were calculated in 2003 and again in 2005. In 2003, TMH costs were US$6000 more than in-person interviews. In 2005, TMH costs were US$8000 less. The same pattern was found for established clinics. The cost of high-quality VTC continues to decline markedly. Therefore, many of the cost-effectiveness studies, such as those conducted before 2005, are likely irrelevant to today's health-care economy.

The proliferation of relatively low-cost, high-quality consumer-grade VTC technology may radically alter cost-effectiveness studies in TMH. As with other financial analyses involving technology, the estimates of cost may become obsolete over the time lapsed between the start and completion of a particular study. Nonetheless, given the radical changes occurring in health-care policy, such data, even when dated, are essential. This rapid development of technology combined with the possibility of major health-care reform may provide the final push needed to integrate TMH into mainstream health care.

Future Directions and Conclusion

Research in TMH has matured beyond the initial stages of establishing feasibility and satisfaction. More research is needed to test effectiveness, particularly in TMH psychotherapy. Cost analyses, though initially promising, are likely to be more persuasive in favor of TMH as technology costs decline and health-care systems become more open to system redesign in response to major health-care reform. Each of these novel lines of research also addresses the questions and concerns of those who remain skeptical about TMH. Though continuing to address these skeptical concerns is essential, the field is ready to take on more nuanced questions that address how TMH can best be delivered.

One important question is whether there are patient characteristics that predict responsiveness to TMH or indicate when TMH is contraindicated. This question is already beginning to be addressed in the *e*-Therapy with minimal or no real-time therapist interaction. Findings such as those by Andersson, Carlbring, and Grimlund (2008) regarding agoraphobic avoidance predicting negative outcome in same-room care could be replicated and expanded upon.

More work like this need to be done in real-time TMH research. Studies of moderators and mediators of treatment response will (i) help determine if VTC TMH is ever contraindicated and the conditions where this would be true, (ii) point to potential shortcomings of TMH that the field can subsequently try to address, and (iii) help to better understand paradoxical findings like the lower ratings of therapeutic alliance combined with weaker associations between alliance and group differences in treatment response in TMH. These questions could be addressed within standard randomized controlled trials for effectiveness if there is a large enough sample size and assessment beyond just measures of outcomes and satisfaction.

As already stated, TMH cost-effectiveness analyses would benefit from more input on design from health economists. However, it would also be helpful to develop more metrics to quantify exactly how TMH reduces barriers to care and subsequently affects costs. Rabinowitz et al. (2010) calculated travel cost, gasoline cost, and time savings for both patients and providers. Such innovative assessment of all the resources involved in a health-care visit will better demonstrate the contribution of TMH in containing these costs. As health-care investigators aim to quantify health-care access, such metrics can be incorporated easily into TMH research.

Finally, more exploration of innovative ways of combining TMH, e-Health, and same-room interventions is needed. The use of mobile and e-Health technologies in conjunction with same-room psychotherapy is growing and may maximize the effectiveness of treatments. This model can be expanded to include innovative models that combine same-room consultations, VTC consultations, possibly VTC consultation directly to patients' homes, and mobile applications to enhance and reinforce therapeutic practices between formal health-care sessions. Dismantling designs combined with comparative effectiveness methods make the most sense for this type of research, in which technologic adjuncts are added to established same-room treatments.

This line of research will bring TMH beyond the defensive stance of being "as-good-as" same-room care. Patients are using more technology, particularly VTC technology, in their personal lives. In the future, patients may expect it to be harnessed in health care so that it can increase their access to care and reduce burden. The current imperative for all care to have an evidence-base means that proactive anticipation of patients' needs and technology's potential should inform our current research on how best to practice TMH.

References

Altman, D. G., Schulz, K. F., Moher, D., Egger, M., Davidoff, F., Elbourne, D., et al. (2001). The revised CONSORT statement for reporting randomized trials: Explanation and elaboration. *Annals of Internal Medicine*, *134*, 663–694.

Andersson, G. (2009). Using the internet to provide cognitive behaviour therapy. *Behaviour Research and Therapy*, *47*, 175–180.

Andersson, G. (2010). The promise and pitfalls of the internet for cognitive behavioral therapy. *BioMed Central Medicine*, *8*, 1–5.

Andersson, G., Carlbring, P., & Grimund, A. (2008). Predicting treatment outcome in internet versus face to face treatment of panic disorder. *Computers in Human Behavior*, *24*, 1790–1801.

Andersson, G., & Cuijpers, P. (2009). Internet-based and other computerized psychological treatments for adult depression: A meta-analysis. *Cognitive Behaviour Therapy, 38*, 196–205.

Andrews, G., Davies, M., & Titov, N. (2011). Effectiveness randomized controlled trial of face to face versus internet cognitive behaviour therapy for social phobia. *Australian and New Zealand Journal of Psychiatry, 45*, 337–340.

Antonacci, D. J., Bloch, R. M., Saeed, S. A., Yildirim, Y., & Talley, J. (2008). Empirical evidence on the use and effectiveness of telepsychiatry via videoconferencing: Implications for forensic and correctional psychiatry. *Behavioral Sciences and the Law, 26*, 253–269.

Barak, A., Hen, L., Boniel-Nissim, M., & Shapira, N. (2008). A comprehensive review and a meta-nalysis of the effectiveness of internet-based psychotherapeutic interventions. *Journal of Technology in Human Services, 26*, 109–160.

Blackmon, L. A., Kaak, H. O., & Ranseen, J. (1997). Consumer satisfaction with telemedicine child psychiatry consultation in rural Kentucky. *Psychiatric Services, 48*, 1464–1466.

Blanchard, E. B., Jones-Alexander, J., Buckley, T. C., & Forneris, C. A. (1996). Psychometric properties of the PTSD Checklist (PCL). *Behaviour Research and Therapy, 34*, 669–673.

Bouchard, S., Paquin, B., Payeur, R., Allard, M., Rivard, V., Fournier, T., et al. (2004). Delivering cognitive-behavior therapy for panic disorder with agoraphobia in videoconference. *Telemedicine Journal and e-Health, 10*, 13–25.

Callahan, E. J., Hilty, D. M., & Nesbitt, T. S. (1998). Patient satisfaction with telemedicine consultation in primary care: Comparison of ratings of medical and mental health applications. *Telemedicine Journal, 4*, 363–369.

Carlbring, P., Maurin, L., Torngren, C., Linna, E., Eriksson, T., Sparthan, E., et al. (2011). Individually-tailored, internet-based treatment for anxiety disorders: A randomized controlled trial. *Behaviour Research and Therapy, 49*, 18–24.

Chambless, D. L., Caputo, G. C., Bright, P., & Gallagher, R. (1984). Assessment of fear of fear in agoraphobics: The body sensations questionnaire and the agoraphobic cognitions questionnaire. *Journal of Consulting and Clinical Psychology, 52*, 1090–1097.

Christensen, H., Griffiths, K. M., Mackinnon, A. J., & Brittliffe, K. (2006). Online randomized controlled trial of brief and full cognitive behaviour therapy for depression. *Psychological Medicine, 36*, 1737–1746.

Cook, J. E., & Doyle, C. (2002). Working alliance in online therapy as compared to face-to-face therapy: Preliminary results. *Cyberpsychology and Behavior: The Impact of the Internet, Multimedia and Virtual Reality on Behavior and Society, 5*, 95–105.

Crow, R., Gage, H., Hampson, S., Hart, J., Kimber, A., Storey, L., et al. (2002). The measurement of satisfaction with healthcare: Implications for practice from a systematic review of the literature. *Health Technology Assessment, 6*, 1–244.

Cucciare, M. A., Weingardt, K. R., & Humphreys, K. (2009). How internet technology can improve the quality of care for substance use disorders. *Current Drug Abuse Reviews, 2*, 256–262.

Day, S. X., & Schneider, P. L. (2002). Psychotherapy using distance technology: A comparison of face-to-face, video, and audio treatment. *Journal of Counseling Psychology, 49*, 499–503.

Doze, S., Simpson, J., Hailey, D., & Jacobs, P. (1999). Evaluation of a telepsychiatry pilot project. *Journal of Telemedicine and Telecare, 5*, 38–46.

Egede, L. E., Frueh, C. B., Richardson, L. K., Acierno, R., Mauldin, P. D., Knapp, R. G., et al. (2009). Rationale and design: Telepsychology service delivery for depressed elderly veterans. *Trials, 10*, 22.

Ertelt, T. W., Crosby, R. D., Marino, J. M., Mitchell, J. E., Lancaster, K., & Crow, S. J. (2011). Therapeutic factors affecting the cognitive behavioral treatment of bulimia nervosa via telemedicine versus face-to-face delivery. *The International Journal of Eating Disorders, 44*, 687–691.

Ferguson, H., Myles, B. S., & Hagiwara, T. (2005). Using a personal digital assistant to enhance the independence of an adolescent with Asperger syndrome. *Education and Training in Mental Retardation and Developmental Disabilities, 40*, 60–67.

Fortney, J. C., Maciejewski, M. L., Tripathi, S. P., Deen, T. L., & Pyne, J. M. (2011). A budget impact analysis of telemedicine-based collaborative care for depression. *Medical Care, 49*, 872–880.

Fortney, J. C., Pyne, J. M., Edlund, M. J., Williams, D. K., Robinson, D. E., Mittal, D., et al. (2007). A randomized trial of telemedicine-based collaborative care for depression. *Journal of General Internal Medicine, 22*, 1086–1093.

Frueh, B. C., Deitsch, S. E., Santos, A. B., Gold, P. B., Johnson, M. R., Meisler, N., et al. (2000). Procedural and methodological issues in telepsychiatry research and program development. *Psychiatric Services, 51*, 1522–1527.

Frueh, B. C., Henderson, S., & Myrick, H. (2005). Telehealth service delivery for persons with alcoholism. *Journal of Telemedicine and Telecare, 11*, 372–375.

Frueh, B. C., Monnier, J., Grubaugh, A. L., Elhai, J. D., Yim, E., & Knapp, R. (2007). Therapist adherence and competence with manualized cognitive-behavioral therapy for PTSD delivered via videoconferencing technology. *Behavior Modification, 31*, 856–866.

Frueh, B. C., Monnier, J., Yim, E., Grubaugh, A. L., Hamner, M. B., & Knapp, R. G. (2007). A randomized trial of telepsychiatry for post-traumatic stress disorder. *Journal of Telemedicine and Telecare, 13*, 142–147.

Gainsbury, S., & Blaszczynski, A. (2011). A systematic review of internet-based therapy for the treatment of addictions. *Clinical Psychology Review, 31*, 490–498.

Garcia-Lizana, F., & Munoz-Mayorga, I. (2010). Telemedicine for depression: A systematic review. *Perspectives in Psychiatric Care, 46*, 119–126.

Grady, B., Myers, K. M., Nelson, E. L., Belz, N., Bennett, L., Carnahan, L., et al. (2011). Evidence-based practice for telemental health. *Telemedicine Journal and e-Health, 17*, 131–148.

Graham, M. A. (1996). Telepsychiatry in Appalachia. *American Behavioral Scientist, 39*, 602–615.

Grassi, A., Preziosa, A., Villani, D., & Riva, G. (2007). A relaxing journey: The use of mobile phones for well-being improvement. *Annual Review of Cyber Therapy and Telemedicine, 5*, 123–131.

Greene, C. J., Morland, L. A., Macdonald, A., Frueh, B. C., Grubbs, K. M., & Rosen, C. S. (2010). How does tele-mental health affect group therapy process? Secondary analysis of a noninferiority trial. *Journal of Consulting and Clinical Psychology, 78*, 746–750.

Gros, D. F., Yoder, M., Tuerk, P. W., Lozano, B. E., & Acierno, R. (2011). Exposure therapy for PTSD delivered to veterans via telehealth: Predictors of treatment completion and outcome and comparison to treatment delivered in person. *Behavior Therapy, 42*, 276–283.

Grubaugh, A. L., Cain, G. D., Elhai, J. D., Patrick, S. L., & Frueh, B. C. (2008). Attitudes toward medical and mental health care delivered via telehealth applications among rural and urban primary care patients. *Journal of Nervous and Mental Disease, 196,* 166−170.

Hilty, D. M., Luo, J. S., Morache, C., Marcelo, D. A., & Nesbitt, T. S. (2002). Telepsychiatry: An overview for psychiatrists. *CNS Drugs, 16,* 527−548.

Hilty, D. M., Yellowlees, P. M., & Nesbitt, T. S. (2006). Evolution of telepsychiatry to rural sites: Changes over time in types of referral and in primary care providers' knowledge, skills and satisfaction. *General Hospital Psychiatry, 28,* 367−373.

Holden, D., & Dew, E. (2008). Telemedicine in a rural gero-psychiatric inpatient unit: Comparison of perception/satisfaction to onsite psychiatric care. *Telemedicine Journal and e-Health, 14,* 381−384.

Jenkinson, C., Coulter, A., Bruster, S., Richards, N., & Chandola, T. (2002). Patients' experiences and satisfaction with health care: Results of a questionnaire study of specific aspects of care. *Quality and Safety in Health Care, 11,* 335−339.

Kaltenthaler, E., Parry, G., Beverley, C., & Ferriter, M. (2008). Computerised cognitive-behavioural therapy for depression: Systematic review. *British Journal of Psychiatry: The Journal of Mental Science, 193,* 181−184.

Kennedy, C. A. (2005). The challenges of economic evaluations of remote technical health interventions. *Clinical and Investigative Medicine, 28,* 71−74.

Kessler, D., Lewis, G., Kaur, S., Wiles, N., King, M., Weich, S., et al. (2009). Therapist-delivered internet psychotherapy for depression in primary care: A randomised controlled trial. *Lancet, 374,* 628−634.

King, V. L., Stoller, K. B., Kidorf, M., Kindbom, K., Hursh, S., Brady, T., et al. (2009). Assessing the effectiveness of an internet-based videoconferencing platform for delivering intensified substance abuse counseling. *Journal of Substance Abuse Treatment, 36,* 331−338.

Knaevelsrud, C., & Maercker, A. (2006). Does the quality of the working alliance predict treatment outcome in online psychotherapy for traumatized patients? *Journal of Medical Internet Research, 8,* e31.

Kraemer, H. C., Wilson, G. T., Fairburn, C. G., & Agras, W. S. (2002). Mediators and moderators of treatment effects in randomized clinical trials. *Archives of General Psychiatry, 59,* 877−883.

Luxton, D. D., Sirotin, A. P., & Mishkind, M. C. (2010). Safety of telemental healthcare delivered to clinically unsupervised settings: A systematic review. *Telemedicine Journal and e-Health, 16,* 705−711.

Mair, F. S., Haycox, A., May, C., & Williams, T. (2000). A review of telemedicine cost-effectiveness studies. *Journal of Telemedicine and Telecare, 6*(Suppl. 1), S38−S40.

McCrone, P., Knapp, M., Proudfoot, J., Ryden, C., Cavanagh, K., Shapiro, D. A., et al. (2004). Cost-effectiveness of computerised cognitive-behavioural therapy for anxiety and depression in primary care: Randomised controlled trial. *British Journal of Psychiatry: The Journal of Mental Science, 185,* 55−62.

Mechling, L. C., Gast, D. L., & Seid, N. H. (2009). Using a personal digital assistant to increase independent task completion by students with autism spectrum disorder. *Journal of Autism and Developmental Disorders, 39,* 1420−1434.

Mekhjian, H., Turner, J. W., Gailiun, M., & McCain, T. A. (1999). Patient satisfaction with telemedicine in a prison environment. *Journal of Telemedicine and Telecare, 5,* 55−61.

Mitchell, J. E., Crosby, R. D., Wonderlich, S. A., Crow, S., Lancaster, K., Simonich, H., et al. (2008). A randomized trial comparing the efficacy of cognitive-behavioral therapy for bulimia nervosa delivered via telemedicine versus face-to-face. *Behaviour Research and Therapy, 46,* 581−592.

Mobile App: PTSD Coach. <www.PTSD.VA.Gov/Public/Pages/PTSDCoach.asp>.

Monnier, J., Knapp, R. G., & Frueh, B. C. (2003). Recent advances in telepsychiatry: An updated review. *Psychiatric Services, 54*, 1604–1609.

Morgan, R. D., Patrick, A. R., & Magaletta, P. R. (2008). Does the use of telemental health alter the treatment experience? Inmates' perceptions of telemental health versus face-to-face treatment modalities. *Journal of Consulting and Clinical Psychology, 76*, 158–162.

Morland, L. A., Greene, C. J., Rosen, C., Mauldin, P. D., & Frueh, B. C. (2009). Issues in the design of a randomized noninferiority clinical trial of telemental health psychotherapy for rural combat veterans with PTSD. *Contemporary Clinical Trials, 30*, 513–522.

Morland, L. A., Greene, C. J., Rosen, C. S., Foy, D., Reilly, P., Shore, J., et al. (2010). Telemedicine for anger management therapy in a rural population of combat veterans with posttraumatic stress disorder: A randomized noninferiority trial. *The Journal of Clinical Psychiatry, 71*, 855–863.

Myers, K. M., Sulzbacher, S., & Melzer, S. M. (2004). Telepsychiatry with children and adolescents: Are patients comparable to those evaluated in usual outpatient care? *Telemedicine Journal and e-Health, 10*, 278–285.

Nelson, E. L., Barnard, M., & Cain, S. (2003). Treating childhood depression over videoconferencing. *Telemedicine Journal and e-Health, 9*, 49–55.

O'Reilly, R., Bishop, J., Maddox, K., Hutchinson, L., Fisman, M., & Takhar, J. (2007). Is telepsychiatry equivalent to face-to-face psychiatry? Results from a randomized controlled equivalence trial. *Psychiatric Services, 58*, 836–843.

Picker Survey (1999). *Implementation manual*. Boston, MA: Picker Institute.

Porcari, C. E., Amdur, R. L., Koch, E. I., Richard, D. C., Favorite, T., Martis, B., et al. (2009). Assessment of post-traumatic stress disorder in veterans by videoconferencing and by face-to-face methods. *Journal of Telemedicine and Telecare, 15*, 89–94.

Proudfoot, J., Ryden, C., Everitt, B., Shapiro, D. A., Goldberg, D., Mann, A., et al. (2004). Clinical efficacy of computerised cognitive-behavioural therapy for anxiety and depression in primary care: Randomised controlled trial. *British Journal of Psychiatry: The Journal of Mental Science, 185*, 46–54.

Rabinowitz, T., Murphy, K. M., Amour, J. L., Ricci, M. A., Caputo, M. P., & Newhouse, P. A. (2010). Benefits of a telepsychiatry consultation service for rural nursing home residents. *Telemedicine Journal and e-Health, 16*, 34–40.

Ruskin, P. E., Silver-Aylaian, M., Kling, M. A., Reed, S. A., Bradham, D. D., Hebel, J. R., et al. (2004). Treatment outcomes in depression: Comparison of remote treatment through telepsychiatry to in-person treatment. *American Journal of Psychiatry, 161*, 1471–1476.

Schopp, L., Johnstone, B., & Merrell, D. (2000). Telehealth and neuropsychological assessment: New opportunities for psychologists. *Professional Psychology, Research and Practice, 31*, 179–183.

Schopp, L. H., Johnstone, B. R., & Merveille, O. C. (2000). Multidimensional telecare strategies for rural residents with brain injury. *Journal of Telemedicine and Telecare, 6* (Suppl. 1), S146–S149.

Sharp, I. R., Kobak, K. A., & Osman, D. A. (2011). The use of videoconferencing with patients with psychosis: A review of the literature. *Annals of General Psychiatry, 10*, 1–14.

Sheeran, T., Rabinowitz, T., Lotterman, J., Reilly, C. F., Brown, S., Donehower, P., et al. (2011). Feasibility and impact of telemonitor-based depression care management for geriatric homecare patients. *Telemedicine Journal and e-Health, 17*, 620–626.

Shore, J. H., Brooks, E., Savin, D. M., Manson, S. M., & Libby, A. M. (2007). An economic
    evaluation of telehealth data collection with rural populations. *Psychiatric Services*, *58*,
    830−835.

Shore, P. (2011). *Home-based telemental health (HBTMH) standard operating procedures
    manual*. Portland, OR: VA Northwest Health Network Office (VISN 20).

Shores, M. M., Ryan-Dykes, P., Williams, R. M., Mamerto, B., Sadak, T., Pascualy, M.,
    et al. (2004). Identifying undiagnosed dementia in residential care veterans: Comparing
    telemedicine to in-person clinical examination. *International Journal of Geriatric
    Psychiatry*, *19*, 101−108.

Simpson, S. (2001). The provision of a telepsychology service to Shetland: Client and thera-
    pist satisfaction and the ability to develop a therapeutic alliance. *Journal of
    Telemedicine and Telecare*, *7*(Suppl. 1), 34−36.

Spaulding, R., Belz, N., DeLurgio, S., & Williams, A. R. (2010). Cost savings of telemedi-
    cine utilization for child psychiatry in a rural Kansas community. *Telemedicine Journal
    and e-Health*, *16*, 867−871.

Trott, P., & Blignault, I. (1998). Cost evaluation of a telepsychiatry service in northern
    Queensland. *Journal of Telemedicine and Telecare*, *4*(Suppl. 1), 66−68.

Williams, T. L., May, C. R., & Esmail, A. (2001). Limitations of patient satisfaction studies
    in telehealthcare: A systematic review of the literature. *Telemedicine Journal and
    e-Health*, *7*, 293−316.

Wilson, J. A., Onorati, K., Mishkind, M., Reger, M. A., & Gahm, G. A. (2008). Soldier atti-
    tudes about technology-based approaches to mental health care. *Cyberpsychology &
    Behavior: The Impact of the Internet, Multimedia and Virtual Reality on Behavior and
    Society*, *11*, 767−769.

Yellowlees, P., Shore, J., Roberts, L., & American Telemedicine Association Guidelines
    Workgroup (2010). Practice guidelines for videoconferencing-based telemental health—
    October 2009. *Telemedicine Journal and e-Health*, *16*, 1074−1089.

Zarate, C. A., Jr., Weinstock, L., Cukor, P., Morabito, C., Leahy, L., Burns, C., et al. (1997).
    Applicability of telemedicine for assessing patients with schizophrenia: Acceptance and
    reliability. *Journal of Clinical Psychiatry*, *58*, 22−25.

20 Conclusions

Carolyn L. Turvey[a,b] and Kathleen Myers[c,*]

[a]Department of Psychiatry, University of Iowa Carver College of Medicine, Iowa City, IA, [b]Comprehensive Access and Delivery Research and Evaluation (CADRE) Center, Iowa City VA Healthcare System, Iowa City, IA, [c]Department of Psychiatry and Behavioral Sciences, University of Washington School of Medicine, Telemental Health Service, Seattle Children's Hospital, Seattle, WA

Telemental health (TMH) has arrived. One of the main goals in developing the proposal for this textbook was to provide a resource that thoroughly reviews the research on TMH and its status in clinical practice. One of the rewards of writing this book was learning of the diverse populations participating in TMH, the models of care provided, and the rapid pace of technological developments that are making TMH more available to varied populations as well as a viable option for practitioners. An unexpected reward was learning of the vastness of this evolving evidence base to include areas that are beyond standard videoconferencing in the provision of care, such as online therapies, and the potential of newer platforms, such as social networking, to further influence how mental health care can be provided. Though much work is needed to understand the untapped scope of TMH, the current evidence justifies its widespread use for rectifying disparities in health care, as well as for improving care and outcomes for those who already enjoy access to care.

Any drawback to TMH, any chinks in the armor, discussed in this text should serve as an impetus to further development and dissemination through technical and/or clinical innovations. The field of TMH gives new definition to the term multidisciplinary and in that, such solutions often require the input of health-care professionals, computer technologists, clinical administrators, and policy makers. The clinical and technical contributors to this text have provided the foundation to inform those who have the power to influence how health care is delivered and reimbursed.

*Corresponding Author: Kathleen Myers, Department of Psychiatry and Behavioral Sciences, University of Washington School of Medicine, Telemental Health Service, Seattle Children's Hospital, Seattle, WA. Tel.: +1-206-987-1663, Fax: +1-206-987-2246, E-mail: Kathleen.myers@seattlechildrens.org

Telemental Health. DOI: http://dx.doi.org/10.1016/B978-0-12-416048-4.00020-8

As mentioned in the introduction, both authors are optimistic about the future of TMH and are fortunate to be part of this exciting development in health care. Though we both are early adopters, our academic training and the constant scrutiny of journal and grant reviews have forced us to hold a temperate view of the strengths and weaknesses of TMH, and we tried to convey that tone throughout the text. Nonetheless, the range and depth of current work presented here warrants strong enthusiasm about TMH. The research is sound, the technology is user friendly, patients are waiting, and health-care reform is at the doorstep. Let us cross the threshold to better mental health care for all Americans.

Appendix I: Glossary

The following provides a listing of commonly used words or phrases to describe telehealth activities, equipment, or requirements. Further information regarding terminology can be found at the websites for each of the federally funded telehealth resource centers listed in Appendix II.

Telemedicine/Telehealth Terms

Digital camera (still images) A digital camera is typically used to take still images of a patient. General uses for this type of camera include dermatology and wound care. This camera produces images that can be downloaded to a personal computer (PC) and sent to a provider/consultant over a network.

Distant site The Centers for Medicare and Medicaid Services (CMS) define the distant site as the telehealth site where the provider/specialist is seeing the patient at a distance or consulting with a patient's provider. Other common names for this term include hub site, specialty site, provider/physician site, and referral site.

Document camera A camera that can display written or typed information (e.g., lab results), photographs, graphics (e.g., electrocardiogram (EKG) strips), and in some cases X-rays.

Originating site CMS defines originating site as the site where the patient and/or the patient's physician is located during the telehealth encounter or consult. Other common names for this term include spoke site, patient site, remote site, and rural site.

Patient examination camera (video) This is the camera typically used to examine the general condition of the patient. Types of cameras include those that may be embedded with set-top videoconferencing units, handheld video cameras, gooseneck cameras, camcorders, etc. The camera may be analog or digital depending upon the connection to the videoconferencing unit.

Presenter (patient presenter) Telehealth encounters require the distant provider to perform an examination of a patient or client from many miles away. In order to assist the provider, an individual at the patient (originating) site is often needed to coordinate tasks, such as use of the equipment or obtaining vital signs. Many providers also prefer that a staff with a clinical background (e.g., licensed practical nurse (LPN) and registered nurse (RN)) at the patient site "presents" the patient, manages the cameras, and performs any "hands-on" activities to successfully complete the examination. For example, a neurological diagnostic exam usually requires a nurse capable of testing a patient's reflexes and other manipulative activities. It should be noted that in certain cases (e.g., some dermatology or mental health encounters) a presenter with a clinical background is not always necessary, because the encounter may only require camera-management skills. Sometimes, especially for psychiatric or other medically oriented examinations, the clinical staff will attend the entire session.

Store and forward (S&F) or asynchronous telemedicine S&F is a type of telehealth encounter or consult that uses still digital images of a patient for the purpose of rendering a medical opinion or diagnosis. Common types of S&F services include radiology, pathology, dermatology, and wound care. S&F also includes the asynchronous transmission of clinical data, such as blood glucose levels and electrocardiogram (ECG) measurements, from one site (e.g., patient's home) to another site (e.g., home health agency, hospital, and clinic). Recent work in telemental health has assessed the reliability of conducting and recording a clinical examination of a patient at the patient sites at one point in time and then forwarding the recording to a psychiatrist for review at a later time.

Universal Service Administrative Company (USAC) The USAC administers the Universal Service Fund (USF), which provides communities across the country with affordable telecommunication services. The Rural Health Care Division (RHCD) of USAC manages the telecommunications discount program for health care.

Telecommunication/Networking Terms

Analog Information, electronic or otherwise, that is created and transmitted as a continuous stream, as opposed to small digital packets. Most home telehealth devices require the use of analog lines.

Asynchronous This term is sometimes used to describe S&F transmission of medical images or information because the transmission typically occurs in one direction in time. This is the opposite of synchronous (see below).

Bandwidth The capacity of an electronic transmission to transmit data per unit of time. The higher the bandwidth, the more the data that can be transmitted. Bandwidth is typically measured in kilobits per second (kbps) or megabits per second (Mbps). Standard telephones are low-bandwidth devices. Cable television and T-1 lines are high bandwidth devices.

Baud rate The ring rate or line power of the telephone line providing service into a given structure (e.g., home). Most home telehealth devices require a minimum baud rate of 14,000 to make successful video capture. However, the lower the baud rate, the more likely it is that disconnections will occur.

Broadband Communications (e.g., broadcast television, microwave, and satellite) that are capable of carrying a wide range of frequencies. Broadband refers to transmission of signals in a frequency-modulated fashion, over a segment of the total bandwidth available, thereby permitting simultaneous transmission of several messages.

Codec Acronym for coder–decoder. This is, the videoconferencing device (e.g., Polycom, Tandberg, Sony, and Panasonic) that converts analog video and audio signals to digital video and audio code and vice versa. Codecs typically compress the digital code to conserve bandwidth on a telecommunications path.

Component video This type of video yields better image quality, higher lines of resolution, and better color.

Compressed video Video images that have been processed to reduce the amount of bandwidth needed to capture the necessary information so that the information can be sent over a telephone network.

Digital Information coded in numerical values (bits). Digital data streams are less susceptible to interference than analog streams. They can be more easily integrated with other data streams such as voice/video/data.

Digital camera Captures images (still or motion) digitally and does not require analog to digital conversion before the image can be transmitted or stored in a computer. Most home telehealth equipment uses digital video cameras.

Digital Imaging and Communication in Medicine (DICOM) A standard for communications among medical imaging devices.

DS1 (T1) A digital carrier capable of transmitting 1.544 Mbps of electronic information. The general term used for a digital carrier available for high-value voice, data, or compressed video traffic.

DS3 (T3) A carrier of 45 Mbps. Many systems use only a fraction of this transmission capability "fractional T1 line."

Electronic data interchange (EDI) The sending and receiving of data directly between trading partners without paper or human intervention.

Encryption A mathematical transposition of a file or data stream so that it cannot be deciphered at the receiving end without the proper key. Encryption is a security feature that assures only the appropriate parties participate in a video visit or data transfer.

Firewall A computer connected both to the Internet and a local network (e.g., a hospital) that prevents the passing of Internet traffic to the internal network. It also provides an added security layer.

Frame rate Frames per second displayed on a video unit. A frame rate of 25–30 is considered full motion. A lower frame rate can be associated with a noticeably "jerky" motion on the screen. Slower frame rates may be inadequate for some assessments such as gait and balance activities.

H.320 This is the technical standard for videoconferencing compression standards that allow different equipment to interoperate via connections through T1 lines or an Integrated Services Digital Network (ISDN).

H.323 This is the technical standard for videoconferencing compression standards that allow different equipment to interoperate via the Internet protocol (IP) (see below).

H.324 This is the technical standard for videoconferencing compression standards that allow different equipment to interoperate via plain old telephone service (POTS).

Health level 7 (HL7) data communications protocol A standard interface between hospital information systems. Defines standards for transmitting billing, hospital census, order entries, and other health-related information.

Interactive video/television This is analogous to videoconferencing technologies that allow for two-way, synchronous, interactive video and audio signals for the purpose of delivering telehealth, telemedicine, or distant education services. It is often referred to by the acronyms—ITV, IATV, or VTC (video teleconference).

Internet A loose gathering of thousands of computer networks forming an enormous worldwide area network.

Intranet A "private Internet," or internal web that employs certain communication protocols used over the Internet. The Intranet may be linked to the public Internet through tightly managed gateways.

Integrated services digital network This is a common dial-up transmission path for videoconferencing. Since ISDN services are used on demand by dialing another ISDN-based device, per minute charges accumulate at some contracted rate and then are billed to the site placing the call. This service is analogous to using the dialing features associated with a long-distance telephone call. Whoever dials pays the bill.

ISDN basic rate interface (BRI) This is an ISDN interface that provides 128k of bandwidth for videoconferencing or simultaneous voice and data services. Multiple BRI lines can be linked together using a multiplexer (MUX) (see below) to achieve higher bandwidth levels. For instance, a popular choice among telehealth networks is to combine 3 BRI lines to provide 384k of bandwidth for videoconferencing. It should be noted that BRI services are not available in some rural locations. One should check with their telecommunications providers on the availability of BRI service before ordering video-conferencing equipment that uses this type of service.

ISDN primary rate interface (PRI) This is an ISDN interface standard that operates using 23, 64k channels and one 64k data channel. With the proper multiplexing equipment the ISDN PRI channels can be selected by the user for a video call. For instance, if the user wants to have a videoconference at 384k of bandwidth then they can instruct the MUX to use channels 1 through 6 (6 × 64k = 384k). This is important because the user typically pays charges based on the number of 64k channels used during a videoconference. The fewer the channels used to obtain a quality video signal, the less expensive the call is.

Internet protocol IP is part of the protocols describing the software that tracks the Internet address of outgoing and incoming messages. Most of today's videoconferencing devices have the capability to use IP as a video protocol (see "H.323" above). The IP address of a videoconferencing system is its phone number.

Local area network (LAN) A computer network linking computers, printers, servers, and other equipment within a system. It can support audio, video, and data exchange.

Modem Modulator/demodulator enables transmission of digital data over standard analog phone lines and cable video systems.

Multiplexer A device that combines multiple inputs (ISDN PRI channels or ISDN BRI lines) into an aggregate signal to be transported via a single transmission path.

Multipoint control unit (MCU) A device that can link multiple videoconferencing sites into a single videoconference. An MCU is also often referred to as a "bridge."

Network An assortment of electronic devices (computers, printers, scanners, etc.) connected by wires or wireless for mutual exchange of digital information.

Private branch exchange (PBX) PBX (a.k.a. the switchboard) is a telephone system (i.e., switchboard, telephone lines, and switching computer) within a VHA facility/campus that switches internal phone lines between VHA users, who actually share a certain number of external (outside) phone lines. Having a PBX saves money by reducing the number of lines required to connect all VHA facility telephones to the telephone company's central office.

Peripheral devices Attachments to videoconferencing systems to augment their communications or medical capabilities. Examples include electronic stethoscopes, blood pressure cuffs, glucometers, and weight scales.

Pixel A picture cell with specific color or brightness. The more the pixels an image has, the more the detail or resolution it can display.

POTS Acronym for plain old telephone service. The analog, public-switched telephone network in common use throughout the world. Most home telehealth products rely on POTS.

Real time Sends and receives audio/video/data simultaneously, without more than a fraction of a second delay.

Resolution The level of detail that can be captured or displayed. For video displays, resolution is measured in pixels × lines × bit depth.

Router This is a device that interfaces between two networks or connects subnetworks within a single organization. It routes network traffic between multiple locations and it can find the best route between any two sites. For example, PCs or H.323 videoconferencing devices tell the routers where the destination device is located and the routers find the best way to get the information to that distant point.

Store and forward Captures audio clips, video clips, still images, or data that are transmitted or received at a later time (sometimes no more than a minute).

Switch A switch in the videoconferencing world is an electrical device that selects the path of the video transmission. It may be thought of as an intelligent hub because it can be programmed to direct traffic on specific ports to specific destinations. Hub ports feed the same information to each device.

Synchronous This term is sometimes used to describe interactive video connections because the transmission of information in both directions is occurring at exactly the same period.

Telehealth and telemedicine Telemedicine and telehealth both describe the use of medical information exchanged from one site to another via electronic communications to improve patients' health status. Although these terms are evolving to be more specific, telemedicine is sometimes associated with direct patient clinical services and telehealth sometimes associated with a broader definition of remote health care that may include other health-related services, such as health education and patient-accessed information.

Thumbnail Miniature pictures of images using very small, low-resolution data files. These download for display very quickly.

Transmission control protocol/Internet protocol (TCP/IP) A communications protocol governing data exchanged on the Internet.

Transmission rate Amount of information/unit of time that a technology such as POTS or digital ISDN phone line, satellite or wireless technology, or LAN can transmit.

Wide area network (WAN) A network that is wider in geographic scope than a LAN. It provides digital communications (voice/video/data) over switched or unswitched networks.

Appendix II: Telehealth Resource Centers (TRCs)

Organizations Funded to Help Build and Sustain Telehealth Programs

In 2006, the federal Office for the Advancement of Telehealth (OAT) initiated a regional telehealth resource center grant program to provide support and guidance to telehealth programs. Several geographically dispersed Telehealth Resource Centers (TRCs) have been funded by OAT, Office of Health Information Technology (HIT), the Health Resources and Services Administration (HRSA), and Department of Health and Human Services (DHHS).

The TRCs have a mission to serve as a focal point for advancing the effective use of telehealth and support access to telehealth services in rural and underserved communities. The TRCs have extensive telehealth experience and can provide services, resources, and tools to both developing and operating programs. Each TRC also has an understanding of regional concerns and the climate for telehealth in its geographic region. Their websites offer many tools to assist in program development and success. Below is a list of the TRCs.

Telehealth Resource Centers: Main Website: http://www.telehealthresource-centers.org/—accessed May 17, 2012

Telehealth Technology Assessment Center (Telehealth TAC)
(907) 729-4703
http://www.telehealthtac.org/home—accessed May 17, 2012

Northwest Regional Telehealth Resource Center (NRTRC)
(888) 662-5601
http://www.nrtrc.org/—accessed May 17, 2012

California Telemedicine & eHealth Center (CTEC)
(877) 590-8144
http://www.cteconline.org/—accessed May 17, 2012

Southwest Telehealth Resource Center
(520) 626-4498
http://www.southwesttrc.org/—accessed May 17, 2012

Great Plains Telehealth Resource & Assistance Center
(888) 239-7092
http://www.gptrac.org/—accessed May 17, 2012

Heartland Telehealth Resource Center
(877) 643-4872
http://www.heartlandtrc.org/—accessed May 17, 2012

Upper Midwest Telehealth Resource Center
(855) 283-3734
http://www.umtrc.org/—accessed May 17, 2012

Mid-Atlantic Telehealth Resource Center
(434) 924-5470
http://www.matrc.org/—accessed May 17, 2012

Northeast Telehealth Resource Center
(800) 379-2021
http://www.northeasttrc.org/—accessed May 17, 2012

Southern Telehealth Resource Center
(888) 738-2210
http://www.setrc.us/—accessed May 17, 2012

South Central Telehealth Resource Center
(855) 664-3450
http://learntelehealth.org/—accessed May 17, 2012

Pacific Basin Telehealth Resource Center
(808) 692-1090
http://www.pbtrc.org/—accessed May 17, 2012

Appendix III: Useful Websites Providing Practical Information Regarding Telemental Health Practice

General Information

American Telemedicine Association (ATA) "Quality Healthcare Through Telecommunications Technology"
http://www.americantelemed.org/i4a/pages/index.cfm?pageid = 3331—accessed May 17, 2012
The American Telemedicine Association (ATA) is an international resource and advocate promoting the use of advanced remote medical technologies. ATA, and its diverse membership, works to fully integrate telemedicine into transformed healthcare systems to improve quality, equity, and affordability of health care throughout the world. The ATA website provides comprehensive information on developing standards, technology, applications, vendors, and other needs for telehealth providers.

University of Colorado (UC) Website "Eliminating Mental Health Disparities"
http://www.tmhguide.org/—accessed May 17, 2012
This telemental health guide is a very informative website developed by the UC telemental health group with funding from the Substance Abuse and Mental Health Services Administration (SAMHSA) to provide an overview of telemental health (TMH) for the clinician, administrator, policy maker, consumer, and media. There is a wealth of helpful information addressing TMH across the lifespan, setting, and stakeholder. The section "Clinicians and Administrators" provides excellent information about the practical steps necessary to establish a TMH program. This section covers practical applications for conducting a TMH session, ranging from room setup, billing codes, suggestions on how to support and sustain TMH services, and tools for promoting these services.

Center for Telehealth and e-Health Law (CTeL)
http://ctel.org/—accessed May 17, 2012
Licensure requirements are particularly important, both for interstate and international practice. CTel's mission is to overcome the legal and regulatory barriers that impact the utilization of telehealth and related e-Health services. It has established itself as the "go-to" legal and regulatory telehealth organization—providing vital support to the community on topics such as physician and nurse

licensure; credentialing and privileging; Medicare and Medicaid reimbursement; and private insurance payment policies.

CTel provides a summary of findings regarding malpractice and telemedicine. This publication can be accessed at:

http://www.ctel.org/research/Summary%20of%20Findings%20Malpractice%20and%20Telemedicine.pdf—accessed May 17, 2012

Telehealth Times: Your Authoritative Source on Telemedicine
http://www.telehealthtimes.com/about/—accessed May 17, 2012

TelehealthTimes.com is a source of information about the telehealthcare and telemedicine industry. The sites include telehealth and telemedicine news, reviews of the latest telehealth videoconferencing equipment, software, tools and accessories, active discussion forums, a large selection of sample galleries, a telehealth database and buyers guide, and the most comprehensive database of telehealth and telemedicine software and equipment features and specifications.

Northern Arizona Regional Behavioral Health Authority (NARBHA)
http://www.rbha.net/presentations/RealWorldTelepsychRev/player.html—accessed May 17, 2012

This website contains a slideshow that explores the following topics: provisions of real world telepsychiatry, the practical considerations and of getting organized, telemedicine challenges, how telemedicine works, and diagnostic instruments and exams. The website also has a demonstration of conducting the Abnormal Involuntary Movement Scale (AIMS) through videoteleconferencing.

Telemental Health Institute
http://centerforonlinecounseling.com—accessed May 17, 2012

This website offers online courses in a variety of delivery methods, i.e., webinars, individual courses, and group courses that cover a range of topics such as theory and practice, legal/ethical issues, reimbursement, and advanced clinical telepractice models for success.

Reimbursement Information Relating to Telemedicine and Telemental Health

Center for Medicare and Medicaid Services (CMS)
https://www.cms.gov/Manuals/—accessed May 17, 2012

Telemental health providers should review information at the CMS website prior to any billing to determine any state-specific guidelines.

Some client sites are eligible for Medicare/Medicaid's originating site fees related to the videoteleconferencing coordinator assistance.

The following website managed by CMS provides the definition of telemedicine, telemedicine terms, provider and facility guidelines, reimbursement, and approach to reviewing telemedicine:

http://www.cms.gov/Telemedicine/—accessed May 17, 2012

This information is also helpfully summarized by the Center for Telehealth and e-Health Law (CTeL):

http://ctel.org/expertise/reimbursement/medicare-reimbursement/—accessed May 17, 2012

The following link directs to the Medicare Claims Processing Manual. See #100-04, Chapter 12, #190 (page 7 of 228) regarding "Medicare Payments for Telehealth Services":

http://www.cms.gov/Regulations-and-Guidance/Guidance/Manuals/Downloads/clm104c12.pdf—accessed May 17, 2012

AMD Global Telemedicine

http://www.amdtelemedicine.com/telemedicine-resources/private_payer.html—accessed May 17, 2012

The above link provides a reference to support private payer reimbursement for telemedicine clinical consults. The information contained in this website is the result of a survey jointly sponsored by the American Telemedicine Association and AMD Global Telemedicine. The directory contains a listing of telemedicine providers receiving private payer reimbursement, private payers providing reimbursement, and state legislation mandating private payer reimbursement of telemedicine services.

The following AMD link directs to information regarding private payer reimbursement by state:

http://www.amdtelemedicine.com/telemedicine-resources/PrivatePayersByState.html—accessed May 17, 2012

The AMD link directs to helpful information regarding private payer telemedicine programs.

http://www.amdtelemedicine.com/telemedicine-resources/PrivatePayerTelemedicinePrograms.html—accessed May 17, 2012

Reimbursement Handbooks

http://crihb.org/files/Telemedicine-Reimbursement-Handbook.pdf—accessed May 17, 2012

Some states provide handbooks regarding reimbursement. It is recommended that telemental health providers conduct Internet searches to determine whether there are existing documents relevant to their state's reimbursement guidelines. If these are not in place, reviewing documents by other states can also aid in advocacy efforts within the provider's home state.

The above link to the California Telemedicine and e-Health Center provides information on reimbursement.

Rural Health Care Programs

http://transition.fcc.gov/wcb/tapd/ruralhealth/—accessed May 17, 2012

The Federal Communications Commission supports the Rural Healthcare Program that matches line charges so that rural areas have rates that are competitive with urban rates in that state. Information about this program can be obtained through their website above.

Relevant Publications

American Medical Association. Policy Statement H-480.969: The promotion of quality telemedicine. This policy can be found at:

http://www.ama-assn.org/resources/doc/council-on-med-ed/cme-rep6-a10.pdf—accessed May 17, 2012

American Psychological Association (APA). American Psychological Association ethical principles of psychologists and code of conduct. This can be found at the link below:

http://www.apa.org/ethics/code/index.aspx—accessed May 17, 2012

American Psychological Association Ethics Committee (APA). The APA's statement on services by telephone, teleconferencing, and Internet. This can be found at:

http://www.apa.org/ethics/education/telephone-statement.aspx—accessed May 17, 2012

American Psychological Association. Practice Directorate, Legal & Regulatory Affairs. Telehealth 50-state review. This can be found at:

http://www.apapracticecentral.org/advocacy/state/telehealth-slides.pdf—accessed May 17, 2012

American Telemedicine Association. Medical licensure and practice requirements. This can be found at:

http://www.americantelemed.org/files/public/policy/
ATAPolicy_StateMedicalLicensure.pdf—accessed May 17, 2012

Federal Communication Commission. National Broadband Plan, Chapter 10, Health Care. http://www.broadband.gov/plan/10-healthcare—accessed May 17, 2012

National Association of Social Workers and Association of Social Work Boards Standards for Technology and Social Work Practice:

http://www.socialworkers.org/practice/standards/NASWTechnologyStandards.
pdf—accessed May 17, 2012

American Psychological Association, Task Force on the Delivery of Services to Ethnic Minority Populations. Guidelines for Providers of Psychological Services to Ethnic, Linguistic, and Culturally Diverse Populations. The guidelines can be found at the link below:

http://www.apa.org/pi/oema/resources/policy/provider-guidelines.aspx—
accessed May 17, 2012

Federation of State Medical Boards Public Policy Compendium. Telemedicine and License Portability policy documents 140.001–140.007:

http://www.fsmb.org/pdf/GRPOL_Public_Policy_compendium.pdf—accessed May 17, 2012

Grady, B., Myers, K., Nelson, E. L., Co-Chairs, & the Telemental Health Standards and Guidelines Working Group (October 2009). *Practice guidelines for videoconferencing-based telemental health*. Washington, DC: American

Telemedicine Association. This publication can be accessed via the following link below:

http://www.americantelemed.org/files/public/standards/
PracticeGuidelinesforVideoconferencing-Based   TeleMentalHealth.pdf—accessed May 17, 2012

Grady, B., Myers, K., Nelson, E.L., Co-Chairs, & the Telemental Health Standards and Guidelines Working Group (July 2009). *Evidence-based practice for telemental health*. Washington, DC: American Telemedicine Association. This publication can be accessed via the following link below:
www.americantelemed.org/files/public/standards/EvidenceBasedTelementalHealth_WithCover.pdf—accessed May 17, 2012

Gupta, A., & Soa, D. (2010). The constitutionality of current legal barriers to telemedicine in the United States: Analysis and future directions of its relationship to National and International Health Care Reform. *Health Matrix: Journal of Law Medicine*, Available at Social Science Research Network. This publication can be accessed via the following link below:
http://ssrn.com/abstract = 1549765—accessed May 17, 2012

Printed in the United States
By Bookmasters